Precision Medicine for African Americans

Gregory L. Hall

Precision Medicine for African Americans

A Concise, Evidence-Based Guide to Important Differences and Better Outcomes

Second Edition

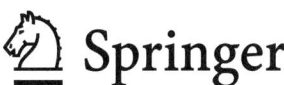

Gregory L. Hall
School of Medicine
Case Western Reserve University
Cleveland, OH, USA

ISBN 978-3-031-95773-4   ISBN 978-3-031-95774-1   (eBook)
https://doi.org/10.1007/978-3-031-95774-1

© The Editor(s) (if applicable) and The Author(s), under exclusive license to Springer Nature Switzerland AG 2020, 2025

This work is subject to copyright. All rights are solely and exclusively licensed by the Publisher, whether the whole or part of the material is concerned, specifically the rights of translation, reprinting, reuse of illustrations, recitation, broadcasting, reproduction on microfilms or in any other physical way, and transmission or information storage and retrieval, electronic adaptation, computer software, or by similar or dissimilar methodology now known or hereafter developed.
The use of general descriptive names, registered names, trademarks, service marks, etc. in this publication does not imply, even in the absence of a specific statement, that such names are exempt from the relevant protective laws and regulations and therefore free for general use.
The publisher, the authors and the editors are safe to assume that the advice and information in this book are believed to be true and accurate at the date of publication. Neither the publisher nor the authors or the editors give a warranty, expressed or implied, with respect to the material contained herein or for any errors or omissions that may have been made. The publisher remains neutral with regard to jurisdictional claims in published maps and institutional affiliations.

This Springer imprint is published by the registered company Springer Nature Switzerland AG
The registered company address is: Gewerbestrasse 11, 6330 Cham, Switzerland

If disposing of this product, please recycle the paper.

This book is dedicated to my wife, Melanie, and our sons, Alex, Nick, and Greg Jr., for all of their sacrifice and unwavering support.

Preface

In the fall of 2002, I was appointed to the Ohio Commission on Minority Health. My name had been submitted to Ohio Governor Bob Taft by Cleveland's Mayor Jane Campbell because they needed a medical professional from the Cleveland area to better balance the representation to the state-wide board. As a Cleveland Clinic-trained internal medicine and primary care provider in an urban practice that was over 90% African American, I could provide in-the-trenches perspectives. Upon joining, I was embarrassed to admit how little I knew about health disparities and how they impacted minorities, but I attended the meetings regularly ... and quietly.

The commission was largely a funding organization and specialized in advancing smaller grants for unique approaches to shrinking health disparities. We also advocated for policies that impact health in the larger scheme. The commission is composed of the directors of key statewide departments including the Departments of Health, Job and Family Services, Education, Medicaid, Developmental Disabilities, and Mental Health and Addiction, in addition to four elected officials and eight governor appointees, of which I was one.

Bringing a "high-end" group like this together was initially intimidating but before long we began to fill our roles appropriately. As a physician, I initially believed that health disparities were almost completely driven by poverty and/or the lack of access to medical services. I also falsely believed that "minorities" had poor health outcomes and the "majority" populations had better health outcomes.

Because of my work with the commission, I soon joined the Medical Care Advisory Committee for Ohio Medicaid. In this capacity, I saw not only the financial burden that poor health outcomes put on a strained state budget but also the disconnect between providers of Medicaid recipients and state agency representatives with good intentions.

My exposure to the breadth of urban healthcare delivery was rounded by my experience as medical director of multiple urban extended care facilities including two with large psychiatric populations, continued inpatient care with patients at an inner-city hospital (St. Vincent Charity Medical Center), and some time as medical director of home health and hospice agencies.

As the years passed, I was elected vice-chair and then chairman of the Ohio Commission on Minority Health. A part of my duties was to prepare an educational chairman's report to be presented at each meeting. As I became familiarized with research articles involving quality outcomes, I was struck by the significant health disparities *between* minority groups and that the specific health issues were not addressed by the same solutions. Problems in the Asian American or Hispanic/Latino communities consisted of issues regarding immigration, communication, language, and access. African American disparities were pervasive across a range of categories: the worst cardiovascular issues, worst cancer outcomes, longest length of hospital stay, lowest referrals for accelerated care, and so on. Put simply, the health-related problems for African Americans were too serious, too unique, and too severe to simply be "bunched" with other racial/ethnic groups.

My second revelation was that physicians, clinicians, and other providers were indirectly contributing to some of these disparities. This perspective was first brought to my attention by the Commission Executive Director Cheryl Boyce, who had noted these differences from both a professional and a personal perspective. I remember initially shrugging off her viewpoint as isolated because variability in care delivery can occur, but when I reviewed the wide-ranging research, the pervasive clinician-driven differences in the care of African Americans were undeniable.

I decided to highlight some of these care differences on my practice website, drgreghall.com, in order to educate the African American community to be better stewards of their medical care. As I composed these short articles with hyperlinks to verified research in PubMed, I was progressively finding more nuances in clinical care.

I realized that my aim to educate about the differences in the clinical care of African Americans was directed to the wrong audience, and I needed to move "upstream" and bring these differences to the notice of medical clinicians. That realization soon led to the process of compiling a collection of best practices for African American clinical care, one that is long overdue and deserving of the medical community's singular attention.

Cleveland, OH, USA Gregory L. Hall
June 18, 2019

With this re-titled second edition, I have been moved by the precision medicine movement, one that considers all aspects of our patients' clinical care. The National Institutes of Health describes precision medicine as "rooted in the belief that since individuals possess nuanced and unique characteristics at the molecular, physiological, environmental exposure, and behavioral levels, they may need to have interventions provided to them for diseases they possess that are tailored to these nuanced and unique characteristics."

The terms "cultural competence" or "cultural humility" always fell short for me in terms of providing a reason that a busy clinician with African American patients should stop what they're doing and learn about African American healthcare differences. To me, the real reason to stop and engage is the clinical differences that contribute to the exact health disparities that we dislike. Admittedly, many cultural differences drive clinical outcomes, but what we were missing was the undeniable genetic differences that have an impact. These "genetic differences" also made everyone so uncomfortable when they were applied to African Americans. Just because there are genetic differences doesn't mean African Americans are inferior in any way. Like everyone else, we are just different, while still remaining over 99.99 percent genetically the same.

Since the publication of the first edition, I have continued to examine the published research on a wide range of African American health topics. As genetic research advances, more and more genetic differences unique to African Americans are reported. These genetic differences are not typically defects but adaptations to environmental challenges. In those other circumstances, these genetic modifications have contributed to the survival of the human species.

African Americans, equipped with past genetic adaptations, now face a new and different environment to navigate. As clinicians working with African American patients, we must equip ourselves with as much information as possible to better illuminate the full landscape of their care.

Cleveland, OH, USA Gregory L. Hall
April 17, 2025

Acknowledgments

This book was definitely a group effort and the culmination of numerous partnerships and affiliations throughout my career. I started the book by interviewing many highly successful physicians who served predominantly African American patient populations. As a provider for African Americans, I knew that my approach to this patient population was different, but I needed to determine if there was a distinct pattern. I particularly appreciate the input of Ronald Adams, MD; Lloyd Cook, MD; Giesele Greene, MD; Carl Jackson, MD; Toye Williams, MD; and Harold James, MD, for their early assistance. I also want to thank my brother, Bill Hall, for introducing me to his physician colleagues for interviews in the Maryland region, including Elmer Carreno, MD; Geoff Mount-Varner, MD; and Don Shell, MD. Another important interview was with my good friend from our Cleveland Clinic residency days, Mark Spears, MD, in Florida.

Randol Kennedy, MD, and Anita Mason-Kennedy, MD, reviewed and added to the entire book with particular contributions to the chapters on cardiology, hematology, and rheumatology. Kim Simpson, MD, and Joan Reeder, MD, were also early reviewers.

I was honored to have the chapters on cardiovascular and renal disease reviewed with significant input from Jackson T. Wright Jr., MD, PhD. Sherrie Dixon-Williams, MD, reviewed and contributed to the pulmonary chapter. I appreciate the ongoing support of Janet Baker, DNP, Associate Dean of Ursuline College School of Graduate Nursing, in reviewing the book. William Tarter Sr. reviewed the chapter on stories and patient counseling, and I value his continued guidance and counsel.

This second edition brought a few new authors with great perspectives on African American health. Staja "Star" Booker, PhD, RN, FAAN, and Simone Jackson, BSN, RN, from the College of Nursing at the University of Florida, added an outstanding review of the treatment of pain in African Americans. Dr. Booker then introduced me to Keesha Roach, PhD, RN, at Rutgers University, and she contributed nicely to the section on sickle cell anemia.

I would also like to express my gratitude to my University Hospitals colleagues Lee Ponsky, MD, David Headen, MD, Randy Vince, MD, and Celina Cunanan, MSN, APRN-CNM, for their unwavering support. I also need to acknowledge the team at the UH Cutler Center for Men as we endeavor to improve all men's health. I am also grateful for receiving the hospital's Edgar B. Jackson, Jr., MD Endowed Chair for Clinical Excellence and Diversity, named after a mentor and true legend in healthcare. That Chair has empowered me with the time to produce this work.

My office practice would not be able to stay afloat without my office manager, Robin Smith, holding everything together. Medical Assistant Damonay Johnson always has a cheerful and caring smile for both my patients and me. My long-term administrative assistant, Katrina Hurt, also deserves recognition for her support over the years. I am also thankful to my patients who have supported my work and encouraged me. My patients are the best in the world, and I treasure their support and commitment.

Having been on the Cuyahoga County Board of Health for over 15 years, I have had the opportunity to see how a world-class public health entity can work. Its former commissioner, Terrence Allan, was instrumental in my initial appointment and has always been supportive and inclusive. As the current board president, I am thankful for a great team at CCBH led by current health commissioner Roderick Harris, DrPH, and my fellow board members Doug Wang, Sherrie Williams, MD, Daniel Richards, JD, and Sonja Rajki, JD.

I also serve as the founder and board chair of the non-profit National Institute for African American Health, which has excellent leadership in Stacey Easterling as its executive director. We continue to support future African American physicians, advocate for better health outcomes, and provide an online resource for trusted health information on NIAAH.org. We enjoy the support of board members Alison Graves-Calhoun, PhD, Patricia A. Ackerman, PhD, Georgia State Senator Emmanuel Jones, Tony Peebles, and Mark Spears, MD.

I speak across the country (and virtually) through the Pri-Med Continuing Medical Education company based in Boston, MA. Their platform has allowed me to meet thousands of clinicians from across the United States while speaking about African American health through our award-winning Bridging the Gap: Conversations with Dr. Greg Hall series. I was honored to be asked to join their Advisory Board and love talking to in-the-trenches clinicians about their continuing educational needs.

Thanks to the team at Springer Nature, including Richard Lansing for his support throughout the publishing process for the first edition and for recognizing the potential of this book, and now Margaret Moore for her guidance in this second edition.

And finally, I want to express my gratitude to the Hall family, particularly my mother and father, Louise and Albert Hall, who supported me unconditionally, and my brothers and sister, Tyrone, Wanda, Bill, and Barry, who always made sure I felt loved and nurtured. With marriage comes my extended family, which has also been supportive, including my sisters-in-law, Robin and Stacie, and my brother-in-law, Sherman, who have consistently provided expert counsel and advice. My wife Melanie's side of the family has been equally supportive and accepting, and I will always cherish my mother-in-law and father-in-law, Mamie and Jesse Coats, along with my brother-in-law, Michael, and sister-in-law, Valeri. I love and thank all our nieces and nephews, as well as the rest of the Hall and Coats families. Other supportive family members include Martin Kelly, Robert "Rusty" Banks, Jeff Johnson, JD, Ethan Coats, James "Terry" Ford, Robert Dennison, Duane Morton, Geovette (GiGi) Simpson, Tony Whitaker, Lonnie Marsh, MD, Cynthia Simpson, Cheryl Staples, Lynette Bennet, Judith Dunn, and our great friends, Paul and Valencia Stephens.

It honestly took a village to get this book written and published.

Contents

1	**Precision Medicine for African Americans**...................	1
	1.1 "Race is Just a Social Construct," But What Does the Evidence Show..	2
	1.2 "Ancestral Genomics" Might Be the Answer	3
	1.3 Who Are African Americans?............................	4
	1.4 Evidence-Based Differences	5
	1.5 Pay for Performance...................................	7
	1.6 Patient-Centered Care	8
	References...	11
2	**Establishing Trust in African American Patients**..............	15
	2.1 The Tuskegee Syphilis Study............................	16
	2.2 Other Examples of Abuse	17
	2.3 Differences in Trust	18
	2.3.1 Trust Improves Health Outcomes	20
	2.4 Explicit and Implicit Biases Impact Our Healthcare	21
	2.5 Building Trust	23
	2.6 Show Competence	25
	References...	27
3	**Delivering Consistent and Equitable Healthcare to African Americans**	31
	3.1 African American Clinical Care and Outcomes Disparities	36
	3.2 Variability in Our Care.................................	40
	References...	42
4	**A Precision Medicine Approach to the Cardiovascular Care of African Americans**	45
	4.1 Hypertension	48
	4.1.1 Salt Sensitivity...................................	48
	4.1.2 Hypertension Control.............................	51

	4.2	Heart Failure	54
		4.2.1 Hereditary Transthyretin Amyloidosis (hATTR)	57
	4.3	Lipids	57
	4.4	Atrial Fibrillation	59
	4.5	Stroke	61
	4.6	Peripheral Vascular Disease	63
	4.7	Abdominal Aortic Aneurysms	65
	4.8	Deep Vein Thrombosis and Pulmonary Embolism	66
	References		69
5	**A Precision Medicine Approach to the Care of Diabetes and Obesity in African Americans**		**81**
	5.1	Obesity	81
	5.2	Type 2 Diabetes	86
		5.2.1 Smoking Drives Up Diabetes Risk	89
		5.2.2 HbA1c Differences	90
		5.2.3 Diabetes Treatment Approaches	91
	5.3	Diabetes Type 1	94
	5.4	Diet Management Approaches	95
	5.5	Marketing Competition	97
	References		98
6	**A Precision Medicine Approach to Cancer in African Americans**		**107**
	6.1	Breast Cancer	109
	6.2	Colon Cancer	112
	6.3	Prostate Cancer	115
	6.4	Lung Cancer	117
		6.4.1 Equitable Tobacco Cessation Advice	119
		6.4.2 African American Smoking Paradox	120
	6.5	Multiple Myeloma	121
	6.6	"Chemotherapy"	123
	References		125
7	**A Precision Medicine Approach to Renal Disease in African Americans**		**133**
	7.1	Hypertensive Nephrosclerosis	136
	7.2	Obesity and Proteinuria	136
	7.3	Kidney Disease Progression	137
	7.4	Treatment and Counseling	137
	7.5	Kidney Transplantation	138
	7.6	Kidney Stones	139
	References		141
8	**A Precision Medicine Approach to Rheumatic Diseases in African Americans**		**145**
	8.1	Osteoarthritis	147
	8.2	Rheumatoid Arthritis	148

	8.3	Systemic Lupus Erythematosus	149
	8.4	Ankylosing Spondylitis	152
	8.5	Primary Sjögren's Syndrome	152
	8.6	Scleroderma (Systemic Sclerosis)	153
	8.7	Polymyalgia Rheumatica and Giant Cell Arteritis	154
	8.8	Gout	154
	References		157
9	**A Precision Medicine Approach to Pulmonary Diseases in African Americans**		165
	9.1	COPD (Emphysema and Chronic Bronchitis)	166
	9.2	Asthma	169
	9.3	Sarcoidosis	171
	9.4	Obstructive Sleep Apnea (OSA)	173
	References		175
10	**A Precision Medicine Approach to Laboratory Results and Hematological Disorders in African Americans**		181
	Gregory L. Hall and Keesha Powell-Roach		
	10.1	Creatinine and GFR Controversy	182
	10.2	Laboratory Results	183
		10.2.1 CBC	183
		10.2.2 Benign Ethnic Neutropenia (Typical Neutrophil Count with Fy(a-b-) Status)	184
		10.2.3 Metabolic Panel	185
		10.2.4 Thyroid-Stimulating Hormone (TSH)	186
		10.2.5 Lipid Profile	187
	10.3	Cancer Markers	187
		10.3.1 Prostate-Specific Antigen (PSA)	187
		10.3.2 Cancer Antigen 125 (CA-125)	188
		10.3.3 Alpha-Fetoprotein (AFP)	189
		10.3.4 Carbohydrate Antigen 19-9 (CA 19-9)	189
	10.4	Vitamin Blood Levels	190
		10.4.1 Vitamin B12	190
		10.4.2 Folate	190
		10.4.3 Vitamin A	191
		10.4.4 Vitamin C	191
		10.4.5 Vitamin E	192
	10.5	Sickle Cell Disease	193
		10.5.1 Renal Complications	194
		10.5.2 Pulmonary Hypertension	195
		10.5.3 Eye Complications	196
		10.5.4 Priapism	196
		10.5.5 Stroke	197
		10.5.6 Aplastic Crisis	197
		10.5.7 Acute Chest Syndrome	198
		10.5.8 Splenic Sequestration	199

		10.5.9 Vaso-Occlusive Pain Management.	200

- 10.6 Thalassemia (Alpha and Beta) 202
- 10.7 Glucose-6-Phosphate Dehydrogenase Deficiency (G6PD) 204
- References. 206

11 A Precision Medicine Approach to Gastrointestinal and Hepatic Diseases in African Americans 219
- 11.1 Hepatitis B 220
- 11.2 Hepatitis C 222
- 11.3 Hepatocellular Carcinoma 225
- 11.4 Inflammatory Bowel Diseases 227
  - 11.4.1 Crohn's Disease and Ulcerative Colitis 227
- 11.5 GERD. 229
- 11.6 Barrett's Esophagus 230
- 11.7 Helicobacter Pylori 231
- 11.8 Gallbladder Disease 232
- References. 234

12 Stress, Mental Illness, Sleep, and Substance Abuse in African Americans 241
- 12.1 Stress 241
  - 12.1.1 Less Educational Opportunities 242
  - 12.1.2 More Unemployment. 242
  - 12.1.3 Less Household Income. 243
  - 12.1.4 Systemic Pressure 243
  - 12.1.5 Stress-Induced Inflammation. 243
  - 12.1.6 Stress Leads to Obesity 244
  - 12.1.7 Stress and Cancer. 244
  - 12.1.8 Stress and Cardiometabolic Disease 245
- 12.2 Mental Illness. 245
  - 12.2.1 Depression 247
  - 12.2.2 Biased Mental Health Diagnoses. 250
  - 12.2.3 Heart Rate Variability, Mental Illness and Stress. . 251
- 12.3 Increased Exposure to Death 252
- 12.4 Sleep Differences. 253
- 12.5 Alcohol and Drug Use 254
- References. 256

13 Pain and Its Management in African Americans: Important Facts, Differences, and Disparities 263
Staja Q. Booker and Simone Jackson
- 13.1 Introduction 263
  - 13.1.1 The Deception of Pain Perception 264
  - 13.1.2 Public Health-Human-Civil Rights Issue 266

	13.2	Differences in the Experience of Pain	267
		13.2.1 Perception and Communication of Pain	267
		13.2.2 Barriers to Care	268
		13.2.3 Cultural Considerations	269
	13.3	Psychosocial Aspects of Pain	271
		13.3.1 Patient Advocacy	272
	13.4	Best Practices for African Americans: Interventions and Treatment Approaches	273
		13.4.1 Pain Affirming Care	273
		13.4.2 Assessment	274
		13.4.3 Diagnosis	274
		13.4.4 Treatment	274
	13.5	Conclusion	277
	13.6	Resources and Tools	277
		13.6.1 Information Sheet	277
		13.6.2 Websites (See Box 13.2)	279
	References		279
14	**Dietary and Nutritional Need Differences in African Americans and Ways to Impact Choices**		285
	14.1	Historical Perspectives	285
	14.2	Dietary Components	286
	14.3	Fried Foods	288
	14.4	Importance of Breakfast	290
		14.4.1 Lactose Intolerance	292
	14.5	Beverage Differences	292
	14.6	Vitamins, Minerals, and Supplements	295
		14.6.1 Vitamin D Deficiency	295
		14.6.2 Other Vitamin Issues	298
		14.6.3 Mineral Deficiencies	299
	References		302
15	**Connecting with African American Patients Using Emotional Intelligence and Stories: Improving Adherence and Compliance**		307
	15.1	Emotional and Cultural Intelligence	307
	15.2	Storytelling	310
		15.2.1 Storytelling Influences Start Early	311
	15.3	Marketing for Good Health	311
		15.3.1 The Patient's Perspective	314
		15.3.2 Hypertension and Diabetes Examples	315
		15.3.3 Worldview = Culture = Cultural Intelligence	317
	References		319

16 An "Oath" and a Responsibility to All Patients.................. 321
    16.1 Foundations of Medical Ethics 323
    16.2 Misunderstandings....................................... 324
    16.3 Recognizing and Correcting Barriers to Good Care 325
    16.4 Small Improvements Within a Population
           Can Yield Impressive Gains............................. 326
    References.. 329

Index... 331

About the Editor and Contributors

Editor

Gregory L. Hall School of Medicine, Case Western Reserve University, Cleveland, OH, USA

Contributors

Staja Q. Booker Department of Biobehavioral Nursing Science, College of Nursing, University of Florida, Gainesville, FL, USA

Simone Jackson Department of Biobehavioral Nursing Science, College of Nursing, University of Florida, Gainesville, FL, USA

Keesha Powell-Roach Rutgers School of Nursing, Nursing Science Division, Rutgers Biomedical and Health Sciences, New Brunswick, NJ, USA

Chapter 1
Precision Medicine for African Americans

Contents

1.1	"Race is Just a Social Construct," But What Does the Evidence Show.	2
1.2	"Ancestral Genomics" Might Be the Answer.	3
1.3	Who Are African Americans?.	4
1.4	Evidence-Based Differences.	5
1.5	Pay for Performance.	7
1.6	Patient-Centered Care.	8
References.		11

The National Institutes of Health defines precision medicine as "an innovative approach that takes into account individual differences in patient's genes, environment, and lifestyles [1]. Another form of "personalized medicine" that is "rooted in the belief that since individuals possess nuanced and unique characteristics at the molecular, physiological, environmental exposure and behavioral levels, they may need to have interventions provided to them for diseases they possess that are tailored to these nuanced and unique characteristics."

Precision medicine was not a widely known concept at the writing of the first edition of this book, but the approach of considering genetic differences (sickle cell, benign ethnic neutropenia, and medication intolerance), environment (lead exposure, urban asthma irritants, and social determinants of health), and lifestyle differences (cultural norms, diet, exercise, and tobacco exposure) with the goal of improving health outcomes was exactly what that and this edition covers.

Pharmacogenomics, which looks at how your DNA affects the way you respond to medication, is one crucial aspect of precision medicine but directing chemotherapy based on tumor genetics or examining an individual's cardiovascular reaction to salt exposure would also easily fit into that mold [2–4].

Within cardiovascular medicine, differences in angiotensin-converting enzyme's ability to control blood pressure, as well as a very high adverse event profile, have been seen in African Americans [5]. An increased tendency to form blood clots in African Americans has a genetic basis and likely drives the highest risk for stroke (blood clot in the brain), heart attack (clot in the heart), and deep vein thrombosis/

© The Author(s), under exclusive license to Springer Nature
Switzerland AG 2025
G. L. Hall, *Precision Medicine for African Americans*,
https://doi.org/10.1007/978-3-031-95774-1_1

pulmonary embolism (blood clots in the legs and lungs) [6]. The ensuing treatment with warfarin is different, requiring higher dosing among African Americans. Hydralazine and isosorbide dinitrate's unique ability to best treat heart failure in this population also has been established [7].

The most frequent cancers including lung, colorectal, breast, prostate, and others have curious differences in occurrence and treatments that can only be best addressed using precision medicine approaches.

1.1 "Race is Just a Social Construct," But What Does the Evidence Show

Richard Lewontin showed in 1972 that approximately 85% of human genetic variation was found within racial groups, compared with only ~15% between groups, and he concluded that race is "of no social value … is positively destructive of social and human relations … [and is] of virtually no genetic or taxonomic significance." [8] This conclusive and frequently replicated finding is not the end of the story, as Jordan and colleagues wrote regarding population pharmacogenomics and drawing conclusions based on race:

> This fundamental result has been replicated many times since, and it is often taken to support the irrelevance of racial classification to human genetic variation. This is consistent with the notion that race and ethnicity are purely social constructs with little or no biological significance. Here, it must be reiterated that observed patterns of pharmacogenomic variation, particularly as they relate to adverse drug reactions, clearly support the clinical relevance of race and ethnicity. In fact, we previously showed that when pharmacogenomic variation is partitioned exactly in the way that Lewontin and others have described, 85% within-group variation and 15% between-group variation, there can be up to 700 excess adverse drug reactions per 1000 patients predicted for the recessive effect mode and as many as 300 adverse reactions predicted for the dominant mode. In other words, a high relative excess of within- versus between-group genetic variation, as is almost always seen for human populations, does not preclude the utility of race and ethnicity for pharmacogenomic risk stratification [9].

In other words, the race-based differences we see in adverse drug reactions, for example, are still statistically possible given the gene variations Lewontin observed. They advocate having a substantially more open mind rather than simply adopting a race-based view … or rejecting it.

> We contend that scientists should be able to accommodate more than one view on the constitution of racial and ethnic groups. Clearly, these groups are socially constructed, given that their boundaries and composition are delineated by humans. Accordingly, they differ with respect to non-genetic factors that are relevant to health outcomes, such as diet, lifestyle, and socioenvironmental factors. And just as clearly, socially defined racial and ethnic groups can and do differ genetically in ways that are relevant to disease treatment decisions. It follows that efforts to eliminate race and ethnicity from genomics research and clinical considerations, however well-intentioned, will ultimately do more harm than good, exacerbating rather than ameliorating existing health disparities. A more nuanced approach to race and ethnicity, one which recognizes both the social and genetic dimensions of these groups,

can be effectively leveraged to support health equity following the roadmap laid out by the United States National Institute on Minority Health and Health Disparities, promoting fairness and opportunity in disease treatments and health outcomes [9].

1.2 "Ancestral Genomics" Might Be the Answer

By looking at specific genes that were passed down from our ancestors, in combination with a consideration of their environment and how that may have influenced the natural selection process, scientists are finding the root cause of many of the human traits as well as disease processes we see. Using ancestry and genetic variations that were created by age-old population migrations, the answers to many questions related to health are much closer to our reach [10].

Constance Hilliard, in her book "Ancestral Genomics: African American Health in the Age of Precision Medicine" discusses our "human" genetics:

> … in the West, the continent of Africa remains marginalized because of its brutal history of colonialism, widespread poverty, and political instability. The genomics of its inhabitants are assumed to be replete with inconsequential and even primitive gene variants. Given the "otherness" associated with African ancestry, it is not surprising that the scientific community reflects the biases of the larger society. But the truth is that the African genome, far from being marginal, is the closest thing we have to a panhuman genome (as it represents the entire ancestral DNA lineage of our species) [11].

The broad variety of the human genome that began in Africa does not negate the migrations and natural selections that ensued based on life on whatever part of the earth various communities landed.

Hilliard also explains the ancestral origins of African Americans that were descendants of African farmers kidnapped during the slave trade. Most of the enslaved were not from coastal West Africa as originally assumed, but instead from arid, low-salt regions hundreds of miles inland. These African farmers' physiology adapted through centuries of very low salt, becoming genetically best suited to thrive with low-salt diets. Once introduced to a higher-salt environment, these descendants developed more hypertension, cardiovascular disease, and kidney failure [11].

The Africans that inhabited the salt-rich coastal African countries show dramatically different health outcomes with much lower salt sensitivity, hypertension, and risk of certain cancers. These differences from within people of African descent may also explain why prostate cancer is ten times more prevalent in African American men compared with West African men and over three times more deadly [12]. As these coastal Africans immigrate to America, their health risks are less consistent with traditional descendants-of-slaves African Americans.

All of the descendants of West Africa were also exposed to the equatorial sun with 12-hour days all year. As farmers, sun exposure was non-negotiable, and vitamin D deficiency was exceedingly rare. Their American descendants show dramatic vitamin D deficiency consistent with much lower sun exposure. Low vitamin D levels have been associated with increased comorbidities, which some researchers suggest are behind many of the disparities we see [13].

> Moderate-to-strong evidence exists that high 25-hydroxyvitamin D levels and/or vitamin D supplementation reduces risk for many adverse health outcomes including all-cause mortality rate, adverse pregnancy and birth outcomes, cancer, diabetes mellitus, Alzheimer's disease and dementia, multiple sclerosis, acute respiratory tract infections, COVID-19, asthma exacerbations, rickets, and osteomalacia. We suggest that people with low vitamin D status, which would include most people with dark skin living at high latitudes, along with their health care provider, consider taking vitamin D3 supplements to raise serum 25-hydroxyvitamin D levels to 30 ng/mL (75 nmol/L) or possibly higher [13].

Genetic science is behind many of the health disparities we see, but surely not all of them. Social determinants drive many, and we need to tease out the root causes and address them as indicated.

1.3 Who Are African Americans?

When we register for almost anything in the United States, we are asked to "self-identify" our race and/or ethnicity. Sometimes, the options are dizzying, but most of the time, there are only a few: non-Hispanic White/Caucasian, non-Hispanic Black/African American, etc. Most of the research information delivered here is based on how patients self-identified. Most research related to patient data starts with a registration form, and then differences can be seen based on demographics by gender, location, profession, etc.

The process of grouping all Americans of African descent together, as is done with most registration forms, neglects to correct for the distinctly different health outcomes seen in native-born African Americans of slave descent and more newly immigrated foreign-born African Americans.

Since 1960, there has been an over 20-fold increase in foreign-born African Americans [14]. Initially, immigration from Caribbean islands was paramount, but since the early 2000s, African nations have contributed the most to that population. Mosi Adesina Ifatunji at the University of Wisconsin wrote about Black nativity and health disparities:

> Our understanding of health disparities is encumbered by overarching disagreements as to whether "race" is defined by or rooted in a social context, group behaviors, or biological endowments ... Although these population trends have resulted in greater diversification in the Black population, most research into population health overlooks this diversity. This practice obscures our ability to analyze and understand the increasing variation in the health status of this rapidly diversifying population. Indeed, disparities between native and foreign-born Blacks are wider than those between other native and foreign-born populations within other racialized groups [15].

A study published in the *Journal of the American Heart Association* by Turkson-Ocran and colleagues compared cardiovascular disease risk factors between African immigrants and African Americans and found consistently lower risk factors in

1.4 Evidence-Based Differences

African immigrants including less hypertension (23% versus 34%), diabetes (8% versus 11%), obesity (60% versus 70%), high cholesterol (4% versus 6%), physical inactivity (53% versus 55%), and current smoking (4% versus 19%) [16].

> We expected differences in hypertension prevalence because both groups have unique cultural backgrounds, values, and lifestyles, although they are considered "blacks." The lower prevalence among African immigrants may be attributed to positive selection processes which allow healthier and more educated individuals to migrate to the United States [16].

Because the legal immigration process is costly, the authors believe the increased financial resources and educational levels seen in African immigrants are skewing the cardiovascular risk factors results in their favor. They also found that immigrants here over 10 years continued to have good cardiovascular profiles and were not negatively impacted by "living in America" [16].

Another review looking at depression in African Americans of Caribbean descent, native African Americans, and European Americans found the following:

> Lifetime MDD (major depressive disorder) prevalence estimates were highest for whites (17.9%), followed by Caribbean blacks (12.9%) and African Americans (10.4%); however, 12-month MDD estimates across groups were similar. The chronicity of MDD was higher for both black groups (56.5% for African Americans and 56.0% for Caribbean blacks) than for whites (38.6%). Fewer than half of the African Americans (45.0%) and fewer than a quarter (24.3%) of the Caribbean blacks who met the criteria received any form of MDD therapy. In addition, relative to whites, both black groups were more likely to rate their MDD as severe or very severe and more disabling [17].

In terms of cancer, Pinheiro and colleagues at the University of Miami School of Medicine looked at cancer variability between African Americans, Afro-Caribbeans, and Africans and found:

> US-born African Americans showed the highest cancer mortality burden, not only for the most common cancers, lung, breast, prostate, and colorectal but also for some infection-related cancers, including stomach and cervical. African immigrants generally had the lowest rates, with notable exceptions for liver and endometrial cancers [18].

A study looking at beliefs associated with cancer screening revealed a 90% lower propensity for African immigrants when compared with African Americans to have completed a colonoscopy [19]. Other reviews also suggested that African immigrants had lower overall cancer screening rates and lower awareness of screening recommendations compared with other populations [20, 21]. Giving precise care means considering these trends and working to improve them.

1.4 Evidence-Based Differences

This book, however, cites "evidence-based" research where "differences" based on race/ethnicity existed however it was defined. When population differences did not achieve statistical significance, it was likely because of the heterogeneity inherent in almost any racial/ethnic group in the United States. In order for differences to exist, a statistical difference had to exist, and with African American health differences (including averaging in the improved outcomes of foreign-born African Americans), many of these differences remained unequivocal.

Many of the important differences in the care of African Americans involve giving more attention to certain details of their care. Screen more vigilantly for cancer, spend more time on smoking cessation, and think about lupus, sarcoidosis, and other rare disorders when you are frustrated by an odd patient presentation. This approach is no different than "thinking of Lyme disease" when a patient presents with complaints after camping in New England. Lyme disease can be transmitted in numerous places across the United States, but providers are trained to particularly look for oddball diseases in these cases because the likelihood is supposed to be higher.

Some of the important differences we see in African Americans are based on genetic differences like sickle cell anemia and others. Other differences are based on diet, environmental exposures, poverty, lifestyle choices, and more. These differences are not to be applied blindly to every African American patient you see, but instead are to be "considered." By simply considering these important differences, improved clinical care outcomes across a population will ensue.

Aside from these crucial considerations, nothing can be accomplished between clinician and patient with effective communication. The Institute of Medicine's *Unequal Treatment: Confronting Racial and Ethnic Disparities in Health Care* section on cross-cultural communication describes the benefits:

> Sociocultural differences between patient and provider influence communication and clinical decision-making. Evidence suggests that provider-patient communication is directly linked to patient satisfaction, adherence, and subsequently, health outcomes. Thus, when sociocultural differences between patient and provider aren't appreciated, explored, understood, or communicated in the medical encounter, the result is patient dissatisfaction, poor adherence, poorer health outcomes, and racial/ethnic disparities in care. And it is not only the patient's culture that matters; the provider's "culture" is equally important. Historical factors for patient mistrust, provider bias, and its impact on physician decision-making have also been documented. Failure to take sociocultural factors into account may lead to stereotyping, and in the worst cases, biased or discriminatory treatment of patients based on race, culture, language proficiency, or social status [22].

After reviewing countless research articles and interviewing numerous physicians, there are clear clinical differences between racial and ethnic communities that allow some generalizations that can be impactful in the clinical setting. Some of these differences are based on poverty, education, or urban environment, while others are more lifestyle-related and based on local community norms (smoking, diet, or lack of exercise). Advances in genetics and epigenetics are also highlighting differences that can impact the course or severity of a number of diseases [23].

Alexis Vick and Heather Burris at Harvard University described the potential impact of social and environmental exposures and the epigenetic pathophysiologic consequences:

> Epigenetic mechanisms, particularly DNA methylation, can be altered in response to exposures such as air pollution, psychosocial stress, and smoking. Each of these exposures has

been linked to the above health states (cardiovascular disease, cancer, and preterm birth) with striking racial disparities in exposure levels. DNA methylation patterns have also been shown to be associated with each of these health outcomes.... Whether DNA methylation mediates exposure-disease relationships and can help explain racial disparities in health is not known. However, because many environmental and adverse social exposures disproportionately affect minorities, understanding the role that epigenetics plays in the human response to these exposures that often result in disease, is critical to reducing disparities in morbidity and mortality [24].

Despite the widespread human genetic similarity described earlier, there are undeniable and statistically significant differences in health outcomes for African Americans. As the root cause of these differences becomes clearer, it is essential for us to stay abreast of the latest trends and distinctions.

1.5 Pay for Performance

Any time spent trying to find ways to better care for patients is advantageous, and now, thanks to clinician "pay-for-performance" outcome measurements, more competently treating individual patients will directly drive our income potential [25–27]. The apparent problem is the potential penalty clinicians pay for having a significant African American patient population. Markovitz and Ryan commented on these "disappointing results":

> There is a pressing need to move from volume-based to value-based payments to health care providers. Theoretically, P4P (pay for performance) presents a clear mechanism by which payers can reward clinical outcomes rather than clinical activity. Empirically, however, P4P presents a murkier picture. Among patient factors, one of the clearest findings was that practices and hospitals that serve poor patients and patients of color fared worse under P4P. Performance did not systematically vary by any other patient factors, including insurance type, gender, age, or patient health.

Using precision medicine to address these disparities and avoid penalties in our pay or outliers in our quality reports is a great first step. If considered selfishly, poor patient outcomes will drag down our "accountability scores," influence our reimbursement and preferred status with insurance, and jeopardize our ability to make a living. More globally, by ignoring potential differences that impact clinical outcomes, we are negatively affecting health disparities and decreasing the quality of the care we provide.

The Agency for Healthcare Research and Quality (AHRQ) looked at hospitalizations by race/ethnicity and then stratified the outcome by income and found that *in all income groups*, the rates of potentially avoidable hospitalizations were higher for African Americans than European Americans. In fact, European Americans in the lowest income groups had lower rates of avoidable hospitalizations than the richest African Americans [28].

Most clinicians acknowledge the existence of health disparities and unequal care when looking outward at the world, the United States, or their immediate community. The problem occurs when individual clinicians have to come to terms with their personal contribution to health disparities [29]. In a sense, many believe unequal care occurs, but *just not when they are around.* Accepting that you might be contributing to unequal care is a big step and can be a professional revelation.

Many minority clinicians falsely believe that because they are minorities, they cannot contribute to health disparities. They believe that through a birthright, they automatically treat everyone appropriately. Not true. A lack of knowledge of clinical differences in patient populations you treat results in inferior care. Anyone of any race or ethnicity can have a lack of knowledge. Learning about the cultural perspective of a patient and the research-verified clinical care differences allows us to better connect, adapt our interventions appropriately, and positively impact clinical outcomes.

The recent expansion of research based on detailed genetic mapping has allowed for significant advances in our understanding of why some medications or clinical approaches work in some patients and not in others. Considerations like salt sensitivity, which impacts less than 50% of the overall American population, affect over 70% of African Americans [30, 31]. These differences offer significantly alternative approaches to population health. Genetic and epigenetic differences that affect the level of kidney disease, severity of cancer, level of cholesterol, risk for stroke or obesity, and much more have all been identified and shown to be significantly different in African Americans.

Knowing about and implementing clinical care that is carefully tailored to your patient population will require additional time and effort, but that energy will be saved in the more efficient control of hypertension, reduction of obesity, anticipation and prevention of cancers, and countless other approaches that will undeniably improve your clinical care.

1.6 Patient-Centered Care

In 1988, the Picker Institute coined the term "patient-centered care" as a way to move medical care back to its roots, where physicians provided compassionate and personalized care to a patient before applying an array of diagnostic technologies that moved the physician away from direct patient involvement [32]. Patient-centered care, as reported by the Institute of Medicine, is one of the six key elements of high-quality care listed in their landmark "Crossing the Quality Chasm" report of 2002 [33]. This medical expert-driven report stresses that healthcare should be:

1. *Safe*—avoiding injuries to patients from the care that is intended to help them
2. *Effective*—providing services based on scientific knowledge to all who could benefit and refraining from providing services to those not likely to benefit (avoiding underuse and overuse)

3. *Patient-centered*—providing care that is respectful of and responsive to individual patient preferences, needs, and values and ensuring that patient values guide all clinical decisions
4. *Timely*—reducing waits and sometimes harmful delays for both those who receive and those who give care
5. *Efficient*—avoiding waste, in particular, waste of resources
6. *Equitable*—providing care that does not vary in quality because of personal characteristics such as gender, ethnicity, geographic location, and socioeconomic status

As healthcare continues to be transformed, placing the patient back into the focus of care has been a central tenet.

With African Americans representing 13% of the total US population and over 45 million people [34], learning about the culturally driven healthcare issues that this population faces is time well spent. African Americans in some urban areas make up greater than 50% of patients at a given hospital. To not spend any time learning about their cultural foundations as a people and their racial or ethnic clinical care idiosyncrasies is a recipe for poor patient outcomes. Having patient-centered care as a quality measure has both simplified and complicated the dilemma that cultural competence presented.

In 1985 the Health and Human Resources Secretary under President Ronald Reagan, Margaret Heckler, formed the Secretary's Task Force on Black and Minority Health [35]. This "Heckler Report" would, for the first time, legitimize the notion that African Americans were suffering from persistent health disparities that accounted for excess morbidity and mortality. This report inspired the formation of the US Office on Minority Health and state-based Commissions on Minority Health.

In 1998 Jeffrey T. Berger wrote "Culture and Ethnicity in Clinical Care" for the Journal of the American Medical Association and stressed the importance of "physician recognition of the cultural context of patients' illnesses (that) can be essential to a successful therapeutic relationship." [36] Soon after, the term cultural competence [37] began to reflect a practitioner's "ability to interact effectively with people of different cultures." It essentially meant being respectful and responsive to the health beliefs and practices—and cultural and linguistic needs—of diverse population groups. Developing cultural competence was seen as an evolving, dynamic process that occurred along a continuum.

Scholars and practitioners questioned the futility of placing any particular patient in a cultural category with any degree of precision [38]. Moreover, anthropologists and sociologists wondered if a person from one culture could truly become "competent" in another culture and maintain it over time. Most agreed that achieving "cultural competence" in multiple cultures was likely futile due to the pure volume of information to master.

Within a couple of years, the concept and benefits of patient-centered care began to take hold. Patient-centered care results in a better perception of the quality of care, improved health status (less discomfort, less concern, and better mental health), and increased efficiency of care (reduced diagnostic tests and referrals), as reported in a study by Stewart et al. [38] They found that patients had the impression of improved health based on "being a full participant in the discussions during the encounter" which led to better trust in their providers.

African Americans have been the recipients of population-centered care. Well-meaning practitioners from across the country have insisted that the American experience culturally provided enough customization for African Americans. One burning question remained. Why were African American clinical outcomes so poor with such significant disparities?

If the cultural experience were the same (or even similar) across Americans, providing cultural care in a standardized fashion would make sense. But from a healthcare standpoint, the cultural differences between African Americans and European Americans are stark. Historically African Americans have not had equal access. Instead, inferior care was accepted, and there was experimentation, exclusions from hospitals, and abuse of African American bodies, both living and dead. These substantive historical differences greatly impact African Americans' perspective of the medical field in general, and of clinicians in particular.

The unequal treatment of the African American poor and disenfranchised throughout the history of slavery, poverty, and civil rights violations is an unfortunate but undeniable part of American history. To ignore that cultural history and the stories of those not-too-distant events and pretend that modern-day African Americans are minimally influenced by those events is wishful thinking at best.

The study and published article "Race and Trust in the Health Care System" looked specifically at the perspectives African Americans had regarding medical research, healthcare, and physicians when compared with European Americans [39]. African Americans were less likely to trust their physicians and more likely to be concerned about personal privacy and harmful experimentation. Thus there are patterns of distrust of our healthcare system among African Americans that impact their acceptance of our advice, comfort with our use of their personal information, and suspicion of our motives to help. This is in stark contrast to European Americans who, by and large, do not come to the table with these concerns [40]. Generally, European Americans have good impressions of the medical care delivered by physicians and nurses, and there is minimal, if any, history of experimentation, collusion, or neglect for this population in America. The two resulting perspectives, one of implicit trust and confidence and the other with mistrust and suspicions of motives, provide a dramatically contrasting patient base that will require differing approaches to establishing a successful patient-physician relationship.

To accept the events of America's medical and clinical past is, at times, painful because we have been trained to believe that our medical profession is the best in the world, and it is. But being the best does not make it flawless. Being the best does not erase the countless indecencies suffered by African Americans. But acknowledging the past and adjusting our care based on that past medical history is a sound and beneficial approach to the care of a historically abused people.

The ensuing chapters will briefly review an approach to the patient-centered care of African Americans that "considers" their cultural and racial past, as well as recent data suggesting best practices in clinical care. These best practices are merely the customization of clinical decisions to the African American race. As researchers find progressively more differences in the genetics and epigenetics of heart disease, specific cancers, approaches to pharmacological therapy, and others that are different in African Americans from European Americans or other ethnicities, thought leaders are now proclaiming (with decreasing health disparities in mind) that there are a number of clear and impactful differences in clinical care that merit all clinicians' notice.

From the genetic mutational profiles of prostate and breast cancers that make them more aggressive to the genomic risk prediction models for common diseases that allow for early detection and more efficient treatment, genetic scientists across the world are uncovering a wealth of clinical nuances that can greatly impact quality care and outcomes in African Americans. Precision clinical care tailored for African Americans will undeniably improve outcomes.

References

1. National Institutes of Health. The Promise of Precision Medicine. https://www.nih.gov/about-nih/what-we-do/nih-turning-discovery-into-health/promise-precision-medicine
2. CDC. Genomics and Your Health. Pharmacogenomics. https://www.cdc.gov/genomics-and-health/about/pharmacogenetics.html
3. The Promise of Precision Medicine. National Institute of Health. https://www.nih.gov/about-nih/what-we-do/nih-turning-discovery-into-health/promise-precision-medicine. Accessed 4 Dec 2024.
4. Richardson SI, Freedman BI, Ellison DH, Rodriguez CJ. Salt sensitivity: a review with a focus on non-Hispanic blacks and Hispanics. J Am Soc Hypertens. 7(2):170–9. https://doi.org/10.1016/j.jash.2013.01.003.
5. Kostis WJ, Mrinali S, Singh CY, Kostis John B. ACE Inhibitor-induced angioedema: a review. Curr Hypertens Rep. 20(7) https://doi.org/10.1007/s11906-018-0859-x.
6. Kuk KH, Tantry US, Hyun-Woong P, Eun-Seok S, Tobias G, Gorog DA, Gurbel Paul A, Young-Hoon J. Ethnic difference of Thrombogenicity in patients with cardiovascular disease: a Pandora box to explain prognostic differences. Korean Circulation Journal. 2021;51(3):202. https://doi.org/10.4070/kcj.2020.0537.
7. Aditi S, Chrisly D, Limdi Nita A. Pharmacogenetics of Warfarin dosing in patients of African and European ancestry. Pharmacogenomics. 19(17):1357–71. https://doi.org/10.2217/pgs-2018-0146.
8. Lewontin RC. Directions in evolutionary biology. Annu Rev Genet. 2002;36(1):1–18.
9. King JI, Shivam S, Leonardo M-R. Population pharmacogenomics for health equity. Genes. 2023;14(10):1840. https://doi.org/10.3390/genes14101840.
10. Sapiens. Padilla-Iglesias, C. Did Humanity Really Arise in One Place? https://www.sapiens.org/archaeology/human-evolution-east-africa/
11. Hilliard CB. Ancestral genomics: African American health in the age of precision medicine. Harvard University Press; 2024.
12. Odedina FT, Ogunbiyi JO, Ukoli FA. Roots of prostate cancer in African-American men. J Natl Med Assoc. 2006;98(4):539–43.
13. Ames BN, Grant WB, Willett WC. Does the high prevalence of vitamin D deficiency in African Americans contribute to health disparities? Nutrients. 2021;13(2):499. https://doi.org/10.3390/nu13020499.

14. Yvonne C-M, Ruth-Alma T-O, Nmezi NA, Manka N, Joycelyn C, Mensah DS, Sarah Y, Sarah M, Nishit P, Eunice A, Justine C, Francoise M-M, George M, Cheryl D-H, Cooper LA. Commentary: engaging African immigrants in research—experiences and lessons from the field. Ethn Dis. 2019;29(4):617–22. https://doi.org/10.18865/ed.29.4.617.
15. Adesina IM, Yanica F, Wendy L, Deshira W. Black nativity and health disparities: a research paradigm for understanding the social determinants of health. Int J Environ Res Public Health. 2022;19(15):9166. https://doi.org/10.3390/ijerph19159166.
16. Turkson-Ocran R-AN, Nmezi NA, Botchway MO, Szanton SL, Hill GS, Cooper LA, Yvonne C-M. Comparison of cardiovascular disease risk factors among African immigrants and African Americans: an analysis of the 2010 to 2016. National Health Interview Surveys. J Am Heart Assoc. 9(5) https://doi.org/10.1161/JAHA.119.013220.
17. Williams David R, González Hector M, Harold N, Randolph N, Abelson Jamie M, Julie S, Jackson James S. Prevalence and distribution of major depressive disorder in African Americans Caribbean blacks and non-Hispanic whites. Arch Gen Psychiatry. 64(3):305. https://doi.org/10.1001/archpsyc.64.3.305.
18. Pinheiro Paulo S, Heidy M, Callahan Karen E, Deukwoo K, Camille R, Recinda S, Kobetz Erin N, Ahmedin J. Cancer mortality among US blacks: variability between African Americans Afro-Caribbeans and Africans. Cancer Epidemiol. 66:66101709. https://doi.org/10.1016/j.canep.2020.101709.
19. Adegboyega A, Wiggins AT, Obielodan O, Dignan M, Schoenberg N. Beliefs associated with cancer screening behaviors among African Americans and sub-Saharan African immigrant adults: a cross-sectional study. BMC Public Health. 2022;22(1):2219. https://doi.org/10.1186/s12889-022-14591-x.
20. Alejandra H-d-M, Minna S, Ocla K, Yvonne J, Ify N, Sheppard Vanessa B. Addressing cancer control needs of African-born immigrants in the US: A systematic literature review. Preventive Med:6789–99. https://doi.org/10.1016/j.ypmed.2014.07.006.
21. Consedine NS, Tuck NL, Ragin CR, Spencer BA. Beyond the black box: a systematic review of breast prostate colorectal and cervical screening among native and Immigrant African-descent Caribbean populations. J Immigr Minor Health. 17(3):905–24. https://doi.org/10.1007/s10903-014-9991-0.
22. Smedley BD, Stith AY, Nelson AR, editors. Unequal treatment: confronting racial and ethnic disparities in health care. Washington: The National Academies Press; 2003. p. 200–1.
23. Andrea SAE, Hedrich Christian M. The role of epigenetics in autoimmune/inflammatory disease. Front Immunol. 2019; https://doi.org/10.3389/fimmu.2019.01525.
24. Vick AD, Burris HH. Epigenetics and health disparities. Curr Epidemiol Rep. 2017;4(1):31–7.
25. Rosenthal MB, Frank RG, Li Z, Epstein AM. Early experience with pay-for-performance: from concept to practice. JAMA. 2005;294:1788–93.
26. Rosenthal MB. Beyond pay for performance--emerging models of provider-payment reform. New Engl J Med 2008;359:1197–1200.
27. Bond AM, Volpp KG, Emanual EJ, et al. Real-time feedback in pay-for-performance: does more information lead to improvement? J Gen Inter Med. 2019;34(9):1737–43. https://doi.org/10.1007/s11606-019-05004-8.
28. 2015 National healthcare quality and disparities report chartbook on health care for blacks. Rockville: Agency for Healthcare Research and Quality. 2016. AHRQ Pub. No 16-0015-1-EF.
29. Kendrick J, Nuccio E, Leiferman JA, Sauaia A. Primary care providers' perceptions of racial/ethnic and socioeconomic disparities in hypertension control. Am J Hypertens. 2015;28(9):1091–7.
30. Luft FC, Grim CE, Higgins JT Jr, Weinberger MH. Differences in response to sodium administration in normotensive white and black subjects. J Lab Clin Med. 1977;90(3):555–62.
31. Madhavan S, Alderman MH. Ethnicity and the relationship of sodium intake to blood pressure. J Hypertens. 1994;12(1):97–103.
32. Frampton Susan B, Sara G, Michael L. Compassion as the foundation of patient-centered care: the importance of compassion in action. J Comp Effective Res. 2(5):443–55. https://doi.org/10.2217/cer.13.54.
33. Institute of Medicine (US). Committee on quality Care in America. Crossing the quality chasm: a new health system for the 21st century. Washington: National Academies Press (US); 2001.

References

34. United States Census Bureau. Retrieved from https://www.census.gov/quickfacts/fact/table/US. Accessed 4 Dec 2024.
35. The heckler report: a force for ending health disparities in America. Retrieved from https://minorityhealth.hhs.gov/heckler30/. Accessed 6 May 2019.
36. Berger J. Culture and ethnicity in clinical care. Arch Intern Med. 1998;158(19):2085–90.
37. Cultural competence. https://www.samhsa.gov/capt/applying-strategic-prevention/cultural-competence. Accessed 6 May 2019.
38. Stewart M, Brown J, Donner A, et al. The impact of patient-centered care on outcomes. J Fam Pract. 2000;49(9):796–804.
39. Boulware L, Cooper L, Ratner L, LaVeist T, Powe N. Race and trust in the health care system. Public Health Rep. 2003;118:358.
40. Halbert C, Armstrong K, Gandy O, Shaker B. Racial differences in trust in health care providers. Arch Intern Med. 2006;166(8):896–901.

Chapter 2
Establishing Trust in African American Patients

Contents

2.1	The Tuskegee Syphilis Study.	16
2.2	Other Examples of Abuse.	17
2.3	Differences in Trust.	18
	2.3.1 Trust Improves Health Outcomes.	20
2.4	Explicit and Implicit Biases Impact Our Healthcare.	21
2.5	Building Trust.	23
2.6	Show Competence.	25
References.		27

Multiple studies over an extended period of time confirm what most clinicians already knew. African Americans are generally not as trusting of medical clinicians as other racial groups [1, 2]. What many of us did not know was why. As clinicians, we spent many years training to help others. Medicine is a service profession. Why would anyone suspect our intentions, question our motives, or assign us collectively as untrustworthy? The answer lies in the historical experience African Americans had with America's doctors, hospitals, and researchers.

Before delving into ways to build trust, it is imperative to have a perspective on why the trust that most of the majority population has for the field of medicine is lost to many African Americans. And why, despite the fact that many of these historical atrocities occurred to people other than today's patients, the stories and suspicions are passed from one generation to the next.

2.1 The Tuskegee Syphilis Study

The U.S. Public Health Service (USPHS) Untreated Syphilis Study at Tuskegee was originally formed to record the natural history of syphilis with the hope of justifying the funding of public treatment programs for African Americans. The study, which began in 1932, included 600 African American men, 399 with syphilis and 201 without the disease [3, 4]. While the study was originally slated to last 6 months, it was extended for over 40 years. Penicillin became widely available in 1942 as an accepted curative treatment for syphilis, but the researchers wanted to gain more information about untreated syphilis, so the participants were neither informed nor treated. Central to the study was the patient's lack of informed consent. None of the patients were told they had syphilis. Instead they were told they had "bad blood" that required ongoing monitoring. In exchange for taking part in the study, the men received free medical exams, free meals, and burial insurance. Many physicians, including African Americans, and national physician societies fully supported the study.

During this government-funded study in the name of public health, researchers not only allowed the disease to progress but actively blocked the men from receiving curable treatment, not just from the study physicians but also from other community physicians. The researchers implemented a coordinated effort ... a verified conspiracy, with area physicians and hospitals to actively block treatment for the study participants if they presented elsewhere for care. While wives and partners were treated, they were not notified of the diagnosis, so the study remained secure, and infected patients remained in the dark. Needless to say, this endeavor required the widespread dissemination of personal health information across an entire region and involving hundreds of people. The names and a stigmatizing diagnosis were circulated widely, and in a way that the patient would not know [2]. The fact that nearly 400 African American men were denied effective treatment for syphilis without their knowledge or consent so that researchers could document the natural history of the disease stands as a singular event that granularly validates the mistrust African Americans have against the medical establishment.

It was not until 1972, when a news article reported the details of the study, that a government review panel finally halted it. The Tuskegee Health Benefit Program was established as a settlement for the class action suit brought against the United States, which agreed to pay all medical and burial expenses for the subjects involved, with added support for their families. During the course of the study, 40 wives contracted the disease, and 19 children were born with congenital syphilis. Many credit the Tuskegee Syphilis Study as the primary reason informed consent regulations exist today. Unfortunately, for many African Americans, the study is a validated reason to not trust doctors, public health, medical research, or the healthcare system.

Some might argue that with the passage of time and lower health literacy among some African Americans, the Tuskegee Syphilis Study is merely a historical footnote for most African Americans. A study done at Johns Hopkins looked at awareness of the Tuskegee Syphilis Study and found an overwhelming number of African

Americans (81%) were aware of the study and its outcomes, while only 28% of European Americans had knowledge of the study [5]. Another study demonstrated widespread misinformation as it relates to the Tuskegee study, but the authors still concluded that the study had tremendous "social power" [6]. With widespread knowledge of this government-sanctioned and funded study among African Americans, mentioning the study as a way to stimulate discussion, and build trust, is a preferable approach to ignoring its existence.

2.2 Other Examples of Abuse

While the Tuskegee Syphilis Study is a "classic example" of abuse based purely on race, unfortunately, the American experience has many more examples of why African Americans mistrust the medical community.

From African Americans' earliest days in this country, abuse based on race was commonplace. Slaves were frequently used as subjects for dissection, surgical experimentation, and medical testing. J. Marion Sims, the so-called father of modern gynecology, perfected many of his surgical techniques on unanesthetized slave girls [7–9]. Stories of doctors kidnapping and killing southern Blacks for experimentation consistently appear in literature throughout American history [10] (see Harriet Washington's book "Medical Apartheid" for a detailed review of this horrendous history).

As medical education expanded in the United States, the need for cadavers for anatomy dissection grew, and grave-robbing African American cemeteries was the unfortunate solution. Medical schools in the South frequently tasked their medical students with "finding" a cadaver to dissect, and the solution was to go to Black or marginalized cemeteries to exhume the recently buried [11].

One account in Philadelphia reported that in the spring of 1883, after the snow had melted, the cemeteries looked as if "they had been subjected to an aerial bombardment" due to grave robbers actively securing specimens for anatomical dissection. The mayor at the time claimed he didn't have sufficient police to guard cemeteries [11]. Another report from the Medical College of Georgia says that they purchased a slave, Grandison Harris, whose principal task was to procure cadavers. Over the years, he became a teaching assistant and frequently appeared in graduating class photos [11]. Who better to sneak into and out of a Black cemetery than a Black man? But imagine having a loved one die, and upon your first visit to the burial site, you find the site desecrated and the body gone, and you know exactly who is responsible: the nearest medical school.

As Vanesa Northington Gamble put it in her article "Under the Shadow of Tuskegee: African Americans and Health Care" tales of "medical student" grave robbers recount the exploitation of southern African Americans as their deceased family members would be stolen and sent to northern medical schools for anatomy dissection [10]. Dr. Gamble writes:

These historical examples clearly demonstrate that African Americans' distrust of the medical profession has a longer history than the public revelations of the Tuskegee Syphilis Study. There is a collective memory among African Americans about their exploitation by the medical establishment [12].

Another book titled "The Organ Thieves: The Shocking Story of the First Heart Transplant in the Segregated South" recounts when the Medical College of Virginia Hospital orchestrated its first heart transplant harvest on a Black man who presented unconscious after a head injury from a fall at a baseball park. No family was contacted and the transplant occurred within a day of his arrival [13]. Events like this negatively impact the perspectives of the family, friends, and co-workers of this man as they undoubtedly tell more in their community. As stories of these real events spread, it negatively impacts the overall African American perspective of hospitals, clinicians, and organ donation.

History shows the first English colonists arrived at Jamestown in 1607, and 12 years later (1619), the first African Americans arrived [14]. The arrival of the first African Americans marked the beginning of a complex and tragic history of slavery and racial discrimination in America. This event set the stage for centuries of systemic inequality and injustice, which had profound social, health, economic, and political implications. It also sparked the long struggle for civil rights and equality that continues to shape American society today. This alignment of arrival in North America negates the suggestion that African Americans were a later add-on to this America as the "New World" histories aligned almost concurrently.

The arrival of African Americans led to the establishment of a racial hierarchy that permeated every aspect of society. This hierarchy justified the exploitation and dehumanization of African Americans, resulting in a legacy of social division and prejudice. Over time, these social implications manifested in segregation, disenfranchisement, and a persistent struggle for civil rights. Trust that health professionals, institutions, and society in general would be fair and equitable in the treatment of African Americans was never established.

2.3 Differences in Trust

Chanita Hughes Halbert published a study in the *Journal of the American Medical Association (JAMA)* in 2006 looking at racial differences in trust in healthcare providers. Her study of almost one thousand European American and African American patients found that "compared with European Americans, African Americans were most likely to report low trust in healthcare providers" [1].

2.3 Differences in Trust

Trust has been described as an expectation that medical care providers (physicians, nurses, and others) will act in ways that demonstrate that the patient's interests are a priority. Trust is a multidimensional construct that includes perceptions of the health care provider's technical ability, interpersonal skills, and the extent to which the patient perceives that his or her welfare is placed above other considerations. Trust is an important determinant of adherence to treatment and screening recommendations and the length and quality of relationships with health care providers [1].

Fortunately, the level of trust a patient has for any specific provider is not stagnant. It can be earned. Increased exposure to providers in general, and to the same provider specifically, has been shown to improve trust.

Studies have also shown that *racial concordance* positively impacts the level of trust for a same-race patient [15]. In simpler terms, African American patients are initially more trustful of African American providers. Those non-African American providers can, and do, achieve high levels of trust with African American patients, but doing so usually takes a little more effort.

A preference for racial/ethnic concordance in clinicians is not restricted to African Americans. Jessica Greene and colleagues surveyed over 13,000 people nationally about trust in their clinician.

Using a large, national survey, we found that almost six in ten adults (59.8%) who had a regular clinician reported having trust in the clinician. White, Black, and Latino participants were similarly likely to report trusting their clinician, while those from other racial and ethnic groups were approximately 15 percentage points less likely to. There was evidence that participants from all racial and ethnic groups were more likely to have a racial/ethnic concordant regular clinician than would be expected given the numbers of doctors currently practicing by race/ethnicity [16].

This study also found that people were more comfortable discussing gender concordance preferences than race or ethnicity as it related to their clinician. Both male and female participants were more likely to have gender-concordant clinicians. Statistical analysis found that participants with racial- and ethnic-concordant clinicians were approximately 7 percentage points more likely to report trust in their clinician than those with non-concordant clinicians (62.4% vs. 55.0%) [16].

Curiously, non-White clinicians are at a trust disadvantage when dealing with White patients and reported lower trust in clinicians of other race or ethnicities [16, 17].

It is not clear the extent to which this pattern is due to cultural connection with clinicians from similar background or racism towards those who are different from them. Since patient trust is related to patient experience scores, white patients' lower trust in non-concordant clinicians has the potential to negatively impact non-white clinicians' compensation and reputation through lower patient experiences ratings [16].

Trust is variable, and dependent on an array of factors, but being intentional about building trust in all of your patients is essential.

2.3.1 Trust Improves Health Outcomes

In 1979 Russell Caterinicchio published what is believed to be the first study attempting to measure trust in patients for their physician and its impact on outcomes [18]. They made a clear distinction between trust and satisfaction, with trust as a condition that characterizes the present and future relationship and satisfaction characterizing past encounters and outcomes. Subsequent studies have confirmed and validated what providers suspected: there is a one-to-one correlation with trust in providers and self-rated health, therapeutic response, adherence to treatments, and decreased cost of care [19].

Conversely, the lack of trust in providers has been associated with lower rates of care-seeking, preventive services, surgical treatment, and overall care. In David Thom's article "Measuring Trust in Physicians When Assessing Quality of Care," "increasing trust generally falls into the categories of competency, communication, caring, honesty, and partnering [20]." He cites prior studies that listed the following components of a trusting relationship:

1. Greater perceived mutual interests
2. Clear communication
3. A history of fulfilled trust
4. Less perceived difference in power with the person being trusted
5. Acceptance of personal disclosures
6. An expectation of a longer-term relationship

African American providers have a distinct advantage over others in the level of trust at the very beginning of their clinician-patient relationship because of their mutual cultural history. As African Americans, there is clearly a perception of comparable mutual interests, as well as a less perceived difference in power. Clearer communication may also come from the better translation of complicated medical concepts into terms and analogies that have a similar cultural basis in the African American experience.

Thom goes on to explain how a provider can achieve these components of trust:

> All of these associations suggest approaches that would be expected to increase patient trust, such as emphasizing mutual interests (the patient's health); checking patients' understanding of communication; taking opportunities to fulfill trust (phoning with test results); reducing power differences (sharing information); responding to patients' self-disclosures in a supportive and nonjudgmental way; and promoting continuity of care [20].

There are also differences in the acceptance of personal disclosures across racial lines, with African American physicians being more tolerant of disclosures that may be more pervasive in their social community. The disclosure that a patient was raised in a single-parent family and has "no idea" what medical problems their father has may flow more smoothly to an African American provider who would be perceived as having a higher likelihood of not stigmatizing that history.

A comprehensive review of racial concordance and patient-physician communication done by Megan Johnson Shen and colleagues showed the following:

Results from this systematic review demonstrate that the association between patient race (black or white) and patient-physician communication varies across studies, but the majority of the studies support the finding that black patients report poorer patient-physician communication than white patients. Namely [21], out of 66 results from analyses show that black patients report lower patient-physician communication quality and satisfaction; less information-giving, partnership building, participatory decision-making, and positive talk; more negative talk; shorter visits; physicians who were more verbally dominant; and worse outcomes on non-verbal communication, respect, and support [22].

These "objective" findings from analyzing actual clinician/patient interactions merely allow an opportunity for improvement in communication and not a reflection on a stagnant and unchangeable problem.

2.4 Explicit and Implicit Biases Impact Our Healthcare

African American patients are also generally on guard for biases, whether conscious or unconscious. More formally known as explicit and implicit biases, researchers have looked at the impact bias can have on the quality of patient encounters. Implicit biases are subconscious, whereas explicit biases are those that the practitioner is fully aware of. Providers may have an explicit bias against patients who were child molesters (as one extreme example) or against patients who are unemployed and presumably not seeking work (a subtler example). When a provider has an explicit bias, one that they admit to themselves and others, they typically work to minimize the effect of the bias on their quality of care. What is presumed is the provider's ability to work through those acknowledged explicit biases and still work for the full benefit of the patient.

Implicit biases are attitudes and stereotypes that impact our care delivery, discussion, and decisions in an unconscious manner. As noted by the Kirwan Institute for the Study of Race and Ethnicity at The Ohio State University, "implicit biases are pervasive. Everyone possesses them, even people with avowed commitments to impartiality such as judges." They go on to propose that "the implicit associations we hold do not necessarily align with our declared beliefs or even reflect stances we would explicitly endorse [23]." So many of us have no idea what our implicit biases may be … what is important is to accept that they exist and to work to get a better understanding of how they impact the care we provide.

The impact of bias on healthcare is more far-reaching than most assume. Monica Vela and associates suggested the following:

> It has been theorized that implicit bias and structural racism mutually reinforce one another—ambient structural racism and its outcomes reinforce an individual's psychological associations between racial identity and poorer outcomes (implicit bias). Inequitable structural determinants have diminished housing, education, health care, and income and have increased exposure to environmental pollutants and chronic stressors for marginalized populations. Structural inequities and discrimination have created stereotypes of marginalized populations or communities and implicit and explicit biases toward them. Health care providers hold negative explicit and implicit biases against racialized minorities. A similar

reinforcing dynamic may exist for marginalized populations such as those who are overweight/obese, use wheelchairs, have limited English proficiency, have mental health illness, and belong to lower socioeconomic classes. These biases can facilitate the creation and perpetuation of discriminatory systems and practices, creating a complex feedback loop that sustains itself [24].

Biases both expedite and influence medical decision-making more than many of us realize. By bringing awareness to how our minds work, we can more easily adapt and minimize negative outcomes in our patients.

In the "Medscape Internist Lifestyle Report 2017," Carol Peckham looked at internist's admitted explicit biases "toward specific types or groups of patients" and found wide differences between racial groups, with 75% of Japanese internists admitting bias versus 29% of Asian (non-Indian) physicians [25]. A little over half (54%) of African American internists admitted to patient biases. Being biased against patients with emotional problems led the list, and over half of internists reported this issue. Physicians also reported biases toward or against patients who are overweight, have low intelligence, speak a different language, lack insurance, have low income, are older, have a different race, are physically unattractive, or are from a different gender (in decreasing occurrence). Providers were clearly biased to the benefit of older patients, but the other biases listed were generally negative or mixed outcome biases. These biases are not mutually exclusive. If a negatively biased clinician sees a poor, undereducated, older, obese, African American woman without insurance, they have a significant number of conscious biases impacting their care. There were also distinct gender differences, with men having more biases than women across the board. The study further examined whether physician bias actually impacted care delivery, and almost one in five providers (18%) admitted that their bias did impact the quality of their care.

Generally these biases are positive toward European American patients and negative toward African American patients as a study by Oliver et al. demonstrated at the University of Virginia [26]. They found providers explicitly preferred European Americans to African Americans with "significantly higher feelings of warmth toward (European Americans)" and also found that European American patients were "more medically cooperative than African Americans." The study found no significant difference in the quality of care between the racial groups. These biases can be consciously counteracted, and admitting the existence of biases is the critical first step in canceling their effect on medical care.

A study done at Johns Hopkins by Lisa Cooper and colleagues found that primary care physicians who hold unconscious racial biases tend to dominate conversations with African American patients during routine visits, paying less attention to patients' social and emotional needs, and making these patients feel less involved in decision-making related to their health [27]. These patients also reported reduced trust in their doctors, less respectful treatment, and a lower likelihood of recommending the physician to a friend.

Louis Penner and colleagues studied the impact bias has on medical interactions with African American patients and found that implicit biases impacted perceptions more dramatically than explicit biases and that these subtly biased behaviors were perceived as more deceitful than overt explicit bias [25]:

> Whereas people are aware of their overt and deliberative (e.g., verbal) behaviors, which relate to explicit measures of their attitudes, they may be unaware of their subtly biased and spontaneous (e.g., nonverbal) behaviors, which relate to implicit measures. As targets of these behaviors, however, (African Americans) and members of other disadvantaged groups attend closely to these subtly biased behaviors, which critically shape their impressions of intergroup interactions [28].

Coming to recognize implicit bias and its impact on medical decision-making, and then sensitizing clinicians regarding their ability to correct for these covert biases, is an important step in providing equitable care. Correcting for biases eliminates unspoken barriers to trust.

2.5 Building Trust

A study by L. Ebony Boulware, in addition to confirming much lower levels of trust in African American patients, also found elevated concerns about personal privacy and the potential for harmful experimentation [29]. This is a culturally driven privacy concern based on historical trust violations suffered by African Americans. While HIPAA laws protect everyone's health information, a patient may not be as aware of these restrictions on sharing patients' information. Making a point of emphasizing the privacy of their information and your discussions, as well as affirming the absence of experimentation, can go a long way to reassuring a skeptical patient.

With the earnest goal of providing high-quality, comprehensive care, many "review-of-systems"-type questions done routinely at an initial visit may strike some patients as overly probing and bordering on obtrusive. Imagine coming in for a hip replacement and having questions regarding a history of erection problems, depression, or prior abortions. While some may view these questions as consistent with being thorough, others could easily see them as invasive, and not pertinent.

When the clinician is aware of the inclination on the part of the patient to "wonder" why they are asking about "unrelated" health problems, it is advisable to explain the rationale or skip sensitive review-of-systems questions that are not clearly pertinent to the diagnosis or discussion at hand until a more trusting rapport can be established.

Trust can be developed over time, but this requires continuity and is negatively impacted by urban clinic environments that have high clinician turnover that may limit access to a consistent primary care clinician. A study by Mark Doescher and colleagues found a disparity in the trust for healthcare providers, and additionally found that low trust levels sink lower when on subsequent visits clinician continuity was not preserved [30].

Although this seems obvious, spending time with patients is an easy approach to establishing trust. Fiscella and colleagues measured patient trust against the time spent with a patient and found a one-to-one correlation: more time spent led to more perceived trust on the part of the patient [31].

Paul Duberstein et al. looked specifically at what impacts patients' "satisfaction" with doctors and found that "openness" was associated with a much higher satisfaction rating than any of the other variables [32]. Openness, or a tendency toward self-revelations, as a way to connect, simply decreases the perceived barriers between patient and provider. The humanizing effects of discussing the provider's personal vulnerabilities while developing a relationship with a patient go a long way to building trust. The patient has come to present their personal or medical deficiencies, and without some small degree of disclosure on the provider's part, the relationship seems overly one-sided. Divulging something as simple as "I'm terrible at typing on computers" will go far to defuse some patients who may feel too large a difference in perceived power and stance. Openness facilitates the transfer of historically pertinent information that could be vital to the accurate diagnosis and treatment of many patients.

When it comes to African Americans specifically, Myra Sabir and Karl Pillemer looked at ways to gain the trust of older African Americans and improve their involvement with research [33]. In their study "An Intensely Sympathetic Awareness: Experiential Similarity and Cultural Norms as Means for Gaining Older African Americans' Trust of Scientific Research," they applied trust-building techniques with great success. By specifically honoring and reinforcing older African Americans' worth and dignity through "high-touch hospitality" measures, they were able to enlist and retain a significantly higher level of participation than the norm. Put simply, they complimented their patients, and the patients appreciated their compliments. The researchers also race-matched the primary researcher with the subjects. In addition to preserving the continuity of the primary researcher from week to week, they also sent birthday and holiday cards, and finally, they took advantage of experiential similarities as a way to bond.

Many older African Americans are annoyed by the use of their first name at an initial encounter while having to address the clinician more formally ("Good morning, Francis, I'm Doctor Smith"). Best practice is to ask how they would like to be addressed before proceeding with the assumption that you can call them by their first name [34]. This approach will avoid getting off to a bad start by annoying a patient with your very first statement.

Because of the struggles of many African Americans, confessing challenges in your own life not only shows openness but a vulnerability that can lead to a trusting connection. By "explicitly emphasizing similarities," you can break down barriers to trust and empathy. While some patients are emboldened by an invincibly intelligent and successful physician, many African Americans identify more with professionals they can identify with … one who struggled and persisted. While a majority patient would likely prefer a physician who has succeeded in all they did, minority patients look to connect through a similar redemptive experience, and the honesty to share that experience.

Walter Lee and Julia Canick compare building trust with patients to all of our earliest human experiences.

> Recognizing that trust is fundamental not only to the practice of medicine but also to every aspect of human interactions and relationships, perhaps we should remind ourselves of how trust is developed in early in life. These foundations can be found in the psychosocial development stages proposed by psychologist Erik Erikson. The first stage of development occurs when infants and toddlers learn about trust in others. Erikson asserts that trust during this phase can be successfully developed through three key components: feeling comfort, meeting immediate needs, and experiencing affection [35].

The authors then fold in the three components of trust as proposed by Dhruv Khullar: competence, transparency, and motive [36].

- Competence: "Do you know what you are doing?"
- Transparency: "Will you tell me what you are doing?"
- Motive: "Are you doing this to help me or yourself?"

When you reflect on these essential trust components (comfort, satisfaction, and affection) while demonstrating the answer to the three simple questions, trust will undoubtedly ensue.

2.6 Show Competence

One final, yet critical, approach to establishing trust or unified rapport is to show competence in your environment, demeanor, and examination. Showing competence is a simple yet undeniable aspect of assuming the care of African American patients. All patients want to know that their physician is competent, but African Americans may need a little more obvious evidence.

This air of competence begins with the environment of the office. Is it clean? Is there objective evidence of competence? Having diplomas and photos demonstrating a high level of competence can improve the early confidence a patient may place in the clinician. For more tech-savvy patients, online biographies and introductory videos can substitute for diplomas on the walls. More patients are doing online "research" on potential clinicians as well as reading reviews by other patients. Letting the patient know where you went to school, or that you volunteer with community organizations, for example, may also boost early confidence.

How do the staff present themselves? What are the other patients in the waiting room saying about the clinician? Answering the phone respectfully, seeing the patient in a timely fashion, and calling the patient with laboratory results or in response to an inquiry all show fundamental interpersonal competence that is both noticed and appreciated by the patient. Your respect for "patients" in general is critically important, and it shows in your environment of care. Due to racial concordance satisfaction outcomes, if your practice has a significant African American population (and you are not African American), it would be beneficial to have staff members who reflect that population.

After a fruitful discussion and thorough history have been obtained, a thoughtful and respectful physical examination can do much to clarify the awareness of your competence. Abraham Verghese, in his article "The Bedside Evaluation: Ritual and Reason" in the *Annals of Internal Medicine*, discusses the art, mastery, and connection forged by the physical exam … as well as potential pitfalls [37].

> By giving permission to be examined, the patient affirms the physician's connection with and commitment to the patient—a transformation of both roles is occurring. The patient accords authority to the physician, but it is a gift of authority that many physicians take for granted. The years of study and a busy practice may get in the physician's way of seeing the therapeutic authority from a patient's standpoint. Conversely, the patient's cultural background might contradict or supersede the authority the physician has presumed. The inherent power imbalance in the examination clearly has the potential to harm. Although the presence of a chaperone, parent, or nurse is an attempt to address these issues, the evaluation can still feel like a violation if not done gently, with careful attention to draping, patient modesty, and comfort. In certain cultures, the ritual could be viewed as a serious breach of trust.

We all fundamentally understand that a patient has the right to refuse certain aspects of the physical exam without retribution. Asking permission for the right to examine certain sensitive areas of the body is completely appropriate and, in some cases, expected. This discussion is best approached during the historical aspect of the visit. For example, many female patients may not intuitively understand why a pelvic exam may be necessary if they only presented with urinary tract symptoms. Explaining the rationale early in the visit can do much to allay confusion.

Once permission to perform a detailed and thoughtful exam has been granted, the examination "ritual," as Dr. Verghese describes, is a key part of "conveying a symbolic centering of attention on the body as a locus of personhood as well as disease." The patient, in a very literal sense, exposes themselves both figuratively and literally to us. This vulnerable and sacred connection between clinician and patient should be treated by both parties as the ultimate demonstration of a sober offering and receiving of trust.

Many African Americans complain that "the doctor never touched me" when much of our diagnostic process involves history and review of studies and laboratories. Some may wrongly assume we don't want to touch them. A person presenting with fever, cough, and an x-ray showing classic pneumonia may not need the attending emergency department physician to listen to their lungs in order to get treatment, but from the patient's perspective, not having it done may seem like a glaring omission.

Do not destroy the sanctity or ritual of the clinician's touch by wearing gloves inappropriately. Competence also means following accepted guidelines. OSHA requirements are clear: gloves should be used during all patient-care activities that may involve exposure to blood and all other body fluids [38]. Yet many younger clinicians have begun to wear gloves throughout a physical exam that does not involve bodily fluids. Clinicians who wear gloves according to current guidelines will be compared to the "constant" glove-wearers and confuse patients as to which is actually appropriate. Many African Americans will assume the glove-wearers "don't want to touch them" when compared to physicians they trust who follow guidelines. Establishing a trusting clinician-patient relationship is much easier in the presence of a healing, comforting, or reassuring touch.

Obtain the trust of your patients. Once trust is given and respectfully accepted, it should be valued and revered as the greatest gift a patient could give to their clinician.

> **Establishing Trust in African American Patients**
> 1. Explore ways to discover *implicit biases* and work to minimize their impact on clinical encounters.
> 2. *Invest time:* set aside slightly more time early on in the provider-patient relationship.
> 3. Make *affirming comments* and compliments.
> 4. Make *personal disclosures*.
> 5. *Emphasize your similarities* with the patient.
> 6. *Acknowledge the unequal care* history but affirm equal care going forward.
> 7. *Reserve "sensitive" historical questions* for issues that are specifically related to the presenting condition.
> 8. Show *competence*.
> 9. Perform a thoughtful and respectful *physical exam*.
> 10. *Touch* your patients.

References

1. Halbert C, Armstrong K, Gandy O, Shaker B. Racial differences in trust in health care providers. Arch Intern Med. 2006;166(8):896–901.
2. Blendon RJ, Buhr T, Cassidy EF, et al. Disparities in physician care: experiences and perceptions of a multi-ethnic America. Health Aff (Millwood). 2008;27(2):507–17.
3. Brawley O. The study of untreated syphilis in the negro male. Int J Ratiat Oncol Biol Phys. 1998;40(1):5–8.
4. U.S. Public Health Service Syphilis Study at Tuskegee. Centers for Disease Control and Prevention. https://www.cdc.gov/tuskegee/index.html.
5. Shavers V, Lynch C, Burmeister L. Knowledge of the Tuskegee study and its impact on the willingness to participate in medical research studies. J Natl Med Assoc. 2000;92(12):563–72.
6. Green B, Li L, Morris J, Gluzman R, Davis J, Wang M, Katz R. Detailed knowledge of the Tuskegee syphilis study: who knows what? A framework for health promotion strategies. Health Educ Behav. 2011;38(6):629–36.
7. Ojanuga D. The medical ethics of the "father of gynaecology", Dr J Marion Sims. J Med Thics. 1993;19(1):28–31.
8. Spettel S, White MD. The portrayal of J Marion Sims' controversial legacy. J Urol. 2011;185(6):2424–7.
9. Sartin JS. J. Marion Sims, the father of gynecology: hero or villain? South Med J. 2004;97(5):500–5.

10. Washington H. Medical apartheid: the dark history of medical experimentation on black Americans from colonial times to the present. 1st ed. Harlem Moon: Doubleday; 2006.
11. World Health Organization. Glove use information leaflet. http://www.who.int/gpsc/5may/Glove_Use_Information_Leaflet.pdf.
12. Gamble V. Under the shadow of Tuskegee: African Americans and health care. Am J Public Health. 1997;87(11):1773–8.
13. Halperin Edward C., The poor the Black and the marginalized as the source of cadavers in United States anatomical education. Clinical Anatomy 20(5) 489–495 10.1002/ca.20445.
14. Delmonico FL. The organ thieves: the shocking story of the first heart transplant in the segregated south Chip Jones New York NY: Gallery Books, 389 pages. American J Transp. 2020;21(3):1338. https://doi.org/10.1111/ajt.16407.
15. Blanchard J, Nayar BA, Lurie N. Patient-provider and patient-staff racial concordance and perceptions of mistreatment in the healthcare setting. J Gen Intern Med. 2007;22(8):1184–9.
16. National Park Service, Historic Jamestown. African Americans at Jamestown. https://www.nps.gov/jame/learn/historyculture/african-americans-at-jamestown.htm
17. Vela MB, Erondu AI, Smith NA, Peek ME, Woodruff JN, Chin MH. Eliminating explicit and implicit biases in health care: evidence and research needs. Annual Rev Public Health. 43(1):477–501. https://doi.org/10.1146/annurev-publhealth-052620-103528.
18. Caterinicchio RP. Testing plausible path models of interpersonal trust in patient-physician treatment relationships. Soc Sci Med Part A. 1979;13:81–99.
19. Cuffee YL, Hargraves JL, Rosal M. Reported racial discrimination, trust in physicians, and medication adherence among inner-city African Americans with hypertension. Am J Public Health. 2013;103(11):e55–62.
20. Thom D, Hall M, Pawlson G. Measuring patients' trust in physicians when assessing quality of care. Health Aff (Millwood). 2004;23(4):124–32.
21. Dhruv K. Building trust in health care—why where and how. JAMA. 322(6):507. https://doi.org/10.1001/jama.2019.4892.
22. Jessica G, Diana S, Erin V, Long Sharon K. Is patients' trust in clinicians related to patient-clinician racial/ethnic or gender concordance? Patient Edu Couns:112107750. https://doi.org/10.1016/j.pec.2023.107750.
23. Kirwan Institute for the Study of Race and Ethnicity. http://kirwaninstitute.osu.edu/.
24. Johnson SM, Peterson Emily B, Rosario C-M, Hunter HM, Jewell Sarah T, Konstantina M, Bylund Carma L. The effects of race and racial concordance on patient-physician communication: a systematic review of the literature. J Racial Ethnic Health Disparities. 5(1):117–40. https://doi.org/10.1007/s40615-017-0350-4.
25. Peckham C. Medscape lifestyle report. Race and ethnicity, bias and burnout. 2017. https://www.medscape.com/features/slideshow/lifestyle/2017/overview.
26. Oliver M, Wells K, Joy-Gaba J, Hawkins C, Nosek B. Do physcians' implicit views of African Americans affect clinical decision making? J Am Board Fam Med. 2014;27(2):177–88.
27. Cooper L, Roter D, Carson K, Beach M, Sabin J, Greenwald A, Inui T. The associations of clinicians' implicit attitudes about race with medical visit communication and patient ratings of interpersonal care. Am J Public Health. 2012;102(5):979–87.
28. Penner L, Dovidio J, West T, Gaertner S, Albrecht T, Daily R, Markova T. Aversive racism and medical interactions with black patients: a field study. J Exp Soc Psychol. 2010;46(2):436–40.
29. Boulware L, Cooper L, Ratner L, LaVeist T, Powe N. Race and trust in the health care system. Public Health Rep. 2003;118(4):358–65.
30. https://www.ncbi.nlm.nih.gov/pmc/articles/PMC1497554/pdf/12815085.pdf.
31. Doescher M, Saver B, Fiscella K, Franks P. Preventive care: does continuity count? J Gen Intern Med. 2004;19(6):632–7.

32. Fiscella K, Meldrum S, Franks P, Shields C, Duberstein P, McDaniel S, Epstein R. Patient trust: is it related to patient-centered behavior of primary care physicians? Med Care. 2004;42(11):1049–55.
33. Duberstein P, Meldrum S, Fiscella K, Shields C, Epstein R. Influences on patients' ratings of physicians: physicians demographics and personality. Patient Educ Couns. 2007;65(2):270–4.
34. Martinez KA, Kaitlin K, Radhika R, Joud R, Adrianne F, Rood Mark N, Rothberg Michael B. The association between physician race/ethnicity and patient satisfaction: an exploration in direct to consumer telemedicine. J Gen Intern Med. 35(9):2600–6. https://doi.org/10.1007/s11606-020-06005-8.
35. Lavin M. What doctors should call their patients. J Med Ethics. 1988;14(3):129–31. https://doi.org/10.1136/jme.14.3.129.
36. Lee W, Julia C. Building trust: Reflecting on the earliest human experience. Am J Otolaryngol. 43(3):103411. https://doi.org/10.1016/j.amjoto.2022.103411.
37. Sabir M, Pillemer K. An intensely sympathetic awareness: experiential similarity and cultural norms as means for gaining older African Americans' trust of scientific research. J Aging Stud. 2014;29:142–9.
38. Verghese A, Brady E, Kapur C, Horwitz R. The bedside evaluation: ritual and reason. Ann Intern Med. 2011;155(8):550–3.

Chapter 3
Delivering Consistent and Equitable Healthcare to African Americans

Contents

3.1 African American Clinical Care and Outcomes Disparities 36
3.2 Variability in Our Care 40
References 42

Being consistent and equitable in your care of African Americans is critical and has been key to decreasing a number of health disparities. Consistency (doing the same thing the same way each time) and equity (providing fair and impartial treatment) can, at times, be at odds because, technically, they are not the same. What modern healthcare strives to do is be more consistent across populations, and this attempt at consistency frequently fails due to variability in access, insurance coverage, provider idiosyncrasies, and patient need. African Americans statistically have worse access and get less clinical intervention in many cancers and chronic diseases [1]. Providing better care to African American patients will require more insight into why their care is currently inferior and a closer look at what has worked to decrease health disparities in this population.

    Modern protocols instituted and mandated at hospitals across the country have seen disparities shrink when these protocols are consistently applied across populations for chest pain, pneumonia, or stroke symptoms, for example, [2–6]. The reality is that if true widespread consistency were achieved, disparities in healthcare would still exist because a consistent approach across different patient populations will invariably lead to unequal outcomes. Clinicians are well aware of "differences" in an approach to care or a predilection for the occurrence of many disorders between patient populations and/or gene pools. Students of medicine learned of a greatly increased risk for breast cancer or colon cancer in Ashkenazi Jews [7, 8], for example, and with increased research and data analysis, a number of differences and idiosyncrasies have been discovered relating to the care and treatment of African American patients as well. A reasonable approach would dictate that we first

© The Author(s), under exclusive license to Springer Nature Switzerland AG 2025
G. L. Hall, *Precision Medicine for African Americans*, https://doi.org/10.1007/978-3-031-95774-1_3

educate ourselves about these differences, and then apply nuanced clinical care when appropriate.

The concept of health equity is fundamental in all of medicine. Provide the medical care that the patient requires … no more and no less. The time that we spend learning about the nuances of diseases in different settings, and expecting variable outcomes in different populations, prepares us for competent care in our clinical practice.

Providing equitable care means all patients would get the care and screening they "need." Using this logic, only smokers would get smoking cessation counseling, not everyone. Patient populations known to get aggressive versions of certain disorders would receive more stringent screening than other populations (i.e., Kawasaki disease in Asian and Pacific Islanders or prostate cancer in African American males). Because of the challenges of unequal care in America, striving for improved widespread consistency is still a goal worth pursuing and will continue to shrink disparities because of the many genetic and physiologic similarities across populations. But health equity is the true ultimate healthcare goal: medical care tailored precisely to the patient.

The US Agency for Healthcare Research and Quality presents an annual National Healthcare Quality and Disparities Report, which tracks health outcomes and the progress in eliminating disparities [9]. Year after year, disparities based on race, income, and other factors are tracked by clinical measures. Outcomes such as time to electrocardiogram after presentation with chest pain or patient satisfaction with physician communication are measured and reported. Hospital scores are publicly presented, and benchmarks are set for comparison. Significant outliers are financially impacted. By having protocols for critical presentations, the process of deciding who gets what medical tests and when has been moved from the clinician to a "knee-jerk" process mediated by the presentation. While this is seen by some to negatively impact the "art" of medicine (and it unquestionably does in some circumstances), it has had a great impact in decreasing a host of racial and gender disparities based on how a person presents.

Our responsibility as clinicians is to provide equitable care regardless of insurance, financial resources, or access. Because we are constantly presented with barriers to equitable care in the form of medication formularies, prior authorizations for studies we order, patients' ability to comply with an order, and our own biases, we frequently acquiesce and settle for the less-than-ideal alternative. A patient with "good insurance" presenting with poorly controlled diabetes can initially get the latest diabetes medication to lower their glucose to target, while a "managed care insurance" patient may have to use a less efficacious diabetes drug first, fail to reach their goal, and then progress to the "better" drug we would have chosen without being "managed." While progressing through this "managed care" process will result in more affordable care and may occasionally reveal success with first-line diabetes medications, prolonging the path to successful glucose lowering will frustrate many patients, jeopardize ongoing compliance due to patients questioning our competence, prolong cardiovascular risk exposure, and impede our ability to reach the targeted control we seek for our patient populations.

As these small impedances to proper care accumulate, foundational barriers are formed that comprise many of the health disparities based on socioeconomic status. When seeing poor patients, we have come to expect that some of our initial choices for medications will not get covered, or a radiologic study approved, and we adjust our care to work around these barriers (whether perceived or real). If we order an MRI of the head for a patient with severe headaches, we generally will see that order denied. After the first few denials, we begin to anticipate the denial and follow the next most appropriate course without first getting the denial. If we see this pattern with a specific insurance, we adjust our orders in response. As these stumbling blocks continue, we begin to categorize the barriers we see based on insurance, ability to pay, access, etc.

With African Americans comprising a higher percentage of the poor (18% for African Americans vs. 8% for European Americans) [10], some providers will categorize all African Americans as poor, and when they see an African American, they "anticipate" the more stringent insurance issues normally seen with the poor. Those adjustments based on anticipated barriers are followed, and the inferior outcomes associated with low income become a barrier to the 82% of African Americans that live above the poverty level. The adjustments that providers make are simply made as an approach to a complex and ever-changing set of clinical rules and restrictions. But put simply, the dynamics and disadvantages of poor patients' care place an additional burden on the care of some nonpoor African Americans. These health disparities extend to outpatient rehabilitation therapy referrals, which, again, are typically not easily approved in a "managed care" environment [11]. There was a "reduced likelihood of an office-based therapy visit for (African) Americans with arthritis when controlled for income, insurance, and education," a study by Sandstrom and Bruns published in the Journal of Racial and Ethnic Health Disparities [12]. This "stereotyping" by healthcare providers contributes to the disparate treatment plans seen when comparing racial outcomes. The preconceptions regarding a particular patient's tendency to follow through with an order, an insurance preference to approve an order, or the effectiveness of a protocol in a particular racial population are merely the clinicians' attempt to simplify a complicated set of conflicting interactions. Joseph Betancourt wrote about this stereotyping phenomenon:

> This is a normal, functional, adaptive, cognitive process that is automatic, and usually centers on characteristics that manifest visually, such as race, gender, and age. Interestingly, we tend to activate stereotypes most when we are stressed, multitasking, and under time pressure—the hallmarks of the clinical encounter.
>
> For example, many medical students and residents are often trained—and minorities cared for—in academic health centers or public hospitals located in socioeconomically disadvantaged areas. As a result, doctors may begin to equate certain races and ethnicities with specific health beliefs and behaviors (i.e., "these patients" engage in risky behaviors, or "those patients" tend to be non-compliant) that are more associated with the social environment (e.g., poverty) than patient's racial/ethnic background or cultural traditions. This stereotyping is a natural and expected—but no less dangerous—phenomenon that may affect the way doctors make decisions and offer specific interventions to different patients based on their race or ethnicity [13].

This stereotyping, confounding, and preconception-forming behavior impacts clinical decision-making to the detriment of African Americans. Specialist referrals [14], advanced treatments for cancer [15], rheumatological condition chemotherapies [16], and other "higher-end" interventions that represent an escalation of care are all decreased in African Americans independent of socioeconomic status [17]. To be clear, these interventions represent clinician-written orders not impacted by patient condition or responsibility. The prospect of disentangling the confounding of race, socioeconomic status, and other preconceptions in African Americans can lead to significantly improved care.

With African Americans tending to live where African Americans live, community barriers to care also impact our ability to deliver consistent and equitable care. The most recent census data show that in the United States, over half of African Americans live in southern states where quality care outcomes are inferior (see Fig. 3.1) [18, 19].

"Hospital care for (African American) patients in the United States is remarkably concentrated in a small percentage of hospitals" studies have confirmed [20]. The 5% of hospitals with the highest volume of African American patients care for nearly half of this demographic.

Studies have also shown that patients without access to primary care providers have higher emergency services utilization. Curiously, in one study of emergency department use among African American HMO enrollees, they found a persistently higher use of the emergency department in African Americans even when they reported having a primary care provider [21]. The same study also found these trends "after controlling for sociodemographic differences." The researchers supposed that the increased use of emergency services, even in the face of presumed primary care access, was likely driven by "dissatisfaction with a usual source of

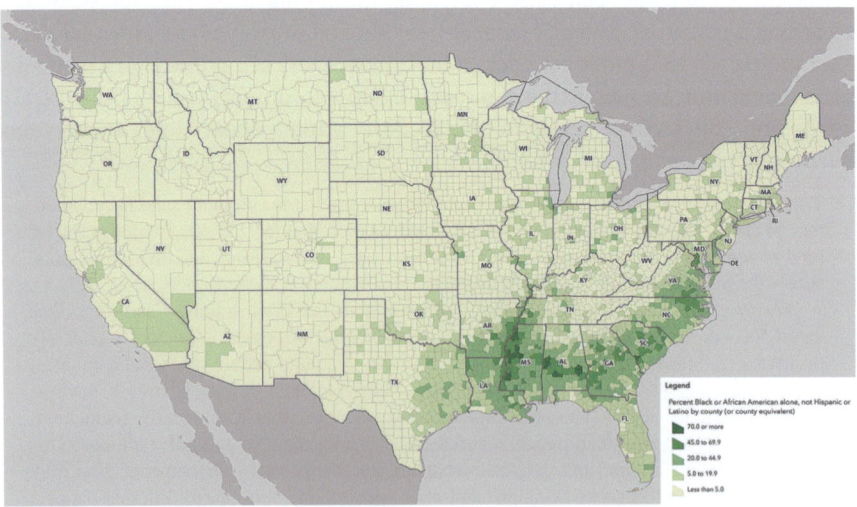

Fig. 3.1 U.S. Census 2020. Percent Black or African American, not Hispanic or Latino by County

care, long waits to schedule appointments, ... belief in the urgency of the condition and the convenience of the emergency room [21]." This increased use of emergency services can stretch resources and impact access for all patients.

Emergency medical care for many in African American communities may actually start in an ambulance on the way to a hospital. Hospitals in highly African American-populated regions are more likely to be on "ambulance diversion," where the emergency services are temporarily closed to ambulance traffic due to overcrowding or a lack of other resources at the hospital (personnel and/or hospital beds) [22]. These diversions delay emergency treatment (intubations, surgeries, catheterizations), medical interventions (antibiotics for sepsis, pharmaceutical cardioversions), and many other diagnostic and lifesaving interventions. Numerous studies have shown the negative impact these delays in care have on clinical outcomes. Diversions were "associated with poorer access to cardiac technology, lower probability of receiving revascularization, and worse long-term mortality outcomes," a study in California reported [22]. Shen and Hsia, the authors of the study, found that racial disparities do exist and "(African American) patients are more likely to be diverted than (European American) patients because the ED closest to them is more likely to be on diversion [22]." In another study, Hsia and colleagues found that in California, "hospitals serving minorities were more likely to divert, even when controlling for hospital ownership, emergency department capacity, and other hospital-level demographic and structural factors" [23]. Having to be diverted to another hospital will definitely impact care in terms of medical history and records access, clinician familiarity, timeliness of care, and countless other factors.

Once at a hospital, African Americans still have worse outcomes. Karen Joynt at the Department of Health Policy and Management at the Harvard School of Public Health looked at the 30-day readmission rate for all fee-for-service Medicare recipients for a 3-year period [13]. Her examination of over three million discharges found a number of adverse quality outcomes based purely on race. She found a trend among *minority-serving hospitals*, which were defined as hospitals in the "highest decile (10%) of proportion of (African American) patients ... while the other 90% of hospitals were categorized as nonminority-serving":

> At minority-serving hospitals, on average, 37% of patients were (African American), compared with 1.4% of patients at non-minority-serving hospitals. Minority-serving hospitals were more often large, public or for-profit hospitals. Seventy percent of the minority-serving hospitals were located in the south, compared with 35% of the non-minority-serving hospitals. Minority-serving hospitals were more often teaching hospitals, and served a higher proportion of Medicaid patients... Minority-serving hospitals had fewer nurses per 1000 patient-days, and had somewhat lower performance on HQA measures. Length of stay was greater at minority-serving hospitals for each condition [13].

Across the board, African American patients were much more likely to be admitted to a minority-serving hospital (40% chance versus a 1.4% chance for Whites) and had 13% higher odds of all-cause 30-day readmission than European Americans. They also found that "(European American) patients at nonminority serving hospitals consistently had the lowest odds of readmission, and (African American) patients at minority-serving hospitals (had) the highest." Interestingly, African

American patients at nonminority-serving hospitals got care essentially equivalent to European American patients at minority-serving hospitals. Overall this analysis found that:

> ... elderly (African American) patients had higher odds of 30-day readmission than (European American) patients for AMI, CHF, and pneumonia. These disparities were related to race itself as well as to the site where care was provided: (African American) patients had a 13% higher odds of readmission than (European American) patients, while patients discharged from minority-serving hospitals had a 23% higher odds of readmission than patients discharged from non-minority-serving hospitals [24].

Health disparities based on where you live and how the community uses healthcare resources like ambulances, hospitals, and emergency departments are difficult to change, but the first step is undoubtedly awareness.

3.1 African American Clinical Care and Outcomes Disparities

The African American racial differences in outcomes while hospitalized are numerous, and disparities driven by the care delivered there have been documented in a number of research articles. Cardiovascular disease is the number one cause of death in the USA [25] and African Americans have the highest rates of myocardial infarctions (MI) and related mortality and are more likely to have heart failure during an MI-associated hospitalization [26]. Similarly, African Americans are less likely to undergo revascularization during an MI-related hospitalization [26]. In a cohort of young and middle-aged post-MI patients, Garcia et al. demonstrated that African American patients have more than a twofold risk of developing adverse cardiovascular events (recurrent MI, heart failure, stroke, or death) compared with non-African American patients [27] (Fig. 3.2).

A review article looking at stroke disparities found that Hispanic and African American patients were at lower risk of receiving tPA (tissue-type plasminogen activator) or thrombectomy treatments, utilized EMS less frequently, had longer emergency department wait times, and were at lower risk of being referred to endovascular-capable centers [28]. African American stroke patients are also less likely to receive thrombolytic treatment [6] at both primary stroke centers and nonprimary stroke centers and less likely to be discharged on secondary prevention measures (including lipid-lowering medications) [29, 30]. While atrial fibrillation occurs curiously less often in African Americans [31], a resultant stroke occurs more often and African Americans are less likely to be treated with warfarin [31, 32].

Cardiovascular disease is, by far, the leading cause of death, and these glaring decision-making disparities by race represent an opportunity for clinicians to make a significant difference because of the sheer magnitude. Better control of hypertension or hyperlipidemia across the African American population would have a vast impact on downstream implications. Yet Safford and colleagues showed that

3.1 African American Clinical Care and Outcomes Disparities

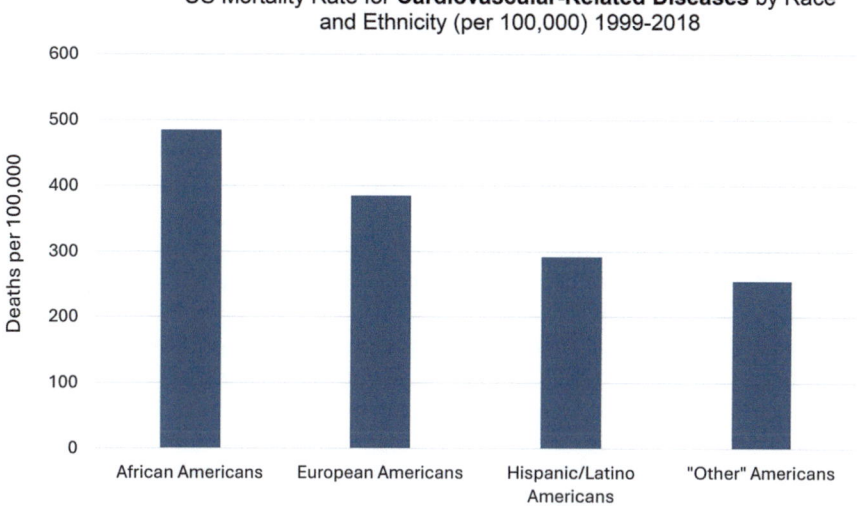

Fig. 3.2 Cardiovascular disease mortality by race/ethnicity

European American men had a marked advantage in the treatment and control of hyperlipidemia when compared with women of European or African descent, or African American men [33]. Diet and exercise improvement is essential to improving cardiovascular health, yet Wilson and others show a lower level of referrals for African Americans to diet, nutritional, or exercise counseling [30].

A summary review of surgical outcomes reflected the same disadvantage for African Americans.

> We demonstrate that Black race, after matching, is associated with an increased odds of adverse events; including morbidity, mortality, readmissions, and reoperations... . Furthermore, we demonstrate that Black patients are particularly vulnerable to an increased risk of serious complications such as re-intubation, difficulty weaning from ventilator, venous thromboembolism, pulmonary embolism, renal failure, postoperative bleeding requiring transfusion, and cardiac arrest. Importantly, these associations held true despite matching for important patient comorbidity confounders relevant to the aforementioned outcome measures [34].

This retrospective analysis of surgical outcomes in over 600,000 patients is stunning because the researchers corrected for many of the non-race-based hypotheses for this well-known disparity, including more advanced disease, late presentations, and more comorbidities (including cardiovascular disease, renal disease, and hypertension) in African Americans [34]. If these increased complications and mortality are not based on "reasonable explanations" like those listed, what are we missing? We need to take a nuanced patient-centered approach that does not ignore differences but embraces them and uses them to the advantage of the patient. By acknowledging and valuing these differences, healthcare clinicians can tailor their communication and treatment plans to better align with each patient's unique genetic, cultural, risk profile, and personal needs. This precision medicine approach can increase patient satisfaction, as individuals feel seen, heard, and respected in their healthcare journey. Moreover, embracing diversity can foster innovation within medical teams, as diverse perspectives often lead to creative problem-solving and more comprehensive care strategies.

Peripheral vascular disease is also increased in African Americans and this results in increased leg amputations [35]. African Americans "comprise 29% of patients undergoing a major lower extremity amputation, but only 12% of those undergoing an open surgical procedure and 10% of those undergoing an endovascular procedure for limb salvage" [36]. Using 13% as a population benchmark, this disparity is painfully high.

Approximately twice as many African American individuals are diagnosed with Alzheimer's disease compared to those with European ancestry [37]. Despite not fully understanding the reasons for the disparity, both genetic and environmental factors contribute. This difference in prevalence has been attributed to factors such as economic disparities, cardiovascular health, education, and biases in diagnosing the disease. Hereditary factors may also contribute to Alzheimer's disease risk differences. Recent studies have identified certain genetic variants that are more prevalent in African American populations, which may contribute to increased risk [37]. For instance, variations in the APOE gene, particularly the APOE ε4 allele, have been associated with a higher likelihood of developing Alzheimer's in African Americans [37]. Combining this gene with other cofactors, including posttraumatic stress or traumatic brain injuries, heightens the risk for more severe dementia [37]. The APOE ε4 allele represents the most significant single Alzheimer's disease genetic risk factor in African Americans, and the effect of this gene is much less if found in European Americans [37]. Understanding these genetic factors is crucial for developing targeted interventions and improving diagnostic accuracy (Fig. 3.3).

Once diagnosed with Alzheimer's disease, African Americans are more likely to be undertreated [38, 39] either through delayed or missed diagnosis or finding a more advanced dementia state. A more recent review found no disparity in the initiation of acetylcholinesterase inhibitors (donepezil, galantamine, and rivastigmine) at diagnosis, but African Americans and Hispanics/Latinos have a higher rate of medication discontinuation [40].

Cancer outcomes also show significant disparities, with African Americans having the worst outcomes in a majority of cancers [41]. Prostate cancer leads the list of new cancer cases in African American men, while lung cancer is the number one killer. For African American women, breast cancer occurs the most and also has the highest mortality, with lung cancer coming in second [41]. Colon cancer has the third most occurrence and mortality for African American men and women [41]. Among African American men, cancer incidence rates are higher overall for several common cancers, including prostate, lung, colon, kidney, liver, and pancreas (Fig. 3.4).

In contrast, African American women have a lower incidence than European American women for a number of common cancers, particularly breast and lung. However, they have a higher incidence of several cancers with low survival rates,

3.1 African American Clinical Care and Outcomes Disparities

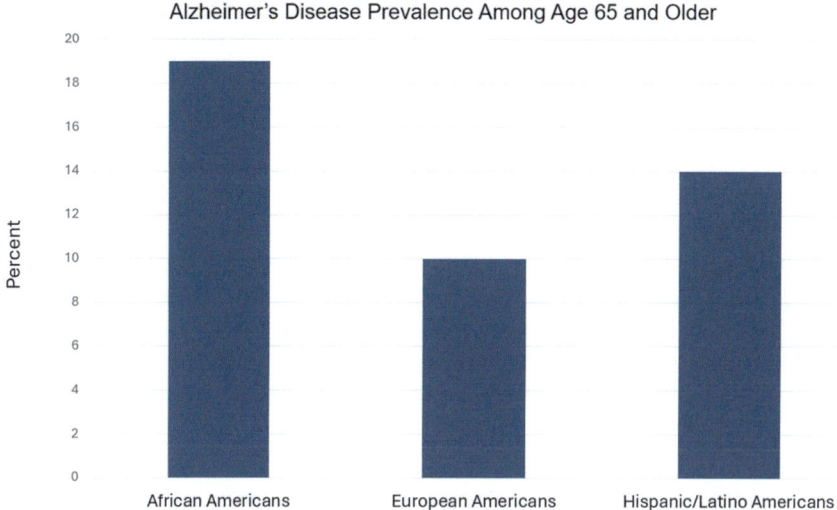

Fig. 3.3 Alzheimer's disease by race/ethnicity

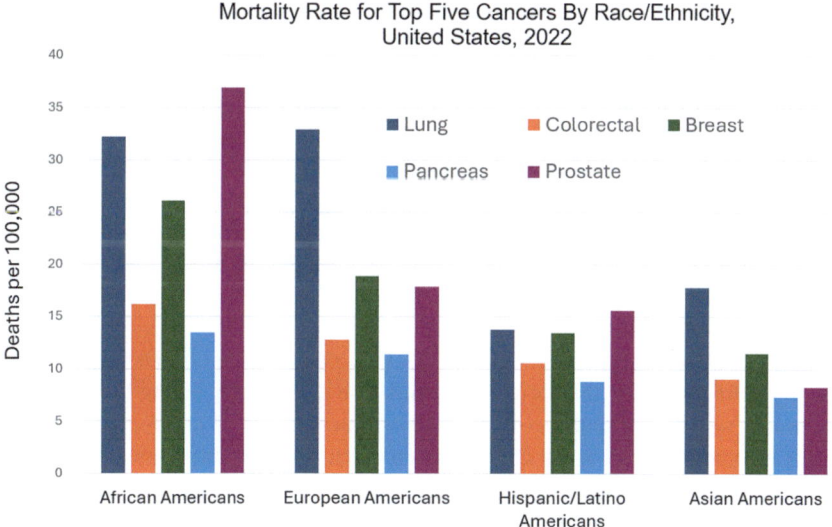

Fig. 3.4 Cancer mortality by race/ethnicity

such as liver, pancreas, and gastric cancers. Overall, African American women are more likely to die from cancer than European American women. These disparities are traditionally explained by a variety of factors, including socioeconomic status, access to healthcare, and environmental exposures. Additionally, genetic predispositions and differences in tumor biology also play a role in the disparities observed in cancer incidence and mortality rates [41].

The 5-year relative survival rate is lower in Black people than in White people for every stage of diagnosis for most cancer sites. Most of this disparity is not genetic but, instead, is caused by socioeconomic differences that influence access to timely, high-quality cancer prevention, detection, and treatment. Because of these barriers, Black people are more likely to be diagnosed with advanced-stage (regional or distant) disease when treatment is usually more costly and less effective. Once diagnosed, Black people are more likely to experience delays in treatment and less likely to receive recommended treatment. Most studies have found that, in equal-access healthcare systems, disparities in treatment and cancer outcomes are reduced [41].

When they refer to "equal access" healthcare systems, they include the absence of biased decision-making in prescriptions and referrals, as well as eliminating screening and insurance allowance barriers. Put simply, many of these poor outcomes are at least partially driven by clinician action … or inaction. The dicey question is always, "Who is contributing to these disparities?" The uncomfortable answer is that we all contribute.

3.2 Variability in Our Care

Care approaches based on what an insurance allows, or an anticipated noncompliance, or a presumed poor outcome, result in unequal care. We assume that unequal care results in superior care for some and inferior care for others, but in the end, we all provide unequal care. If your favorite US president or most admired celebrity presented for medical care in your hospital, you would likely more closely review your clinical decisions. You would spend more time with the patient, order more labs and radiographic studies, and if needed, you would research every aspect of their presenting complaints. In a sense, they would get the best care you could provide. But keep in mind that providing everyone with that level of care is intensive, expensive, impractical, and unadvisable. So do not beat yourself up too badly for adding to health disparities!

But also, do not delude yourself into thinking you provide consistent and equal care. By acknowledging that your care varies, you are actually taking the first critical step to decrease disparities in your own practice. While some clinicians are quick to acknowledge obvious ongoing unequal care, others flatly reject the notion of unequal care … particularly in America.

Let us put racial disparities aside for a moment. My patients that smell bad do not get great care from me. Since I was a child, I always had a weak stomach in response to bad smells. When I walk into an exam room and the patient smells bad of urine or stool, or has very bad breath, I will be acutely aware of, and distracted by, the smell. I will proceed to get as brief a history as I can, do a somewhat distracted exam, and exit as quickly as possible without being overtly disrespectful. In my defense, I will try to compensate by doing more background research, documenting more thoroughly, and making follow-up phone calls to fill in the gaps caused by my weak stomach. These patients get less small talk, less history taking, and a faster exam. I provide different care to that population, and because I haven't learned to control my nasogastric reflexes, I cannot change the basics of the situation. Because I go out of my way to compensate for my weakness, I do not believe this population gets inferior care from me, but I know for sure that they do not get superior care. A good degree of my strength as a physician stems from my personal "connection" with the patient and my intuition of their strengths and weaknesses as sensed during my personal time with them. Being distracted by adverse smells reroutes my thinking, impairs my intuition, and impacts my in-person care.

I assume most clinicians lack my odiferous weakness and have no problem with this aspect of patient care, but I am sure there are other similar examples that some providers could report. Try giving equal care and time to a mean and spiteful person, or a child rapist? During the recent opioid addiction epidemic, caregivers have been treating pregnant and new mothers with high systemic opioid levels in themselves and toxic levels in their baby's systems. The perceived irresponsibility of these situations tests the clinician's tolerance and ability to give complete and compassionate care to mothers that they perceive as abusive to their unborn or newly born child. In short, providers are offended by the irresponsibility of these mothers and have difficulty forging a warm, caring relationship with them. In reality, a forgiving and trusting therapeutic relationship with these addicted patients is the first critical step to the success of their treatment, but many providers struggle with this concept and put forth a more punishing and judgmental demeanor. While these provider reactions are natural and understandable, they are also inefficient and therapeutically counterintuitive.

Delivering consistent and equitable care in a number of clinical scenarios takes education, self-awareness (biases and all), and practice. Realizing that your care frequently varies due to a number of conflicting and compounding variables is the only approach to ultimately minimizing their impact. Acknowledging that your African American patient is prone to worse clinical outcomes and proactively compensating and advocating on your patient's behalf will drive down the clinician-driven disparate outcomes we see.

Delivering Consistent and Equitable Healthcare to African Americans
- Understand that from a racial standpoint and across an array of parameters, African Americans receive the worst clinical care.
- Equitable care means providing interventions that are "needed" and appropriate for the patient.
- Sometimes clinician orders and directives are influenced by presumptions related to socioeconomic status, insurance coverage patterns, and patient idiosyncrasies.
- 60% of African Americans live in only six states, and over half live in southern states.

(continued)

- Hospital care for African American patients in the United States is remarkably concentrated in a small percentage of hospitals. The 5% of hospitals with the highest volume of African American patients care for nearly half of all elderly African American patients.
- African Americans tend to follow community-specific referral patterns and go to hospitals where they feel "welcome."
- Hospitals with more minority patients see increased ambulance diversion and emergency department closures that negatively impact quality and continuity of care.
- Surgery in African Americans brings an increased odds of adverse events, including morbidity, mortality, readmissions, and reoperations.
- African Americans with peripheral vascular disease have a significantly increased risk for amputation and lower odds of receiving limb salvage procedures.
- African Americans have twice the risk for Alzheimer's disease diagnosis, but it is diagnosed at later stages, and they are less likely to stay on medications.
- The APOE ε4 allele puts African Americans at a higher risk for Alzheimer's disease, particularly in patients with PTSD or traumatic brain injury.
- Cancer in African Americans is more likely to be diagnosed with advanced-stage (regional or distant) disease, and mortality is higher.
- Genetic predispositions and differences in tumor biology play a role in the cancer disparities seen, and these variants receive less attention in research.
- We all have biases … both explicit and implicit.

We all provide variable care that is dependent on our biases. The key is to be more self-aware.

References

1. 2015 National healthcare quality and disparities report Chartbook on health care for blacks. Rockville: Agency for Healthcare Research and Quality; 2016. AHRQ Pub. No 16-0015-1-EF.
2. Gomez MA, Anderson JL, Karagounis LA, Muhlestein JB, Mooers FB. An emergency department-based protocol for rapidly ruling out myocardial ischemia reduces hospital time and expense: results of a randomized study (ROMIO). J Am Coll Cardiol. 1996;28:25–33.
3. Pope JH, Aufderheide TP, Ruthazer R, Woolard RH, Feldman JA, Beshansky JR, Griffith JL, Selker HP. Missed diagnoses of acute cardiac ischemia in the emergency department. N Engl J Med. 2000;342:1163–70.
4. Six AJ, Backus BE, Kelder JC. Chest pain in the emergency room: value of the HEART score. Neth Heart J. 2008;16:191–6.
5. Grief SN, Loza JK. Guidelines for the evaluation and treatment of pneumonia. Prim Care. 2018;45(3):485–503. https://doi.org/10.1016/j.pop.2018.04.001.

6. Meschia JF, Bushnell C, Boden-Albala B, et al. Guidelines for the primary prevention of stroke: a statement for healthcare professionals from the American Heart Association/American Stroke Association. Stroke. 2014;45(12):3754–832.
7. Rinella ES, Shao Y, Yackowski L, et al. Genetic variants associated with breast cancer risk for Ashkenazi Jewish women with strong family histories but no identifiable BRCA1/2 mutation. Hum Genet. 2013;132(5):523–36.
8. Jasperson KW, Tuohy TM, Neklason DW, Burt RW. Hereditary and familial colon cancer Gastroenerology. 2010;138960:2044–58.
9. 2023 National Healthcare Quality and Disparities Report. Retrieved from https://www.ahrq.gov/research/findings/nhqrdr/nhqdr23/index.html. 2023. Accessed 24 Nov 2024.
10. Poverty in the United States. 2023. United States Census Bureau. https://www.census.gov/library/publications/2024/demo/p60-283.html. Accessed 24 Nov 2024.
11. Carvalho E, Bettger JP, Goode AP. Insurance coverage, costs, and barriers to care for outpatient musculoskeletal therapy and rehabilitation services. N C Med J. 2017;78(5):312–4.
12. Sandstrom R, Bruns A. Disparities in access to outpatient rehabilitation therapy for African Americans with arthritis. J Racial Ethn Health Disparities. 2016;4(4):599–606.
13. Betancourt JR. Eliminating racial and ethnic disparities in health care: what is the role of academic medicine? Acad Med. 2006;81(9):788–92.
14. Simpson DR, Martínez ME, Gupta S, Hattangadi-Gluth J, Mell LK, Heestand G, et al. Racial disparity in consultation, treatment, and the impact on survival in metastatic colorectal cancer. JNCI: J Natl Cancer Inst. 2013;105(23):1814–20.
15. Murphy MM, Simons JP, Ng SC, Mcdade TP, Smith JK, Shah SA, et al. Racial differences in cancer specialist consultation, treatment, and outcomes for locoregional pancreatic adenocarcinoma. Ann Surg Oncol. 2009;16(11):2968–77. https://doi.org/10.1245/s10434-009-0656-5.
16. Katz JN, Barrett J, Liang MH, Kaplan H, Roberts W, Baron JA. Utilization of rheumatology physician services by the elderly. Am J Med. 1998;105(4):312–8.
17. LaVeist TA, Morgan A, Arthur M, Plantholt S, Rubinstein M. Physician referral patterns and race differences in receipt of coronary angiography. Health Serv Res. 2002;37(4):949–62.
18. Facts About the U.S. Black Population. Pew Research Center. https://pewrsr.ch/39hFVzP. Accessed 24 Nov 2024.
19. Health Coverage and Care in the South: A Chartbook. Kaiser Family Foundation. https://www.kff.org/report-section/health-coverage-and-care-in-the-south-a-chartbook-section-3-health-status/. Accessed 24 Nov 2024.
20. Jha A, Orav E, Li Z, Epstein A. Concentration and quality of hospitals that care for elderly black patients. Arch Intern Med. 2007;167(11):1177–82.
21. Roby D, Nicholson G, Kominski G. African Americans in commercial HMO's more likely to delay prescription drugs and use emergency room. Policy Brief UCLA Cent Health Policy Res. 2009;PB2009-7:1–12.
22. Shen Y, Hsia R. Do patients hospitalized in high-minority hospitals experience more diversion and poorer outcomes? A retrospective multivariate analysis of Medicare patients in California. BMJ Open. 2016;6(3):e010263.
23. Hsia R, Asch S, Weiss R, Zingmond D, Liang L, Han W, McCreath H, Sun B. California hospitals serving large minority populations were more likely than others to employ ambulance diversion. Health Aff (Millwood). 2012;31(8):1767–76.
24. Joynt K, Orav E, Jha A. Patient race, site of care, and 30-day readmission rates among elderly Americans. JAMA. 2011;305(7):675–81.
25. Ahmad FB, Cisewski JA, Anderson RN. Leading Causes of Death in the US 2019–2023. JAMA. 332(12):957. https://doi.org/10.1001/jama.2024.15563.
26. Walker BJ, Safford Monika M, Mefford Matthew T, Elizabeth F, George H, Howard Virginia J, Naftel David C, Brown Todd M, Levitan Emily B. Cardiovascular disease events and mortality after myocardial infarction among black and white adults. Circ Cardiovas Quality Outcomes. 13(12) https://doi.org/10.1161/CIRCOUTCOMES.120.006683.

27. Mariana G, Zakaria A, Kasra M, An Y, Lima Bruno B, Samaah S, Belal K, Lewis Tené T, Muhammad H, Oleksiy L, Lisa E, Douglas BJ, Paolo R, Shah Amit J, Quyyumi Arshed A, Viola V. Racial disparities in adverse cardiovascular outcomes after a myocardial infarction in young or middle-aged patients. J American Heart Assoc. 10(17) https://doi.org/10.1161/JAHA.121.020828.
28. Shelly I, Emilie K, Goldfield U, Waleed B. Evidence-based disparities in stroke care metrics and outcomes in the United States: a systematic review. Stroke. 53(3):670–9. https://doi.org/10.1161/STROKEAHA.121.036263.
29. Cruz-Flores S, Biller J, Elkind M, et al. Racial-ethnic disparities in stroke care: the American experience: a statement for healthcare professionals from the American Heart Association/American Stroke Association. Stroke. 2011;42(7):2091–116.
30. Willson M, Neumiller J, Sclar D, Robison L, Skaer T. Ethnicity/race, use of pharmacotherapy, scope of physician-ordered cholesterol screening, and provision of diet/nutrition or exercise counseling during office-based visits by patients with hyperlipidemia. Am J Cardiovasc Drugs. 2010;10(2):105–8.
31. Patrick B, David G, Baicu Catalin F, Viswanathan R, Spinale Francis G, Zile Michael R, Gold Michael R. Racial difference in atrial size and extracellular matrix homeostatic response to hypertension: Is this a potential mechanism of reduced atrial fibrillation in African Americans? Heart Rhythm O2. 2(1):37–45. https://doi.org/10.1016/j.hroo.2021.01.001.
32. Amponsah M, Benjamin E, Magnani J. Atrial fibrillation and race—a contemporary review. Curr Cardiovasc Risk Rep. 2013;7(5):336. https://doi.org/10.1007/s12170-013-0327-8.
33. Safford MM, Gamboa CM, Durant RW, Brown TM, Glasser SP, Shikany JM, Zweifler RM, George H, Paul M. Race–sex differences in the management of hyperlipidemia. American J Prev Med. 48(5):520–7. https://doi.org/10.1016/j.amepre.2014.10.025.
34. Arash A, Hirpara DH, Sachin D, Chesney TR, Quereshy FA, Chadi SA. Racial disparities in surgery. Annals Sur Open. 2020;1(2):e023. https://doi.org/10.1097/AS9.0000000000000023.
35. Lefebvre K, Chevan J. The persistence of gender and racial disparities in vascular lower extremity amputation: an examination of HCUP-NIS data (2002–2011). Vasc Med. 2015;20(1):51–9.
36. Holman K, Henke P, Dimick J, Birkmeyer J. Racial disparities in the use of revascularization before leg amputation in medicare patients. J Vasc Surg. 2011;54(2):420–6, 426.e1.
37. Logue MW, Shoumita D, Farrer LA. Genetics of Alzheimer's disease in the African American population. J Clin Med. 2023;12(16):5189. https://doi.org/10.3390/jcm12165189.
38. Gilligan A, Malone D, Warholak T, Armstrong E. Racial and ethnic disparities in Alzheimer's disease pharmacotherapy exposure: an analysis across four state Medicaid populations. Am J Geriatr Pharmacother. 2012;10(5):303–12.
39. Ladson H, Duyen T, Kate P, Meyer Oanh L, Quiñones Ana R. Mapping racial and ethnic healthcare disparities for persons living with dementia: a scoping review. Alzheimer's and Dementia. 20(4):3000–20. https://doi.org/10.1002/alz.13612.
40. Natalia O, Daly Allan T, Yingying Z, Rachel B, Cohen Joshua T, Neumann Peter J, Faul Jessica D, Fillit Howard M, Freund Karen M, Pei-Jung L. Alzheimer's disease medication use and adherence patterns by race and ethnicity. Alzheimer's Dementia. 19(4):1184–93. https://doi.org/10.1002/alz.12753.
41. Giaquinto AN, Miller KD, Tossas KY, Winn RA, Ahmedin J, Siegel RL. Cancer statistics for African American/Black People. CA: Cancer J Clin. 2022;72(3):202–29. https://doi.org/10.3322/caac.21718.

Chapter 4
A Precision Medicine Approach to the Cardiovascular Care of African Americans

Contents

4.1	Hypertension.	48
	4.1.1 Salt Sensitivity.	48
	4.1.2 Hypertension Control.	51
4.2	Heart Failure.	54
	4.2.1 Hereditary Transthyretin Amyloidosis (hATTR).	57
4.3	Lipids.	57
4.4	Atrial Fibrillation.	59
4.5	Stroke.	61
4.6	Peripheral Vascular Disease.	63
4.7	Abdominal Aortic Aneurysms.	65
4.8	Deep Vein Thrombosis and Pulmonary Embolism.	66
References.		69

Genetic, environmental, and societal factors influence cardiovascular health in African Americans who have the highest mortality (see Fig. 4.1). Genetic studies have identified correlations between African American populations and specific cardiovascular disease biomarkers. These biomarkers include those related to inflammation [1], thrombosis [2], salt sensitivity [3–5], hypertension [1, 2, 6], lipid profiles [6, 7], arrhythmias [6, 8, 9], and left ventricular mass [10–12]. Genome-wide association studies have explored genetic relationships to cardiac risk factors, including hypertension and inflammation biomarkers, suggesting an inherent predisposition to these conditions. Moreover, hypertension, a critical risk factor for cardiovascular disease, has been shown to have a heritable component, with studies indicating that 15% to 35% of the correlation in hypertension could be inherited [13, 14]. Black children and adolescents are observed to have higher blood pressure levels and a higher prevalence of hypertension compared to other populations. This trend persists into adulthood, further implying a genetic influence [15, 16].

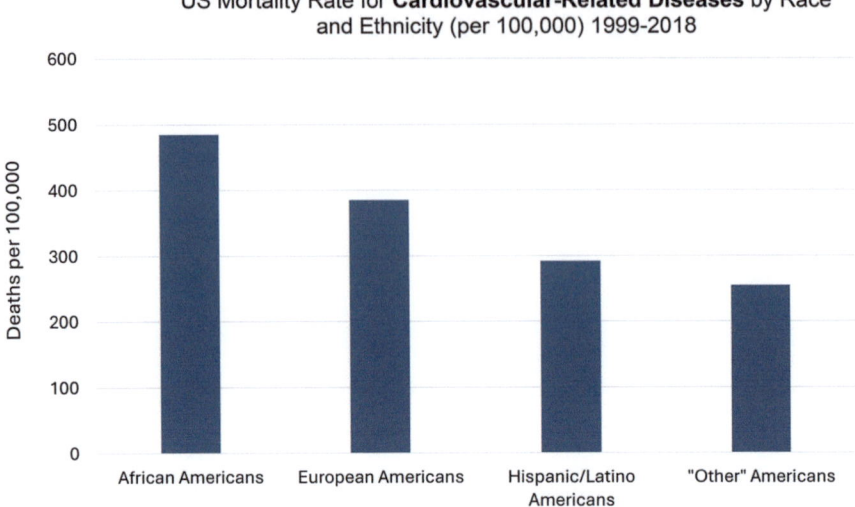

Fig. 4.1 Cardiovascular disease mortality by race and ethnicity

One significant genetic contributor to heart disease is the presence of APOL1 genetic variants, which are associated with an increased risk of chronic kidney disease and atherosclerotic cardiovascular disease in individuals carrying two risk alleles [13, 14]. These variants are more prevalent in African Americans due to their protective effect against *Trypanosoma brucei* rhodesiense infection, known more popularly as African sleeping sickness [17]. This is a largely fatal disease transmitted by an infected tsetse fly. While this APOL1 genetic modification allowed the population with one allele to thrive and avoid sickness, the population with two alleles experiences an increased risk of chronic kidney disease and atherosclerotic cardiovascular disease [9]. This trade-off highlights the complex interplay between genetics and disease susceptibility in different populations; 13% of African Americans (1 in 8) carry two risk alleles, and almost half (46%) have one allele. In comparison, these APOL1 risk alleles are virtually absent in populations of European or Asian descent [13, 14].

Additionally, admixture mapping studies have identified specific chromosomal regions associated with blood pressure phenotypes in African Americans. Blood pressure phenotypes, such as elevated systolic and diastolic blood pressure, are critical indicators of cardiovascular health [18]. Chronic high blood pressure can lead to damage to blood vessels and organs, increasing the risk of heart attack, stroke, and heart failure. In African Americans, specific genetic factors contributing to these phenotypes may exacerbate their susceptibility to cardiovascular diseases, necessitating targeted prevention and treatment strategies. For example, regions 1q21.2–21.3, 4p15.1, 19q12, and 20p13 have been linked to diastolic blood pressure, with certain single nucleotide polymorphisms within these regions showing significant associations [18].

MicroRNA-related polymorphisms also play a role in cardiovascular disease risk factors and can impact the regulation of gene expression, influencing various biological processes linked to cardiovascular health [19]. These small, non-coding RNAs are involved in posttranscriptional regulation, and variations in their sequences can alter their ability to bind target mRNAs, potentially leading to disrupted gene function. Consequently, such disruptions may contribute to the development or progression of hypertension and other cardiovascular diseases in affected individuals. Variants in miRNA genes and their target sites have been associated with serum lipoprotein(a), high-density lipoprotein, and triglyceride levels, which are all significant cardiovascular risk factors[93] [20].

Furthermore, whole genome sequencing has revealed novel genetic determinants of the plasma proteome in African Americans, identifying associations between genetic variants and proteins involved in cardiovascular processes [21]. This includes novel associations at the APOE gene locus and a pleiotropic locus at the HPX gene [21]. The APOE gene locus is significant because it encodes for apolipoprotein E, a key protein involved in lipid metabolism and transport [21]. Variants in this gene have been linked to differences in cholesterol levels and cardiovascular disease risk, particularly influencing the development of atherosclerosis. The HPX gene encodes for hemopexin, a plasma protein that binds free heme, preventing oxidative damage and inflammation. Variants in the HPX gene can affect hemopexin levels and functionality, potentially disrupting the clearance of free heme and contributing to oxidative stress [21]. This oxidative stress is a known factor in the development of cardiovascular diseases, as it can lead to endothelial dysfunction and promote atherosclerosis.

Despite these genetic considerations, the broader social determinants and systemic factors have a much more significant impact on cardiovascular health in African Americans. These genetic influences should make your care more deliberate rather than further establish a "hopeless situation" landscape. By understanding and looking for APOL1 carriers, for example, we can more aggressively anticipate future diseases and benefit entire families with more proactive rather than reactive clinical care. The precision medicine principles of genetics, environment, and culture/lifestyle can significantly improve your understanding of the dynamics influencing your clinical care of African Americans, and in response, your quality care will also improve.

Overall, African Americans are at a higher risk than European Americans for cardiovascular diseases, as evidenced by their:

- Twofold increased risk for stroke [22–24]
- Fourfold increased mortality from stroke [24–26]
- 2.3-fold increased risk for heart failure [22, 27, 28]
- Twofold increased risk for sudden cardiac death [25, 29]
- 1.5-fold increased risk for hypertension [25]
- 1.7-fold increased risk for diabetes [25, 30].

4.1 Hypertension

The prevalence of hypertension in African Americans is the highest in the United States and one of the highest in the world [31, 32], and there has been significant research pertaining to idiosyncrasies unique to this population. Hypertension has been associated with an increased risk of myocardial infarction, heart failure, stroke, and kidney disease. Beginning with a blood pressure at 115/75 mm Hg, an individual's risk of developing cardiovascular disease doubles with every additional rise of 20/10 mm Hg. Recent data regarding the prevalence of hypertension using a threshold of 140/90 reveals a rate of 42% in African American men and 46% in African American women [33]. Other commonly accepted risk factors for hypertension include age, family history, obesity, individual and neighborhood socioeconomic status, and a number of lifestyle factors including activity level, diet, and tobacco use. Digging deeper into the causes of hypertension, Deborah Rohm Young and colleagues found that hypertension rates among African Americans did not vary significantly based on neighborhood socioeconomic status or progressive obesity [34].

> In this large, racially/ethnically and geographically diverse overweight and obese sample, we found that all racial and ethnic minorities, except Hispanics, had higher odds of diagnosed hypertension prevalence across all weight categories and neighborhood education levels compared with whites. In general, although tests for two-way interactions were significant, compared with whites, the magnitude of the odds of hypertension for each racial/ethnic category compared with whites did not substantially vary based on overweight/obese weight category or neighborhood education category. Our results suggest that these factors may not explain the racial/ethnic disparities in hypertension prevalence compared with whites. [34]

The overwhelming evidence in this study curiously found that African Americans living in high socioeconomic neighborhoods and presumably making significantly higher income while having access to healthier foods and exercise opportunities still cannot escape a significantly increased hypertension risk. There must be a genetic predisposition.

4.1.1 Salt Sensitivity

Among the genetic differences getting much attention in hypertensive African Americans is the existence of salt-sensitive genes that may make hypertension worse [3, 35, 36]. Salt sensitivity refers to the body's heightened response to sodium intake, significantly increasing blood pressure. When salt-sensitive individuals consume higher amounts of salt, their blood pressure rises more sharply than those who are not salt-sensitive. Research suggests that genetic factors determine salt sensitivity. Certain gene variants affect how the kidneys handle sodium, potentially influencing blood pressure regulation. The major salt sensitivity genes currently being investigated include:

4.1 Hypertension

- G Protein-Coupled Receptor Kinase 4 (GRK4) variants such as p.Arg65Leu, p.Ala142Val, and p.Val486Ala in the GRK4 gene are associated with impaired sodium excretion and salt-sensitive hypertension [3].
- Epithelial Sodium Channel (ENaC) variants, such as SCNN1B, increase channel activity, leading to sodium and water retention [5].
- The Corin gene variant T555I/Q568P is associated with salt-sensitive hypertension and cardiac hypertrophy. This variant impairs the processing of natriuretic peptides, leading to increased blood pressure in response to dietary salt [37].
- Lysine-Specific Demethylase 1 (LSD-1) gene variants, such as rs587618, are associated with salt sensitivity of blood pressure and aldosterone dysfunction in African Americans. These variants show significant interactions with sex and age, particularly affecting postmenopausal women [35].

These genetic variants are more common and uniquely present in individuals of African descent and remarkably rare in patients of European descent. They also can significantly influence the effectiveness of antihypertensive treatments. For instance, individuals with GRK4 variants may exhibit a reduced response to certain blood pressure medications that target sodium excretion [3]. Those with ENaC variants might require treatments that specifically target sodium retention mechanisms, such as diuretics, to manage their hypertension effectively [5].

Jonathan Williams and colleagues looked specifically at a "lysine-specific demethylase 1" (LSD-1), an epigenetic regulator of salt-sensitive hypertension. The expression of this gene is only seen in the presence of a higher salt dietary load.

> Our results, from animal studies and two hypertensive cohorts of different ethnicities, support LSD-1's role as an epigenetic mediator of dietary sodium's effect on BP. Interestingly, we did not observe this in the (European American) cohort, despite an identical study protocol ... (this) may suggest a relatively intact dietary salt-LSD-1 relationship and/or compensatory mechanisms operating to dampen penetrance in (European Americans). [35]

Research has indicated that LSD-1 plays a pivotal role in the pathophysiology of salt-sensitive hypertension. Elevated salt intake can induce changes in the expression and activity of LSD-1, which in turn affects the methylation status of key genes involved in blood pressure regulation [4, 36]. For example, LSD-1 may regulate the expression of genes related to vascular tone, sodium handling by the kidneys, and inflammation, all of which are critical in the development of hypertension. These findings suggest that targeting LSD-1 could be a potential therapeutic strategy for managing hypertension, particularly in individuals with salt-sensitive hypertension. By modulating LSD-1 activity, it may be possible to mitigate the adverse effects of elevated salt intake on blood pressure and inflammation. Recent advancements in LSD-1 research have focused on developing specific inhibitors that can precisely target its activity [4, 36]. These inhibitors aim to reduce excessive LSD-1 activity, thereby normalizing gene methylation patterns and improving blood pressure regulation. Additionally, studies are exploring the potential of combining LSD-1 inhibitors with other antihypertensive treatments to enhance their efficacy and provide a more comprehensive approach to managing hypertension [4, 36].

Seventy-five percent of all African American patients with hypertension display salt sensitivity compared to 50% across all races with hypertension [38]. The true cause for salt sensitivity in any one patient can be difficult to determine due to a number of comorbid factors that lead to salt sensitivity including obesity, worse renal function, more target organ damage, and lower potassium intake, all of which occur more frequently in African Americans [39]. The combination of these genetic and lifestyle factors gives us the disproportionately high salt sensitivity incidence in African Americans that we see.

There is good evidence that even in the absence of hypertension, elevated dietary sodium can adversely affect multiple target organs and tissues, including the vasculature, kidneys, heart, and brain. For example, increased sodium in patients without hypertension reduced endothelial function, while sodium restriction improved endothelial function. Having adequate endothelial flexibility is critical to preventing adverse cardiovascular events as well as end-organ damage [40, 41]. Increased sodium also leads to increased left ventricular wall thickness (and mass) independent of a patient's hypertension status [42, 43]. Sodium restriction has been shown to decrease protein excretion (thus improving kidney function) and blood pressure in African Americans with hypertension [44]. Finally, there is evidence that chronically elevated dietary sodium affects the brain by way of boosting the sympathetic outflow system, which increases blood pressure variability and can negatively impact end organs [45, 46].

In all, if you have an African American–predominant population, the vast majority of your patients with hypertension are salt sensitive and need counseling related to specific lifestyle modifications they should make. Additionally, salt sensitivity increases with age and is associated with increased mortality independent of a patient's hypertension status [35]. With this in mind, all of your patients need salt restriction counseling.

The good news is that a modest reduction in salt intake (half normal consumption: 5–6 g) for a month has been shown to make significant and sustained reductions in blood pressure [47]. In fact, African Americans showed the most pronounced blood pressure reductions in response to salt restriction, with a drop of 8 mm Hg systolic over 4 mm Hg diastolic averaged across an array of studies. These treatment outcomes in African American patients have long supported a propensity for better responses to salt restrictions. When your African American patient hesitates to start a medication to bring down their mildly elevated blood pressure, spend some time determining how much salt is in their diet, and then explain the great impact a one-half reduction in salt can have. With these nuances in mind, suggesting a decrease in salt in any African American's diet is sound and beneficial advice.

4.1.2 Hypertension Control

Hypertension control is central to primary, secondary, and tertiary interventions aimed at reducing African American mortality and morbidity from hypertension-related complications. Hypertension occurs earlier in African Americans, is more severe, and is more likely to be resistant to therapy [48]. African Americans are also more likely to have "nondipping blood pressure" (blood pressure that does not decrease by >10% from daytime to nighttime) and nighttime hypertension on ambulatory blood pressure monitoring [31].

It is also interesting to note that hypertension prevalence was higher among US-born African Americans than among either foreign-born non-Hispanic Blacks or all African-born immigrants of any race or ethnicity. In addition, "being born outside the United States, speaking a language other than English at home, and living fewer years in the United States were each associated with a decreased prevalence of hypertension [31]."

The American College of Cardiology/American Heart Association Task Force on Clinical Practice Guidelines issued a major reset in hypertension management in 2017 by lowering the systolic and diastolic levels for both the diagnosis of hypertension and treatment targets. Data has consistently shown an increase in cardiovascular events with progressively elevated blood pressure.

> Observational studies have demonstrated graded associations between higher systolic blood pressure (SBP) and diastolic blood pressure (DBP) and increased CVD risk. In a meta-analysis of 61 prospective studies, the risk of CVD increased in a log-linear fashion from SBP levels <115 mm Hg to >180 mm Hg and from DBP levels <75 mm Hg to >105 mm Hg. In that analysis, 20 mm Hg higher SBP and 10 mm Hg higher DBP were each associated with a doubling in the risk of death from stroke, heart disease, or other vascular disease. [49]

In addition, systematic reviews of hypertension treatment trials, including the findings from the Systolic Blood Pressure Intervention Trial (SPRINT) led by prominent African American researcher and physician Jackson Wright, Jr., clearly documented the benefit of treating systolic blood pressure targets well below previously recommended levels in preventing cardiovascular events and all-cause mortality including in African Americans and even in patients over age 75 years of age [50–52]. Thus, a new classification system was proposed, which set parameters for blood pressure categories of normal, elevated, stage 1 hypertension, and stage 2 hypertension (Fig. 4.2).

This reset of the parameters significantly increases the percentage of African Americans with hypertension to 59% for men and 56% for women overall [49]. Being more aggressive with blood pressure control in African Americans makes sense from a number of perspectives given the poor outcomes data for stroke, heart attack, congestive heart failure, and more [53, 54].

When it comes to pharmacotherapy, there are a number of important differences in the African American population that significantly alter your approach to blood pressure control. Evidence from multiple trials suggests that African Americans

Blood Pressure Category	Systolic Blood Pressure		Diastolic Blood Pressure
Normal	< 120 mm Hg	and	< 80 mm Hg
Elevated	120 -129 mm Hg	and	< 80 mm Hg
Hypertension			
Stage 1	130 - 139 mm Hg	or	80 - 89 mm Hg
Stage 2	$\geq$ 140 mm Hg	or	$\geq$ 90 mmHg

Fig. 4.2 Blood pressure categories. (By author)

respond well to thiazide diuretics and calcium channel blockers, and they should be used early and often in hypertensive African Americans [49, 55–57]. Thiazide-type diuretics (chlorthalidone in this study) were better at reducing blood pressure and preventing cardiovascular events than an ACE inhibitor (lisinopril) or an alpha-adrenergic blocker (doxazosin) in African Americans, as found in the "Antihypertensive and Lipid-Lowering Treatment to Prevent Heart Attack" (ALLHAT) trial [48].

For ideal blood pressure control, the thiazide-type diuretic dose should be equivalent to chlorthalidone 12.5–25 mg/day or hydrochlorothiazide 25–50 mg/day because lower doses have not been found to be as effective [48]. Overall, calcium channel blockers (amlodipine) and thiazide diuretics are best in African Americans.

Angiotensin-converting enzyme (ACE) inhibitors are less effective in African Americans for blood pressure control as monotherapy [58, 59]. A large cohort of over 400,000 patients done at the New York University School of Medicine compared outcomes in African Americans and European Americans with three distinct groups:

1. ACE inhibitors vs. calcium channel blockers
2. ACE inhibitors vs. thiazide diuretics
3. ACE inhibitors vs. beta-blockers

Their study showed that ACE inhibitors were associated with poorer control of blood pressure in African Americans and observationally associated with a significant increase in stroke, heart failure, and combined cardiovascular disease when compared with calcium channel blockers or thiazide diuretics. The inferior outcomes with angiotensin-converting enzyme inhibitors were largely similar to those of beta blockers in this population [58].

Because ACE inhibitors are commonly listed as "first-line" medications for blood pressure control in national and international guidelines and recommendations, it should be noted that this principally is based on their response in European American populations. Based on these large African American-inclusive studies and a number of considerations (including cost, comorbid conditions, and disease propensities), most guideline recommendations suggest a diuretic and/or a calcium channel blocker as first-line antihypertensive therapy in African Americans.

These large studies also confirmed that African Americans, along with Asian-Pacific Islanders, have a greater incidence of ACE-related cough and a higher rate of discontinuation due to cough compared to all other racial groups. African Americans were also more prone to develop ACE-associated angioedema [49, 58]. African Americans have a three to four times higher incidence of angiotensin-converting enzyme inhibitor-induced angioedema than European Americans [60]. This allergic reaction frequently results in an emergency department visit and shakes the patient's confidence in your medication selection. Given the availability of Angiotensin II receptor blocker (ARB) alternatives, it is prudent to consider these for African American patients to minimize the risk of angioedema and cough.

The renal-sparing benefits of ARB medications are critical when used to slow renal function decline (particularly in hypertensive renal disease), and they should still be used prophylactically in African American patients with diabetes with proteinuria [61, 62]. ACE inhibitors, because of their high side effect profile in African Americans, should be avoided.

Beta-blockers have long been shown to be significantly less effective in most African Americans and are now not recommended as first-line therapy (in the absence of coronary heart disease or heart failure or unless combined with a diuretic or calcium channel blocker) for blood pressure control [61].

Beta-blockers regain their widespread clinical significance in African Americans in the treatment of myocardial infarctions and systolic heart failure according to guidelines across all other populations [63].

It is important to note that these nuances in the pharmacologic care of hypertensive African Americans are based on the outcomes of multiple well-designed studies over a number of years and truly represent the "standard of care" for this population. A study by Yazdanshenas and colleagues looked at the prescribing patterns of clinicians seeing older African Americans and found that the "(t)reatment of hypertension appears to be inconsistent with the prevailing treatment guidelines for nearly one-third of the aged African Americans." Most of the mismanaged patients were on beta-blockers and ACE inhibitors as monotherapy for hypertension control [64].

Studies have also confirmed that even less intensive interventions (than pharmacotherapy) have helped high-risk African American patients attain better blood pressure control and medication compliance, including:

- Culturally competent provider
- Team-based patient education including providers and allied health professionals
- Appropriate referrals for health conditions and social needs
- Incremental steps approach [65]

These measures help by improving the understanding of the cardiovascular condition, and as trust-building measures that lead to better medication adherence and office follow-up compliance.

Seeing the same provider has also been found to be positively correlated with successful hypertension control. Hypertensive African Americans are significantly less likely than hypertensive European Americans to see the same provider consistently. Setting up clinical visit protocols that encourage provider continuity will improve a number of critical quality measures, including hypertension [65].

4.2 Heart Failure

African Americans have greater incidence and worse outcomes than other racial groups with heart failure. According to the American College of Cardiology, American Heart Association, and Heart Failure Society of America guidelines, African Americans have the highest risk of incident heart failure and a higher prevalence of nonischemic heart failure (see Fig. 4.3). African Americans also exhibit more heart failure risk factors, including hypertension, obesity, and diabetes, compared with the majority population [27].

Disparities in heart failure outcomes are significant. African American patients experience higher rates of heart failure-related hospitalizations and mortality. For instance, the age-adjusted heart failure-related cardiovascular disease death rate for African American men was 1.43-fold higher than for European American men. For African American women, it was 1.54-fold higher than for European American women [27]. These disparities are more pronounced among younger adults (35–64 years) compared with older adults (65–84 years) [66].

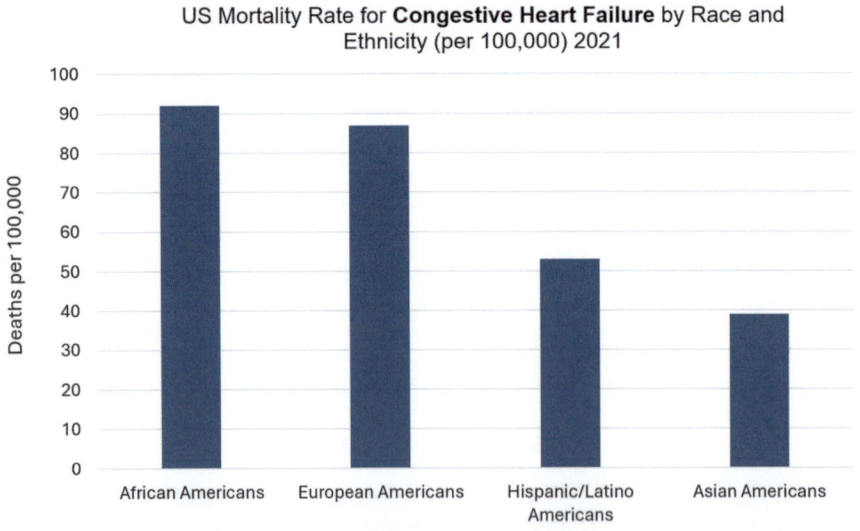

Fig. 4.3 United States mortality rate for congestive heart failure by race and ethnicity (per 100,000) 2021

4.2 Heart Failure

Unlike hypertension, the pharmacological approach to systolic heart failure has not been significantly stratified by race, even though this disease is more predominant in the African American population. Racial disparities in the management of heart failure in African Americans are well-documented and multifaceted. Experts emphasize the importance of guideline-directed medical therapy (GDMT) for all patients with heart failure, including African Americans. This includes the use of angiotensin receptor-neprilysin inhibitors (ARNIs), beta-blockers, mineralocorticoid receptor antagonists (MRAs), and sodium-glucose cotransporter-2 (SGLT2) inhibitors [27]. Additionally, for African American patients with persistent symptoms despite optimal GDMT, the combination of hydralazine and isosorbide dinitrate (HYD/ISDN) is recommended [27].

The combination of hydralazine and isosorbide dinitrate plays a significant role in treating heart failure in African Americans, particularly those with heart failure with reduced ejection fraction [27]. Cardiologists recommend this combination for African American patients who remain symptomatic despite optimal therapy with Angiotensin Receptor Blockers (ARB), beta-blockers, and mineralocorticoid receptor antagonists (spironolactone, for example) [27]. The efficacy of this combination was demonstrated in the African-American Heart Failure Trial (A-HeFT), which showed that adding hydralazine and isosorbide dinitrate to standard therapy significantly improved survival and reduced hospitalizations in African American patients with reduced ejection fraction [67, 68]. The trial was terminated early due to the clear benefits observed, including a 43% reduction in mortality and a 33% reduction in first hospitalization for heart failure [67]. The rationale for this recommendation is based on the unique pathophysiological characteristics of heart failure in African Americans, who often have a lower response to conventional approaches alone. The combination of hydralazine and isosorbide dinitrate works better for heart failure in African Americans due to several key factors; hydralazine acts as a vasodilator, primarily affecting arteries, which reduces afterload and decreases the workload on the heart [69, 70]. On the other hand, isosorbide dinitrate mainly dilates veins, reducing preload and decreasing the amount of blood returning to the heart [69, 70]. African Americans have a reduced ability to produce endogenous nitric oxide, which is crucial for vascular function [69]. Isosorbide dinitrate, a nitrate, increases nitric oxide availability, thereby improving vasodilation and reducing cardiac workload [69]. Hydralazine also acts as an antioxidant, preventing the development of nitrate tolerance, which can occur with continuous nitrate use [69]. This synergistic effect ensures sustained hemodynamic benefits. The G-protein beta-3 subunit genotype (GNB3 TT) is more prevalent in African Americans and is associated with enhanced alpha-adrenergic tone [71]. This genotype predicts a more significant therapeutic response to the hydralazine and isosorbide dinitrate combination [71]. This complementary combination leads to significant improvements in cardiac function, including increased left ventricular ejection fraction and reduced ventricular remodeling [69, 70]. Combination therapy in this way addresses African American-specific needs, providing a more effective treatment option and highlighting the importance of precision medicine in managing heart failure in diverse populations.

Despite these consensus recommendations, African Americans are less likely to receive these medical regimens or more advanced heart failure therapies such as cardiac resynchronization therapy (CRT), ventricular assist devices (VADs), and heart transplants compared with the majority population [72]. They are also less likely to be admitted to cardiology services, which leads to better outcomes [28]. Bias on the clinician's part drives many of these disparities.

The pharmacological management of heart failure with preserved ejection fraction in African Americans involves several key strategies. First, blood pressure control is essential [27]. Diuretics are also added to manage volume overload, and angiotensin receptor blockers, along with beta-blockers, are recommended for persistent hypertension [27]. Second, SGLT2 inhibitors have shown benefits in reducing heart failure hospitalizations and cardiovascular mortality in these patients [27]. Third, mineralocorticoid receptor antagonists may be considered to decrease hospitalizations, particularly in patients with marginally lower ejection fractions [27].

Finally, it should be noted that there are also significant differences in cardiovascular marker laboratory levels between patients of European American and African American backgrounds. The natriuretic peptides, BNP and NT-pro-BNP, are counterregulatory hormones involved in volume homeostasis and cardiovascular remodeling [73]. B-type natriuretic peptide (BNP) levels have been shown to reliably facilitate diagnosis and predict overall prognosis in patients with acute and chronic heart failure. Elevated levels of both markers are predictive of worse cardiovascular disease. African Americans tend to have *lower* levels of BNP and NT-proBNP compared with White individuals [73–75]. This has been consistently observed across multiple studies. For instance, the REGARDS study found that NT-proBNP levels were up to 27% lower in African Americans compared with European Americans, even after adjusting for various clinical factors [74]. Similarly, the Dallas Heart Study reported that NT-proBNP levels were significantly lower in African Americans compared with European and Hispanic-Latino individuals, with a 39% reduction in NT-proBNP levels in African Americans after multivariable adjustments [75]. These findings suggest that traditional biomarkers for heart failure may be less reliable in African Americans, potentially leading to underdiagnosis and undertreatment. Therefore, alternative diagnostic criteria and therapeutic strategies may be necessary to effectively manage heart failure in this population.

The increased risk for mortality stratification that occurs when BNP and NT-proBNP levels increase is still valid across all racial groups, but the baseline level disparities can present potential clinical issues.

> (African American) individuals have a higher prevalence of CV disease; therefore, intuitively they should have higher NTproBNP levels than (European American) individuals, suggesting possible non-hemodynamic mechanisms (eg, decreased production) as a cause for lower NTproBNP levels in (African American) individuals. Taken collectively, the findings of paradoxically low NP levels suggest the likelihood of a primary deficiency among (African American) individuals. [73]

With that deficiency, researchers suggest that lower-level natriuretic peptide results in African Americans may convey the wrong assumption regarding cardiac stability in this population. In other words, early heart failure could exist in the presence of "normal-looking" NT-pro-BNP levels.

4.2.1 Hereditary Transthyretin Amyloidosis (hATTR)

Hereditary transthyretin amyloidosis (hATTR) is another cause of heart failure and occurs substantially more in African Americans. hATTR is a multisystem disease caused by changes in the transthyretin (TTR) gene, with the V122I (Val122Ile) mutation being particularly prevalent among African Americans [23]. Cardiomyopathy and heart failure are associated with this mutation in approximately 3–4% of African Americans [76–78]. A V122I mutation causes misfolding of the TTR protein, resulting in amyloid fibril deposition in the heart, causing an autosomal dominant form of cardiomyopathy that manifests in the sixth decade of life or later [79, 80]. There is a substantial morbidity and mortality associated with this condition, which is often underdiagnosed. Heart failure, polyneuropathy, and carpal tunnel syndrome are common clinical manifestations of hATTR in African Americans with the V122I mutation [77, 81, 82]. Also, due to its association with hATTR, African Americans with bilateral carpal tunnel syndrome might benefit from screening for the V122I mutation [59]. Early diagnosis and treatment are crucial. Tafamidis, a TTR stabilizer, has been shown to reduce mortality and hospitalizations in patients with TTR amyloidosis-associated cardiomyopathy [83]. Given the high prevalence and significant impact of the V122I mutation in African Americans, increased awareness and early screening are essential for improving outcomes in this population.

4.3 Lipids

With all of the cardiovascular bad news reviewed earlier in this chapter, African Americans have more favorable lipid profiles than matched European Americans including having higher HDL cholesterol levels, lower triglycerides, and lower LDL cholesterol levels, multiple studies have confirmed [84–86]. With disproportionately higher cardiovascular disease in African Americans, researchers have wondered how these better lipid profiles coincide with the documented worse outcomes and whether the lipid profile is an "underidentifier" of African Americans at risk for cardiovascular events. The variability seen based on race and ethnicity is yet another curiosity given the clinician's accepted strict association of bad lipids equaling worse outcomes and good lipids leading to improved outcomes.

> It is clear that there is further complexity in this relationship among African Americans, who have, on average, a more favorable lipid profile compared to European Americans, yet they do not experience an associated decrease in diseases that are expected to be responsive to reduction in this key risk factor. [84]

There are both genetic and metabolic reasons for this difference. African Americans have a higher frequency of genetic variants influencing lipid metabolism. For example, the LPL (lipoprotein lipase) gene variant rs328 is associated with higher HDL and lower triglycerides in African Americans [87–89]. Additionally, the hepatic lipase gene (LIPC) -514 T allele, more common in African Americans, is associated with higher HDL levels and larger HDL particle size [87–89]. These genetic variants, however, are not exclusive to African Americans and are present in varying frequencies in other populations. For instance, the LPL gene variant rs328 is also found in European and Asian populations, though it may affect lipid metabolism differently [89]. African Americans exhibit distinctive features in lipoprotein metabolism, including increased postheparin lipoprotein lipase activity, which enhances triglyceride-rich lipoprotein clearance [89]. This results in lower triglyceride levels and higher HDL cholesterol levels [88].

Despite being more insulin-resistant, African Americans have lower visceral adipose tissue and hepatic triglyceride content compared to European Americans [90, 91]. This leads to lower free fatty acid release and reduced substrate availability for very low-density lipoprotein (VLDL) assembly and secretion, contributing to lower triglyceride levels [90, 91].

Attempts to drill down to why good lipids do not lead to better outcomes in African Americans have continued to baffle providers, but the assumption is the impact of other cardiovascular risk factors (hypertension, obesity, and diabetes) overwhelms the beneficial impact of the improved lipid profile.

There are also racial differences in response to diet modifications, with African Americans' lipid profiles being less responsive to an unsaturated fat diet than European Americans. A study by Furtado and colleagues found that African Americans' lipid profiles were less responsive to an unsaturated fat diet compared with European Americans [86]. This difference in response is highlighted in the OmniHeart Trial, which found that dietary interventions aimed at lowering triglycerides and apolipoprotein C-III (apo C-III) were more effective in European Americans than in African Americans. Specifically, while unsaturated fat and protein diets significantly lowered plasma apo C-III and triglycerides in European Americans, these effects were not observed in African Americans [86]. Additionally, a study on the balanced high-fat diet (BHFD) showed that European American women had greater reductions in visceral adipose tissue, fasting insulin levels, and HOMA-IR scores compared to African American women [92]. European Americans also experienced more significant improvements in VLDL particle size, apolipoprotein B levels, serum triglycerides, and LDL cholesterol. In contrast, African American women showed improvements primarily in HDL particle size and the number of large HDL particles [92].

Diet modifications do still work in African Americans with salt sensitivity (already discussed) and for LDL cholesterol lowering, which can still have a dramatic effect on cardiovascular risk. The overall message is to have a lower threshold for cardiovascular prophylaxis in spite of a beneficial-looking lipid profile. Any opportunity to lower or eliminate risk factors in African Americans should never be overlooked.

4.4 Atrial Fibrillation

Atrial fibrillation is the most prevalent arrhythmia in the United States and is associated with significant adverse outcomes that include stroke, heart failure, and increased mortality [93]. Surprisingly, studies also confirm a decreased atrial fibrillation incidence in African Americans (41% lower risk of being diagnosed than European Americans, Fig. 4.4) but a greatly increased occurrence of stroke and sudden death in African Americans with atrial fibrillation [94–96]. Some have suggested the decreased incidence is actually underdiagnosis, but others have called it a "racial paradox" where despite atrial fibrillation being a sequelae of increased hypertension, diabetes, obesity, heart failure, and myocardial infarctions, all of which are higher in African Americans, the incidence of atrial fibrillation is paradoxically lower.

Potential genetic factors influencing the lower incidence of atrial fibrillation (AF) in African Americans include several key elements including Single Nucleotide Polymorphisms (SNPs). The study by Roberts and colleagues identified that the SNP rs10824026 on chromosome 10q22 mediates a modest proportion of the increased risk of atrial fibrillation among European Americans compared with African Americans, potentially through an effect on gene expression levels of MYOZ1 [97]. This suggests that certain genetic variants associated with atrial fibrillation in European Americans may not be as prevalent or impactful in African Americans. Delaney found that while the genomic regions 1q21, 4q25, and 16q22 are associated with atrial fibrillation in African Americans, the specific SNPs within these regions differ from those identified in European-descent populations [98]. This indicates that the genetic architecture contributing to atrial fibrillation risk

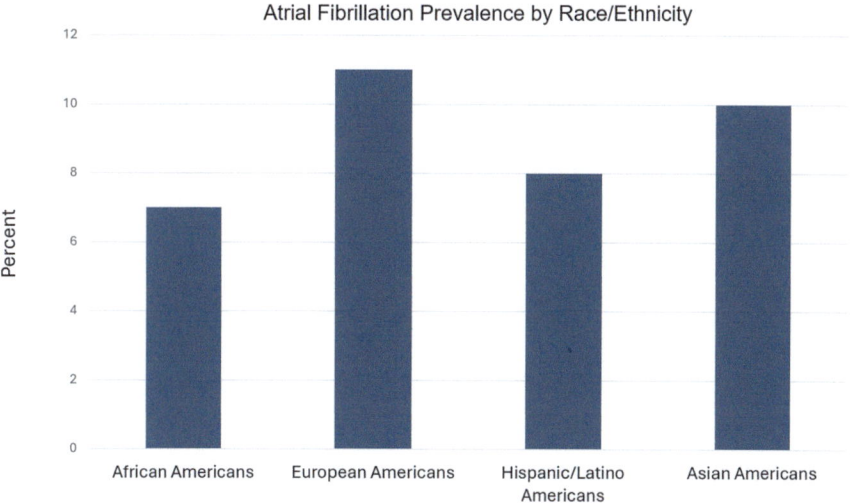

Fig. 4.4 Atrial fibrillation by race/ethnicity

varies between races. Aldosterone synthase polymorphism also plays a part, and the CYP11B2 -344 T > C genotype has been shown to be a significant independent predictor of atrial fibrillation in African Americans with heart failure [99]. Increased West African ancestry was associated with decreased serum aldosterone levels, which may contribute to the lower risk of atrial fibrillation observed in this population [99]. In contrast, researchers at the University of California, San Francisco, demonstrated that increased European ancestry was associated with a higher risk of atrial fibrillation *in African Americans* [100]. This suggests that genetic factors linked to European ancestry may contribute to the higher incidence of atrial fibrillation in European Americans.

When it occurred, African Americans were also less likely to be aware they have atrial fibrillation, and much less likely to be treated with warfarin, and these findings were independent of insurance and socioeconomic class [95]. Significant disparities relating to stroke prevention in a stroke-prone population were found in a study by Meschia and colleagues who looked at over 30,000 patients:

> We also found that among those who were aware that they had AF (atrial fibrillation) and who had confirmation of the diagnosis of AF, (African Americans) were about one quarter as likely to be treated with warfarin as (European Americans). In striking contrast, risk of stroke as stratified by the CHADS$_2$ score was not a predictor of warfarin use. The fact that risk of future stroke did not significantly alter the likelihood of warfarin use would seem to reflect an evidence-practice gap. [101]

The risk for death in the presence of atrial fibrillation in the first 4 months after diagnosis was very high, with CAD, heart failure, and stroke accounting for the majority of deaths, the study also found. Their risk for hospitalization from atrial fibrillation doubled as did the risk for recurrent stroke and related multiinfarct dementia [101].

Overall, African Americans are less likely to receive any oral anticoagulant therapy compared with European Americans [102]. This disparity persists even after adjusting for clinical and socioeconomic factors. Specifically, African Americans are less likely to be prescribed direct oral anticoagulants (DOACs) compared to European Americans [102]. Additionally, the REACH-AF study highlighted significant facility-level variation in anticoagulant prescribing, with some facilities showing a marked disparity in the initiation of any anticoagulant including DOAC therapy between African American and European American patients [103]. The Veterans Health Administration study also found that African Americans were less likely to initiate any anticoagulant therapy and DOACs specifically, compared with European American patients [104]. Moreover, the quality of anticoagulation management is often lower in African Americans. For instance, African Americans treated with warfarin had a lower median time in the therapeutic range compared with European American patients, and those treated with DOACs were more likely to receive inappropriate dosing [102].

4.5 Stroke

As a quarter of all strokes occur in the presence of atrial fibrillation and while representing 13% of the US population [105], African Americans experience almost twice that percentage of all strokes as shown in Fig. 4.5 [106]. And when a stroke occurs, African Americans have them earlier in life and present with more severe and disabling conditions [106, 107].

Several studies have identified genetic variants associated with stroke risk in African Americans. One significant finding is the association of the HNF1A gene with stroke. A genome-wide association study meta-analysis identified a single nucleotide polymorphism near the HNF1A gene that reached genome-wide significance in individuals of African descent [24]. This gene has been previously linked to lipid metabolism and inflammation, which are critical pathways in stroke pathogenesis. Another study highlighted the APOL1 gene variants, particularly the G1 and G2 risk alleles, which are more prevalent in African Americans and have been associated with an increased risk of ischemic stroke, especially small vessel disease [108]. These variants are also known for their role in kidney disease, which can contribute to stroke risk through hypertension and other vascular complications. Additionally, the COX-2 G-765C polymorphism has been associated with an increased risk of incident stroke in African Americans, suggesting a role for inflammation-related genetic polymorphisms in stroke susceptibility [109]. Furthermore, a meta-analysis identified several other loci, including those near the SFXN4 and TMEM108 genes, which represent potential novel ischemic stroke loci in African Americans [24].

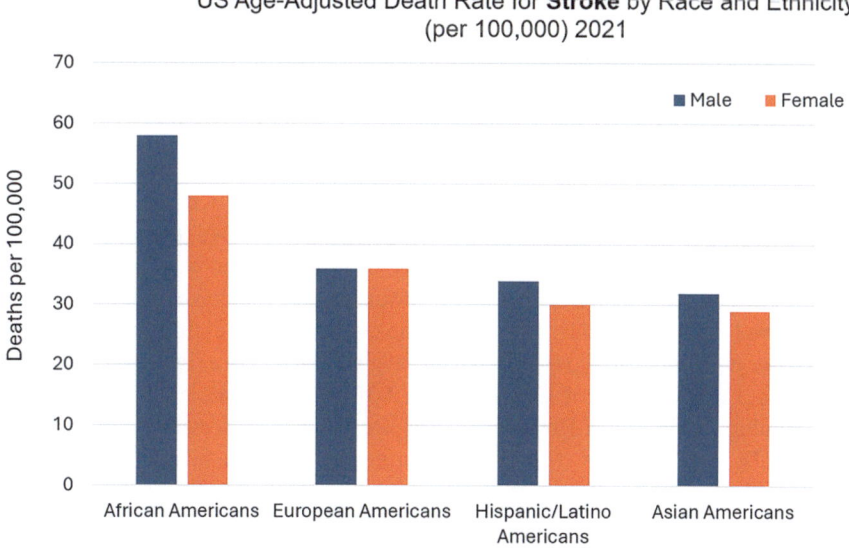

Fig. 4.5 Stroke mortality by race/ethnicity

Poststroke outcomes also differ significantly. African Americans tend to have worse functional and cognitive outcomes at 90 days poststroke compared to European Americans [110]. This includes significant limitations in activities of daily living and more severe stroke symptoms [111]. Additionally, African Americans have a higher risk of long-term mortality after acute ischemic stroke (AIS), even after adjusting for age, sex, and comorbidities [110]. Several factors contribute to these disparities. African Americans are less likely to receive timely emergency medical services and are less likely to arrive at the hospital promptly, which impacts the timely administration of treatments like tissue plasminogen activator (tPA) and endovascular thrombectomy [112]. Moreover, African Americans are less likely to receive these advanced treatments compared with their European American counterparts [113].

The "Cardiovascular Quality and Outcomes" group concluded that "compared with other race/ethnicity groups, (African American) patients were less likely to receive IV tissue-type plasminogen activator <3 hours, early antithrombotics, antithrombotics at discharge, and lipid-lowering medication prescribed at discharge," a study looking at over 200,000 patients showed [114]. Not surprisingly, with these prescriptive deficiencies in play, data analysis also showed a persistently increased rehospitalization rate in African Americans at both 30 days and 1 year for all causes. African Americans also have a 2.4 times higher rate of recurrent strokes than European Americans in the face of lower secondary prevention measures, and the highest burden of mortality than any racial group [115].

Stroke patients overseen by neurologists were 3.7 times more likely to receive intravenous thrombolysis than those attended to by nonneurologists for all races and ethnicities (study from the Baylor College of Medicine), but unfortunately, African Americans were half as likely as European Americans to be seen by a neurologist when presenting with a stroke [115].

Socioeconomic factors, including lower income and insurance status, also play a role in these disparities. African Americans from lower-income backgrounds are less likely to receive an endovascular thrombectomy and have poorer outcomes posttreatment [116].

Prophylactic aspirin.

For secondary prevention, prophylactic aspirin is effective in reducing the risk of recurrent strokes. The African American Antiplatelet Stroke Prevention Study (AAASPS) demonstrated that aspirin is a viable option for secondary stroke prevention in African Americans, with a trend towards better outcomes compared with ticlopidine [117]. For primary prevention, the evidence is more nuanced. The study by Glasser et al. indicated that prophylactic aspirin use was not significantly associated with a reduced risk of first stroke in African Americans after adjusting for confounding factors [118]. However, aspirin use for primary prevention in high-risk individuals, such as those with multiple cardiovascular risk factors, may still be considered on a case-by-case basis, particularly after a thorough discussion of the risks and benefits with a healthcare provider. The American Heart Association (AHA) and the American College of Cardiology (ACC) guidelines recommend considering low-dose aspirin (75–100 mg daily) for primary prevention in adults aged

40–70 years who are at higher cardiovascular risk but not at increased bleeding risk [119]. This recommendation applies universally, including to African Americans, who may benefit from tailored risk assessments and discussions about aspirin therapy.

Overall, the US Preventive Services Task Force (USPSTF) recommends referring adults who have cardiovascular disease risk factors and are obese to intense behavioral counseling interventions to promote a healthful diet and physical activity [120]. The CDC reports that 44% of African American men and 48% of African American women have some form of cardiovascular disease, thus making almost half of your African American patient population eligible for lifestyle modification counseling [121]. Most insurances pride themselves on covering USPSTF preventive recommendations, so there should be no barriers to referring your African American patients to these proven lifestyle modification counselors.

4.6 Peripheral Vascular Disease

Racial and ethnic disparities in the treatment, management, and outcomes for patients with peripheral vascular disease (PVD) are significant, particularly for African Americans as shown in Fig. 4.6. African Americans have a higher prevalence of PVD compared with all other racial/ethnic groups, and this disparity increases with age. African Americans also present with more advanced disease stages including chronic limb-threatening ischemia [122, 123].

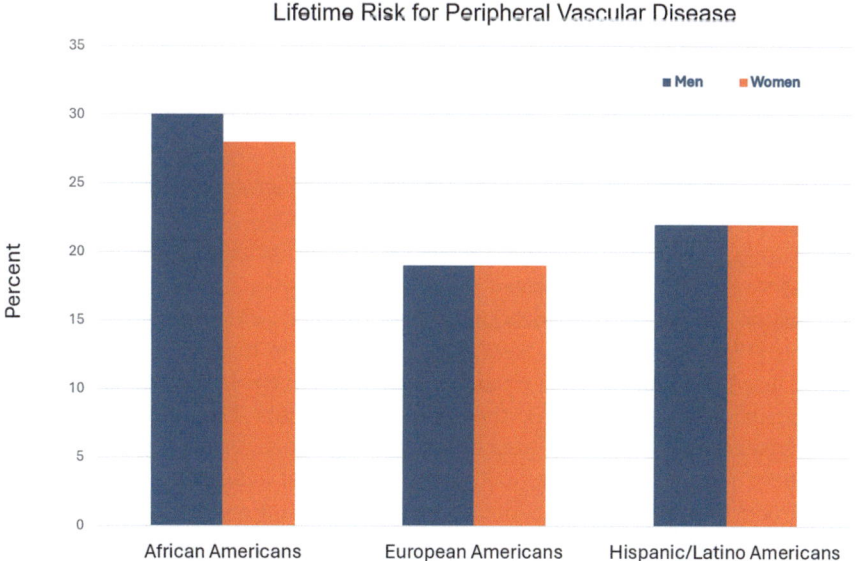

Fig. 4.6 Peripheral vascular disease lifetime risk

Several studies have identified genetic factors associated with PVD in African Americans. For instance, admixture mapping has identified a region on chromosome 11 associated with low ankle-brachial index, a marker of PVD, in African Americans. Specific single nucleotide polymorphisms such as rs12289502 and rs9665943 within this region have been significantly associated with low ankle-brachial index, indicating a genetic predisposition to PVD [124]. Additionally, the APOL1 gene variants, particularly the G1 and G2 risk alleles, have been associated with an increased risk of PVD in African Americans. These variants are also linked to chronic kidney disease, which exacerbates vascular complications [2, 125]. Genome-wide association studies (GWAS) have further identified multiple loci associated with PVD. For example, the largest available GWAS on PVD identified 19 genome-wide significant loci, including genes responsible for circulating lipoproteins and clotting factors, which are implicated in the development of PVD [126]. Moreover, the ABO blood group has been associated with PVD in African Americans. Specifically, the A allele has been linked to a lower ankle-brachial index (ABI) and a higher prevalence of PVD [127].

African Americans are less likely to receive guideline-directed medical therapy, including antiplatelet and statin therapy, and have lower participation in supervised exercise therapy [122, 128–131]. They are also less likely to undergo revascularization procedures and more likely to undergo limb amputation compared with European Americans [122, 132]. This is partly due to disparities in healthcare access, insurance coverage, and the availability of experienced healthcare centers. Outcomes for African Americans with PVD are generally worse [133]. They experience higher rates of major adverse limb events, including limb amputation, and cardiovascular events such as myocardial infarction and stroke. Functional decline and mobility loss are also more pronounced in African Americans with PVD. The American College of Cardiology and the American Heart Association emphasize the need for targeted interventions to address these disparities. These interventions include clinician and patient education, improved access to high-quality healthcare, and policy changes to reduce nontraumatic limb amputations.

Compared to European American patients, several studies have found that African Americans with peripheral vascular disease are more likely to have amputations of limbs and less likely to have their lower limb correctively revascularized either surgically or via an endovascular approach [134–136]. In another study, African Americans were estimated to be at a 77% higher risk of lower extremity amputation versus revascularization when compared with European American patients [135]. Researchers looked at the differences in treatment of patients and found that European American patients sought treatment in the earlier stages of their peripheral vascular disease than African Americans. They added that having more advanced disease at the time of hospital admission, evidenced by a planned outpatient admission versus an emergency department admission, was associated with worse outcomes. African Americans tended toward more emergency department admissions and outpatient-generated admissions [137]. The presumption was that the lack of provider access in minorities drove the majority of the difference.

A study of African Americans in the Jackson Heart Study determined that cigarette smoking was directly linked to peripheral vascular disease, and the correlation of severity was directly linked to the number of cigarettes smoked per day [138]. Moreover, the study determined that African Americans who smoke were at twice the risk for peripheral artery disease that matched European American controls.

> Among current smokers, there was a dose-dependent response whereby those smoking ≥20 cigarettes per day and higher pack-year smoking exposure demonstrated considerably higher odds of subclinical PAD compared with those smoking 1–19 cigarettes per day. [138]

The negative effects of smoking also showed a dose-dependent association with abdominal aorta and aorto-iliac calcification that could lead to obstruction or aneurysmal formation.

4.7 Abdominal Aortic Aneurysms

Racial and ethnic disparities in the treatment, management, and outcomes for African American patients with abdominal aortic aneurysms (AAAs) are significant and multifaceted. African American patients with AAAs tend to present with more severe disease and a greater burden of comorbidities, such as hypertension, diabetes, and chronic kidney disease, which contribute to less favorable outcomes [133]. They have higher rates of postoperative complications, including new postoperative dialysis and return to the operating room, and longer hospital stays after both elective and nonelective endovascular aneurysm repair [139]. Despite these challenges, in-hospital mortality rates for African American patients with AAAs are not significantly different from those of European American patients after adjusting for baseline characteristics [133, 140–142]. However, it is important to note that these findings do not diminish the need for targeted interventions to address the disparities in treatment and management. Further research is required to understand the underlying factors contributing to these disparities and to develop strategies to improve outcomes for African American patients with AAAs. Genome-wide association studies have identified several genetic loci associated with AAAs. For instance, a study identified risk variants proximal to genes such as PSRC1-CELSR2-SORT1, PCIF1-ZNF335-MMP9, RP11-136O12.2/TRIB1, ZNF259/APOA5, IL6R, PCSK9, LPA, and APOE, which were associated with plasma protein levels and AAA incidence in patients of both African and European descent [143]. Specifically, low levels of neogenin and kit ligand were found to be novel risk factors for AAA development, suggesting these proteins may play a role in the pathogenesis of AAAs [143].

Additionally, the APOL1 gene variants, particularly the G1 and G2 risk alleles, have been associated with an increased risk of cardiovascular diseases, including AAAs, in African Americans. These variants have been linked to chronic kidney disease, hypertension, stroke, and others that exacerbate vascular complications [2]. Furthermore, genetic ancestry studies have shown that African Americans with lower percentages of European ancestry have a higher prevalence of subclinical atherosclerosis . . . which is a risk factor for AAAs. This suggests that genetic factors related to ancestry may contribute to the higher burden of AAAs in this population [144]. African American patients are less likely to undergo elective endovascular aneurysm repair compared with European Americans. They are more prone to present with ruptured AAAs and undergo emergent surgical repair, which is associated with higher morbidity and mortality. Additionally, African American patients are less likely to receive timely transfers to specialized centers for ruptured abdominal aortic aneurysms [145, 146]. African American patients have higher rates of 5-year aneurysm rupture, reintervention, and mortality following elective endovascular aneurysm repair compared to other populations. They also experience higher rates of loss-to-imaging follow-up, which is critical for monitoring and managing potential complications [142].

4.8 Deep Vein Thrombosis and Pulmonary Embolism

Health disparities related to Deep Vein Thrombosis (DVT) and Pulmonary Embolism (PE) in African American populations are well-documented in the medical literature. African Americans have a significantly higher incidence of venous thromboembolism (VTE), which includes both DVT and PE, compared with other racial groups, as shown in Fig. 4.7 [147, 148]. As the third leading cause of vascular death behind myocardial infarction and stroke, venous thromboembolism represents a serious threat to clinical outcomes in the African American community. African

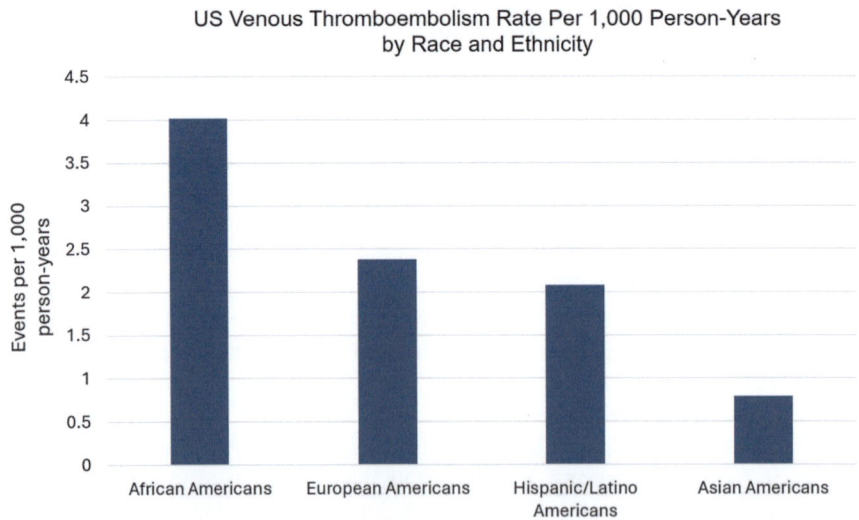

Fig. 4.7 US venous thromboembolism rate by race/ethnicity

4.8 Deep Vein Thrombosis and Pulmonary Embolism

Americans have the highest incidence of both provoked (caused by an identifiable risk factor) and unprovoked venous thromboembolism and the highest short-term mortality [148, 149]. To complicate the situation further, African Americans also have higher major bleeding events when treated for thromboembolism [148].

This increased risk is attributed to a combination of genetic, socioeconomic, and healthcare access factors. Genetic predispositions that are prevalent in African Americans and increase the risk of DVT and Pulmonary Embolism include single-nucleotide polymorphisms (SNPs) on chromosome 20 that are associated with a 2.3-fold greater risk of venous thromboembolism [147, 150]. These variants are more common in African Americans, with a frequency greater than 20%, compared to less than 10% in other racial/ethnic groups. A genome-wide association study found the single-nucleotide polymorphisms LEMD3 rs138916004, LY86 rs3804476, and LOC100130298 rs142143628 that all have been shown to significantly increase venous thromboembolism risk, with LEMD3 and LOC100130298 being specific to populations of African descent [151]. The presence of long (L) alleles (≥ 34 repeats) in the Heme oxygenase-1 (HMOX1) gene promoter is associated with a significantly increased risk of provoked and recurrent venous thromboembolism events in African Americans [152]. The deletion/deletion (D/D) polymorphism in the Angiotensin I-converting enzyme (ACE) gene polymorphism is also associated with a moderate increase in venous thromboembolisms, particularly in African American men [153].

It has been hypothesized that African Americans have a prothrombotic state that may increase susceptibility to DVT and PE due to higher serum concentrations of von Willebrand factor and Factor VIII [154]. Elevated serum concentrations of von Willebrand factor and factor VIII contribute to a prothrombotic state by enhancing platelet adhesion, aggregation, and thrombin generation, thereby increasing susceptibility to clot formation [155]. There are distinct differences in anticoagulation, with African Americans requiring higher warfarin dosing and having more difficulty staying within a therapeutic range [156, 157]. African Americans have unique genetic markers that influence warfarin metabolism and dose requirements. Variants such as CYP2C9 *5, 6, 8, 11*, and rs12777823 are more prevalent in African Americans and significantly affect warfarin dosing [158–163]. These variants are associated with altered enzyme activity, leading to differences in warfarin metabolism and dose requirements. Currently, there are no adjustments in therapy or duration of anticoagulation after thromboembolism specific to African Americans, but this is mainly due to the lack of research containing a significant number of African Americans to study. Like other disparities in care, racial differences in anticoagulation exist as well.

> (European Americans) generally are more likely to receive anticoagulation than (African Americans) and other racial and ethnic minorities. A retrospective study of a heart failure database showed that (African Americans) were less likely to receive anticoagulation compared to (European Americans) after adjustment for multiple variables including age, sex, history of AF, liver disease, and alcohol use. Analysis of in-hospital mortality among approximately 400,000 patients showed that (African Americans) were less likely to be treated with anticoagulants for AF (OR 0.84; 95% CI: 0.75–0.94). In a population-based

study, the odds of (African Americans) being treated with warfarin were only one-fourth as great as (European Americans) (OR 0.28; 95% CI: 0.13–0.60). The racial differences in anticoagulation practice are unexplained and a profound demonstration of racial disparities. [93]

The key is to be vigilant with recommendations for anticoagulation in all indicated disorders, know that African Americans may well be prothrombotic, be prepared to use higher doses of warfarin, and err on the side of anticoagulation when in doubt. When on warfarin, checking an INR more frequently initially should help avoid problems with under- or overanticoagulation.

A Precision Medicine Approach to the Cardiovascular Care of African Americans
- Studies suggest that obesity and low-potassium diet contribute to the higher prevalence of salt sensitivity and show this characteristic can be reversed with weight loss and greater potassium intake.
- Salt sensitivity has been linked to blunted nocturnal blood pressure dipping, decreased endothelial function, proteinuria, and target end-organ damage in African Americans.
- Hypertension therapy should be initiated with a thiazide-type diuretic or a calcium channel blocker that has been proven to have better blood pressure reduction and is better at preventing cardiovascular events.
- ACE inhibitors are less effective at reducing blood pressure and are associated with more side effects and an increased risk for angioedema. They should be avoided in African Americans, and ARBs should be substituted.
- Hydralazine and isosorbide dinitrate have proven mortality benefits in African Americans with heart failure with reduced ejection fraction.
- Elevated BNP and NT-pro-BNP are positively associated with a worsened prognosis in all races, but African Americans have a significantly lower baseline NT-pro-BNP.
- African Americans have more favorable lipid profiles but with disproportionately higher cardiovascular disease. Because of this, clinicians should have a lower threshold for cardiovascular prophylaxis.
- African Americans have a greatly increased risk for stroke and recurrent stroke.
- African Americans have a decreased risk for atrial fibrillation, and because of the increased risk for stroke when atrial fibrillation occurs, this is referred to as a "racial paradox."
- Clinicians should be aware that African Americans have an increased susceptibility to venous thromboembolism (and pulmonary embolism) and they should err on the side of using anticoagulation.

References

1. Wu J, Ma Z, Raman A, Beckerman P, Dhillon P, Mukhi D, Palmer M, Chen HC, Cohen CR, Dunn T, Reilly JP, Meyer NJ, Shashaty MGS, Arany Z, Haskó G, Laudanski K, Hung A, Susztak K. APOL1 risk variants in individuals of African genetic ancestry drive endothelial cell defects that exacerbate sepsis. Immunity. 2021;54(11):2632–2649.e6. https://doi.org/10.1016/j.immuni.2021.10.004.
2. Mukamal KJ, Tremaglio J, Friedman DJ, Ix JH, Kuller LH, Tracy RP, Pollak MR. Arterioscler Thromb Vasc Biol. 2016;36(2):398–403. https://doi.org/10.1161/ATVBAHA.115.305970.
3. Rayner B, Ramesar R. The importance of G protein-coupled receptor kinase 4 (GRK4) in pathogenesis of salt sensitivity salt sensitive hypertension and response to antihypertensive treatment. Int J Mol Sci. 2015;16(3):5741–9. https://doi.org/10.3390/ijms16035741.
4. Parksook WW, Heydarpour M, Gholami SK, Luther JM, Hopkins PN, Pojoga LH, Williams JS. Salt sensitivity of blood pressure and aldosterone: interaction between the lysine-specific demethylase 1 gene sex and age. J Clin Endocrinol Metab. 2022;107(5):1294–302. https://doi.org/10.1210/clinem/dgac011.
5. Jones E, Rayner B. The importance of the epithelial sodium channel in determining salt sensitivity in people of African origin. Pediatr Nephrol. 2021;36(2):237–43. https://doi.org/10.1007/s00467-019-04427-z.
6. Ito K, Bick AG, Flannick J, Friedman DJ, Genovese G, Parfenov MG, Depalma SR, Gupta N, Gabriel SB, Taylor HA Jr, Fox ER, Newton-Cheh C, Kathiresan S, Hirschhorn JN, Altshuler DM, Pollak MR, Wilson JG, Seidman JG, Seidman C. Circ Res. 2014;114(5):845–50. https://doi.org/10.1161/CIRCRESAHA.114.302347.
7. Hassan MO, Duarte R, Dickens C, Dix-Peek T, Naidoo S, Vachiat A, Grinter S, Manga P, Naicker S. APOL1 genetic variants are associated with serum-oxidized low-density lipoprotein levels and subclinical atherosclerosis in south African CKD patients. Nephron. 2020;144(7):331–40. https://doi.org/10.1159/000507860.
8. Avery CL, Sethupathy P, Buyske S, He Q, Lin D-Y, Arking DE, Carty CL, Duggan D, Fesinmeyer MD, Hindorff LA, Jeff JM, Klein L, Patton KK, Peters U, Shohet RV, Sotoodehnia N, Young AM, Kooperberg C, Haiman CA, Mohlke KL, Whitsel EA, North KE, Schork NJ. Fine-mapping and initial characterization of QT interval loci in African Americans. PLoS Genet. 2012;8(8):e1002870. https://doi.org/10.1371/journal.pgen.1002870.
9. Ingelfinger JR, Lee CD, Vivante A. Genetics of chronic kidney disease. N Engl J Med. 2024;391(7):627–39. https://doi.org/10.1056/NEJMra2308577.
10. Irvin MR, Aggarwal P, Claas SA, Fuentes L d l, Do AN, Gu CC, Matter A, Olson BS, Patki A, Schwander K, Smith JD, Srinivasasainagendra V, Tiwari HK, Turner AJ, Nickerson DA, Rao DC, Broeckel U, Arnett DK. Whole-exome sequencing and hiPSC cardiomyocyte models identify MYRIP TRAPPC11 and SLC27A6 of potential importance to left ventricular hypertrophy in an African ancestry population. Front Genet. 2021;12:588452. https://doi.org/10.3389/fgene.2021.588452.
11. Arnett DK, Meyers KJ, Devereux RB, Tiwari HK, Gu CC, Vaughan LK, Perry RT, Patki A, Claas SA, Sun Yan V, Broeckel U, Kardia SL. Genetic variation in NCAM1 contributes to left ventricular wall thickness in hypertensive families. Circ Res. 2011;108(3):279–83. https://doi.org/10.1161/CIRCRESAHA.110.239210.
12. Jones AC, Patki A, Claas SA, Tiwari HK, Chaudhary NS, Absher DM, Lange LA, Lange EM, Zhao W, Ratliff SM, Kardia SLR, Smith JA, Irvin MR, Arnett DK. Differentially methylated DNA regions and left ventricular hypertrophy in African Americans: a HyperGEN study. Genes. 2022;13(10):1700. https://doi.org/10.3390/genes13101700.
13. Nadkarni GN, Galarneau G, Ellis SB, Nadukuru R, Zhang J, Scott SA, Schurmann C, Li R, Rasmussen-Torvik LJ, Kho AN, Hayes MG, Pacheco JA, Manolio TA, Chisholm RL, Roden DM, Denny JC, Kenny EE, Bottinger EP. Apolipoprotein L1 variants and blood pressure traits in African Americans. J Am Coll Cardiol. 2017;69(12):1564–74. https://doi.org/10.1016/j.jacc.2017.01.040.

14. Robinson TW, Freedman BI. The impact of APOL1 on chronic kidney disease and hypertension. Adv Chronic Kidney Dis. 2019;26(2):131–6. https://doi.org/10.1053/j.ackd.2019.01.003.
15. Reidy KJ, Hjorten R, Parekh RS. Genetic risk of APOL1 and kidney disease in children and young adults of African ancestry. Curr Opin Pediatr. 2018;30(2):252–9. https://doi.org/10.1097/MOP.0000000000000603.
16. Jeong S, Hunter SD, Cook MD, Grosicki GJ, Robinson AT. Salty subjects: unpacking racial differences in salt-sensitive hypertension. Curr Hypertens Rep. 2024;26(1):43–58. https://doi.org/10.1007/s11906-023-01275-z.
17. Kennedy PG. Clinical features diagnosis and treatment of human African trypanosomiasis (sleeping sickness). Lancet Neurol. 2013;12(2):186–94. https://doi.org/10.1016/S1474-4422(12)70296-X.
18. Liu Z, Shriner D, Hansen NF, Rotimi CN, Mullikin JC, Wang H. Admixture mapping identifies genetic regions associated with blood pressure phenotypes in African Americans. PLoS One. 2020;15(4):e0232048. https://doi.org/10.1371/journal.pone.0232048.
19. Li C, Grove ML, Yu B, Jones BC, Morrison A, Boerwinkle E, Liu X. Genetic variants in microRNA genes and targets associated with cardiovascular disease risk factors in the African-American population. Hum Genet. 2018;137(1):85–94. https://doi.org/10.1007/s00439-017-1858-8.
20. Shih PB, O'Connor DT. Hereditary determinants of human hypertension. Hypertension. 2008;51(6):1456–64. https://doi.org/10.1161/HYPERTENSIONAHA.107.090480.
21. Katz DH, Tahir UA, Bick AG, Pampana A, Ngo D, Benson MD, Yu Z, Robbins JM, Chen ZZ, Cruz DE, Deng S, et al. Whole genome sequence analysis of the plasma proteome in black adults provides novel insights into cardiovascular disease. Circulation. 2022;145(5):357–70. https://doi.org/10.1161/CIRCULATIONAHA.121.055117.
22. 2015 National Healthcare Quality and Disparities Report Chartbook on Health Care for Blacks. Rockville: Agency for Healthcare Research and Quality; 2016. AHRQ Pub. No 16-0015-1-EF.
23. Goyal A, Lahan S, Dalia T, Ranka S, Bhattad VB, Patel RR, Shah Z. Clinical comparison of V122I genotypic variant of transthyretin amyloid cardiomyopathy with wild-type and other hereditary variants: a systematic review. Heart Fail Rev. 2022;27(3):849–56. https://doi.org/10.1007/s10741-021-10098-6.
24. Keene KL, Hyacinth HI, Bis JC, Kittner SJ, Mitchell BD, Cheng Y-C, Pare G, Chong M, O'Donnell M, Meschia JF, Chen W-M, Sale MM, Rich SS, Nalls MA, Zonderman AB, Evans MK, Wilson JG, Correa A, Markus HS, Traylor M, Lewis CM, Carty CL, Reiner A, Haessler J, Langefeld CD, Gottesman R, Mosley TH, Woo D, Yaffe K, Liu YM, Longstreth WT, Psaty BM, Kooperberg C, Lange LA, Sacco R, Rundek T, Lee J-M, Cruchaga C, Furie KL, Arnett DK, Benavente OR, Grewal RP, Peddareddygari LR, Dichgans M, Malik R, Worrall BB, Fornage M. Genome-wide association study meta-analysis of stroke in 22 000 individuals of African descent identifies novel associations with stroke. Stroke. 2020;51(8):2454–63. https://doi.org/10.1161/STROKEAHA.120.029123.
25. Carnethon M, Pu J, Aalbert M, et al. Cardiovascular health in African Americans: a scientific statement from the American Heart Association. Circulation. 2017;136:e393–423.
26. Chandra A, Skali H, Claggett B, Solomon SD, Rossi JS, Russell SD, Matsushita K, Kitzman DW, Konety SH, Mosley TH, Chang PP, Shah AM. Race- and gender-based differences in cardiac structure and function and risk of heart failure. J Am Coll Cardiol. 2022;79(4):355–68. https://doi.org/10.1016/j.jacc.2021.11.024.
27. Heidenreich PA, Bozkurt B, Aguilar D, Allen LA, Byun JJ, Colvin MM, Deswal A, Drazner MH, Dunlay SM, Evers LR, Fang JC, Fedson SE, Fonarow GC, Hayek SS, Hernandez AF, Khazanie P, Kittleson MM, Lee CS, Link MS, Milano CA, Nnacheta LC, Sandhu AT, Stevenson LW, Vardeny O, Vest AR, Yancy CW. AHA/ACC/HFSA guideline for the management of heart failure: a report of the American College of Cardiology/American Heart Association Joint Committee on clinical practice guidelines. Circulation. 2022;145(18):e895. https://doi.org/10.1161/CIR.0000000000001063.

28. Nayak A, Hicks AJ, Morris AA. Understanding the complexity of heart failure risk and treatment in black patients. Circ Heart Fail. 2020;13(8):e0072642020. https://doi.org/10.1161/CIRCHEARTFAILURE.120.007264.
29. Zhao D, Post WS, Blasco-Colmenares E, Cheng A, Zhang Y, Deo R, Pastor-Barriuso R, Michos ED, Sotoodehnia N, Guallar E. Racial differences in sudden cardiac death. Circulation. 2019;139(14):1688–97. https://doi.org/10.1161/CIRCULATIONAHA.118.036553.
30. Brancati FL, Kao WH, Folsom AR, Watson RL, Szklo M. Incident type 2 diabetes mellitus in African American and white adults. JAMA. 2000;283(17):2253. https://doi.org/10.1001/jama.283.17.2253.
31. Cooper R, Wolf-Maier K, et al. An international comparative study of blood pressure in populations of European vs. African descent. BMC Med. 2005;3:2.
32. Samanic CM, Barbour KE, Liu Y, Fang J, Lu H, Schieb L, Greenlund KJ. Prevalence of self-reported hypertension and antihypertensive medication use among adults — United States 2017. MMWR Morb Mortal Wkly Rep. 2020;69(14):393–8. https://doi.org/10.15585/mmwr.mm6914a1.
33. Whelton PK, Carey RM, Aronow WS, Casey DE, Collins KJ, Himmelfarb CD, DePalma SM, Gidding S, Jamerson KA, Jones DW, MacLaughlin EJ, Muntner P, Ovbiagele B, Smith SC, Spencer CC, Stafford RS, Taler SJ, Thomas RJ, Williams KA, Williamson JD, Wright JT. ACC/AHA/AAPA/ABC/ACPM/AGS/APhA/ASH/ASPC/NMA/PCNA guideline for the prevention detection evaluation and management of high blood pressure in adults: a report of the American College of Cardiology/American Heart Association Task Force on clinical practice guidelines. Circulation. 2017;138(17) https://doi.org/10.1161/CIR.0000000000000596.
34. Young D, Fischer H, Arterburn D, et al. Associations of overweight/obesity and socioeconomic status with hypertension prevalence across racial and ethnic groups. J Clin Hypertens (Greenwich). 2018;20(3):532–40.
35. Williams J, Chamarthi B, Goodarzi M, et al. Lysine-specific demethylase 1: an epigenetic regulator of salt-sensitive hypertension. Am J Hypertens. 2012;25(7):812–7.
36. Williams JS, Chamarthi B, Goodarzi MO, Pojoga LH, Sun B, Garza AE, Raby BA, Adler GK, Hopkins PN, Brown NJ, Jeunemaitre X, Ferri C, Fang R, Leonor T, Cui J, Guo X, Taylor KD, Chen Y-DI, Xiang A, Raffel LJ, Buchanan TA, Rotter JI, Williams GH, Shi Y. Lysine-specific demethylase 1: an epigenetic regulator of salt-sensitive hypertension. Am J Hypertens. 2012;25(7):812–7. https://doi.org/10.1038/ajh.2012.43.
37. Zhang Y, Li H, Zhou J, Wang A, Yang J, Wang C, Liu M, Zhou T, Zhu L, Zhang Y, Dong N, Wu Q. A corin variant identified in hypertensive patients that alters cytoplasmic tail and reduces cell surface expression and activity. Sci Rep. 2014;4(1) https://doi.org/10.1038/srep07378.
38. Richardson S, Freedman B, Ellison D, et al. Salt sensitivity: a review with a focus on non-Hispanic blacks and Hispanics. J Am Soc Hypertens. 2013;7(2):170–9.
39. Wright J, Rahman M, et al. Determinants of salt sensitivity in black and white normotensive and hypertensive women. Hypertension. 2003;42:1087–92.
40. Gates P, Tanaka H, Hiatt W, et al. Dietary sodium restriction rapidly improves large elastic artery compliance in older adults with systolic hypertension. Hypertension. 2004;44:35–41.
41. Todd A, Macginley R, Schollum J, et al. Dietary salt loading impairs arterial vascular reactivity. Am J Clin Nutr. 2010;91:557–64.
42. Jin Y, Kuznetsova T, Maillard M, et al. Independent relations of left ventricular structure with the 24-hour urinary excretion of sodium and aldosterone. Hypertension. 2009;54:489–95.
43. Rodriguez CJ, Bibbins-Domingo K, Jin Z, et al. Association of sodium and potassium intake with left ventricular mass: coronary artery risk development in young adults. Hypertension. 2011;58:410–6.
44. Swift PA, Markandu ND, Sagnella GA, et al. Modest salt reduction reduces blood pressure and urine protein excretion in black hypertensives: a randomized control trial. Hypertension. 2005;46:308–12.

45. Stocker SD, Monahan KD, Browning KN. Neurogenic and sympatho-excitatory actions of NaCl in hypertension. Curr Hypertens Rep. 2013;15:538–46.
46. Parati G, Ochoa JE, Lombardi C, et al. Assessment and management of blood-pressure variability. Nat Rev Cardiol. 2013;10:143–55.
47. He F, Li J, Macgregor G. Effect of longer term modest salt reduction on blood pressure: Cochrane systematic review and meta-analysis of randomized trials. BMJ. 2013;346:f1325.
48. Wright J, Probstfield JJ, Cushman W, et al. ALLHAT findings revisited in the context of subsequent analyses, other trials, and meta-analyses. Arch Intern Med. 2009;169(9):832–42.
49. Whelton PK, Carey RM, Aronow WS, et al. 2017 ACC/AHA/AAPA/ABC/ACPM/AGS/APhA/ASH/ASPC/NMA/PCNA guideline for the prevention, detection, evaluation, and management of high blood pressure in adults. J Am Coll Cardiol. 2018;71(6):1269–324.
50. Wright J, Williams J, Whelton P, SPRINT Research Group, et al. A randomized trial of intensive versus standard blood pressure control. N Engl J Med. 2015;373(22):2103–16.
51. Williamson J, Supiano M, Applegate W, et al. Intensive vs standard blood pressure control and cardiovascular disease outcomes in adults aged ≥75 years: a randomized clinical trial. JAMA. 2016;315:2673–82.
52. Still C, Rodriguez C, Wright J, et al. Clinical outcomes by race and ethnicity in the systolic blood pressure intervention trial (SPRINT): a randomized clinical trial. Am J Hypertens. 2017;31(1):97–107.
53. Muacevic A, Adler J, Asad A, et al. American Heart Association high blood pressure protocol 2017: a literature review. Cureus. 2018;10(8):e3230.
54. Wright J, Dunn J, Cutler J, et al. Outcomes in hypertensive black and nonblack patients treated with chlorthalidone, amlodipine, and lisinopril. JAMA. 2005;293(13):1595–608.
55. Materson B, Reda D, Cushman W, et al. Single-drug therapy for hypertension in men—a comparison of six antihypertensive agents with placebo. N Engl J Med. 1993;328:914–21.
56. Trunbull F. Effects of different blood-pressure-lowering regimens on major cardiovascular events: results of prospectively-designed overviews of randomized trials. Lancet. 2003;362(9395):1527–35.
57. Solomon CG, Taler SJ. Initial treatment of hypertension. N Engl J Med. 2018;378(7):636–44. https://doi.org/10.1056/NEJMcp1613481.
58. Bangalore S, Ogedegbe G, Gyamfi J, et al. Outcomes with angiotensin-converting enzyme inhibitors vs other antihypertensive agents in hypertensive blacks. Am J Med. 2015;128(11):1195–203.
59. Helmer A, Slater N, Smithgall S. A review of ACE inhibitors and ARBs in black patients with hypertension. Ann Pharmacother. 2018;52(11):1143–51. https://doi.org/10.1177/1060028018779082.
60. Davis CM, Apter AJ, Casillas A, Foggs MB, Louisias M, Morris EC, Nanda A, Nelson MR, Ogbogu PU, Walker-McGill CL, Wang J, Perry TT. Health disparities in allergic and immunologic conditions in racial and ethnic underserved populations: a work group report of the AAAAI Committee on the underserved. J Allergy Clin Immunol. 2021;147(5):1579–93. https://doi.org/10.1016/j.jaci.2021.02.034.
61. National Clinical Guideline Centre. Hypertension: the clinical management of primary hypertension in adults: update of clincal guidlines 18 and 34. London: Royal College of Physicians (UK) - National Clinical Guideline Centre; 2011.
62. Williams S, Nicholas S, Vaziri N, Norris K. African Americans, hypertension and the renin angiotensin system. World J Cardiol. 2014;6(9):878–89.
63. Rizos C, Elisaf M. Antihypertensive drug therapy in patients with African ancestry. Expert Opin Pharmacother. 2014;15(8):1061–4.
64. Yazdanshenas H, Bazargan M, Orum G, et al. Original reports: cardiovascular disease and risk factors. Prescribing patterns in the treatment of hypertension among underserved African American elderly. Ethn Dis. 2014;24(4):431–7.
65. Scisney-Matlock M, Bosworth H, Giger J, et al. Strategies for implementing and sustaining therapeutic lifestyle changes as part of hypertension management in African Americans. Postgrad Med. 2009;121(3):147–59.

66. Richard JN, Sama J, Onwuanyi A, Ilonze OJ. Top five considerations for improving outcomes in black patients with heart failure: a guide for primary care clinicians. J Natl Med Assoc. 2024;116(5):499–507. https://doi.org/10.1016/j.jnma.2023.11.008.
67. Taylor AL, Ziesche S, Yancy C, Carson P, D'Agostino R Jr, Ferdinand K, Taylor M, Adams K, Sabolinski M, Worcel M, Cohn JN. Combination of isosorbide dinitrate and hydralazine in blacks with heart failure. N Engl J Med. 2004;351(20):2049–57. https://doi.org/10.1056/NEJMoa042934.
68. Anand IS, Win S, Rector TS, Cohn JN, Taylor AL. Effect of fixed-dose combination of isosorbide dinitrate and hydralazine on all hospitalizations and on 30-day readmission rates in patients with heart failure. Circ Heart Fail. 2014;7(5):759–65. https://doi.org/10.1161/CIRCHEARTFAILURE.114.001360.
69. Cheng JWM. A review of isosorbide dinitrate and hydralazine in the management of heart failure in black patients with a focus on a new fixed-dose combination. Clin Ther. 2006;28(5):666–78. https://doi.org/10.1016/j.clinthera.2006.05.007.
70. Ferdinand KC. African American heart failure trial: role of endothelial dysfunction and heart failure in African Americans. Am J Card Imaging. 2007;99(6):S3–6. https://doi.org/10.1016/j.amjcard.2006.12.013.
71. McNamara DM, Taylor AL, Tam SW, Worcel M, Yancy CW, Hanley-Yanez K, Cohn JN, Feldman AM. G-protein beta-3 subunit genotype predicts enhanced benefit of fixed-dose isosorbide dinitrate and hydralazine. JACC Heart Fail. 2014;2(6):551–7. https://doi.org/10.1016/j.jchf.2014.04.016.
72. Bansal N, Alharbi A, Qiu S, Wang L. Racial and ethnic disparities in the outcomes and treatment of patients admitted with heart failure: a nationwide analysis. J Clin Med. 2024;14(1):18. https://doi.org/10.3390/jcm14010018.
73. Bajaj N, Gutierrez O, Arora G, et al. Racial differences in plasma levels of N-terminal pro-B-type natriuretic peptide and outcomes: the reasons for geographic and racial differences in stroke (REGARDS) study. JAMA Cardiol. 2018;3(1):11–7.
74. Patel N, Cushman M, Gutiérrez OM, Howard G, Safford MM, Muntner P, Durant RW, Prabhu SD, Arora G, Levitan EB, Arora P. Racial differences in the association of NT-proBNP with risk of incident heart failure in REGARDS. JCI. Insight. 2019;4(13) https://doi.org/10.1172/jci.insight.129979.
75. Gupta DK, de Lemos JA, Ayers CR, Berry JD, Wang TJ. Racial differences in natriuretic peptide levels. JACC Heart Fail. 2015;3(7):513–9. https://doi.org/10.1016/j.jchf.2015.02.008.
76. Parker MM, Damrauer SM, Tcheandjieu C, Erbe D, Aldinc E, Hawkins PN, Gillmore JD, Hull LE, Lynch JA, Joseph J, Ticau S, Flynn-Carroll AO, Deaton AM, Ward LD, Assimes TL, Tsao PS, Chang K-M, Rader DJ, Fitzgerald K, Vaishnaw AK, Hinkle G, Nioi P. Association of the transthyretin variant V122I with polyneuropathy among individuals of African ancestry. Sci Rep. 2021;11(1):11645. https://doi.org/10.1038/s41598-021-91113-6.
77. Shije JZ, Bautista MAB, Smotherman C. The frequency of V122I transthyretin mutation in a cohort of African American individuals with bilateral carpal tunnel syndrome. Front Neurol. 2022;13:949401. https://doi.org/10.3389/fneur.2022.949401.
78. Akinboboye O, Shah K, Warner AL, Damy T, Taylor HA, Gollob J, Powell C, Karsten V, Vest J, Maurer MS. Amyloid. 2020;27(4):223–30. https://doi.org/10.1080/13506129.2020.1764928.
79. Quarta CC, Buxbaum JN, Shah AM, Falk RH, Claggett B, Kitzman DW, Mosley TH, Butler KR, Boerwinkle E, Solomon SD. The amyloidogenic V122I transthyretin variant in elderly black Americans. N Engl J Med. 2015;372(1):21–9. https://doi.org/10.1056/NEJMoa1404852.
80. Damrauer SM, Chaudhary K, Cho JH, Liang LW, Argulian E, Chan L, Dobbyn A, Guerraty MA, Judy R, Kay J, Kember RL, Levin MG, Saha A, Van Vleck T, Verma SS, Weaver JE, Abul-Husn NS, Baras A, Chirinos JA, Drachman B, Kenny EE, Loos RJF, Narula J, Overton J, Reid J, Ritchie M, Sirugo G, Nadkarni G, Rader DJ, Do R. Association of the V122I hereditary transthyretin amyloidosis genetic variant with heart failure among individuals

of African or Hispanic/latino ancestry. JAMA. 2019;322(22):2191. https://doi.org/10.1001/jama.2019.17935.
81. Buxbaum JN, Ruberg FL. Transthyretin V122I (pV142I)* cardiac amyloidosis: an age-dependent autosomal dominant cardiomyopathy too common to be overlooked as a cause of significant heart disease in elderly African Americans. Genet Med. 2017;19(7):733–42. https://doi.org/10.1038/gim.2016.200.
82. Shah KB, Mankad AK, Castano A, Akinboboye OO, Duncan PB, Fergus IV, Maurer MS. Transthyretin cardiac amyloidosis in Black Americans. Circ Heart Fail. 2016;9(6):e002558. https://doi.org/10.1161/CIRCHEARTFAILURE.115.002558.
83. Ruberg FL, Maurer MS. Cardiac amyloidosis due to transthyretin protein. JAMA. 2024;331(9):778. https://doi.org/10.1001/jama.2024.0442.
84. Bentley A, Rotimi C. Inter-ethnic variation in lipid profiles: implications for under-identification of African Americans at risk for metabolic disorders. Expert Rev Endocrinol Metab. 2012;7(6):659–67.
85. Pan Y, Pratt C. Metabolic syndrome and its association with diet and physical activity in US adolescents. J Am Diet Assoc. 2008;108(2):276–86.
86. Furtado J, Campos H, Summer A, Appel L, Cary V, Sacks F. Dietary interventions that lower lipoproteins cantaining apolipoprotein C-III are more effective in whites than in blacks: results of the OmniHeart trial. Am J Clin Nutr. 2010;92(4):714–22.
87. Bentley AR, Chen G, Shriner D, Doumatey AP, Zhou J, Huang H, Mullikin JC, Blakesley RW, Hansen NF, Bouffard GG, Cherukuri PF, Maskeri B, Young AC, Adeyemo A, Rotimi CN. Gene-based sequencing identifies lipid-influencing variants with ethnicity-specific effects in African Americans. PLoS Genet. 2014;10(3):e1004190. https://doi.org/10.1371/journal.pgen.1004190.
88. Miljkovic-Gacic I, Bunker CH, Ferrell RE, Kammerer CM, Evans RW, Patrick AL, Kuller LH. Lipoprotein subclass and particle size differences in Afro-Caribbeans African Americans and white Americans: associations with hepatic lipase gene variation. Metabolism. 2006;55(1):96–102. https://doi.org/10.1016/j.metabol.2005.07.011.
89. Nie L, Niu S, Vega GL, Clark LT, Tang A, Grundy SM, Cohen JC. Three polymorphisms associated with low hepatic lipase activity are common in African Americans. J Lipid Res. 1998;39(9):1900–3.
90. Jacobson TA, Maki KC, Orringer CE, Jones PH, Kris-Etherton P, Sikand G, La Forge R, Daniels SR, Wilson DP, Morris PB, Wild RA, Grundy SM, Daviglus M, Ferdinand KC, Vijayaraghavan K, Deedwania PC, Aberg JA, Liao KP, McKenney JM, Ross JL, Braun LT, Ito MK, Bays HE, Brown WV. National lipid association recommendations for patient-centered management of dyslipidemia: Part 2. J Clin Lipidol. 2015;9(6):S1–S122.e1. https://doi.org/10.1016/j.jacl.2015.09.002.
91. Després JP, Couillard C, Gagnon J, Bergeron J, Leon AS, Rao DC, Skinner JS, Wilmore JH, Bouchard C. Race visceral adipose tissue plasma lipids and lipoprotein lipase activity in men and women. Arterioscler Thromb Vasc Biol. 2000;20(8):1932–8. https://doi.org/10.1161/01.ATV.20.8.1932.
92. Niswender KD, Fazio S, Gower BA, Silver HJ. Balanced high fat diet reduces cardiovascular risk in obese women although changes in adipose tissue lipoproteins and insulin resistance differ by race. Metabolism. 2018;82:125–34. https://doi.org/10.1016/j.metabol.2018.01.020.
93. Amponash M, Benjamin E, Magnani J. Atrial fibrillation and race—a contemporary review. Curr Cardiovasc Risk Rep. 2013;7(5):336. https://doi.org/10.1007/s12170-013-0327-8.
94. Alonso A, Agarwal SK, Soliman EZ, Ambrose M, Chamberlain AM, Prineas RJ, Folsom AR. Incidence of atrial fibrillation in whites and African-Americans: the Atherosclerosis Risk in Communities (ARIC) study. Am Heart J. 2009;158(1):111–7. https://doi.org/10.1016/j.ahj.2009.05.010.
95. Heckbert SR, Austin TR, Jensen PN, Chen LY, Post WS, Floyd JS, Soliman EZ, Kronmal RA, Psaty BM. Differences by race/ethnicity in the prevalence of clinically detected and

monitor-detected atrial fibrillation. Circ Arrhythm Electrophysiol. 2020;13(1):e007698. https://doi.org/10.1161/CIRCEP.119.007698.
96. Jensen PN, Thacker EL, Dublin S, Psaty BM, Heckbert SR. Racial differences in the incidence of and risk factors for atrial fibrillation in older adults: the cardiovascular health study. J Am Geriatr Soc. 2013;61(2):276–80. https://doi.org/10.1111/jgs.12085.
97. Roberts JD, Hu D, Heckbert SR, Alonso A, Dewland TA, Vittinghoff E, Liu Y, Psaty BM, Olgin JE, Magnani JW, Huntsman S, Burchard EG, Arking DE, Bibbins-Domingo K, Harris TB, Perez MV, Ziv E, Marcus GM. Genetic investigation into the differential risk of atrial fibrillation among black and white individuals. JAMA Cardiol. 2016;1(4):442. https://doi.org/10.1001/jamacardio.2016.1185.
98. Delaney JT, Jeff JM, Brown NJ, Pretorius M, Okafor HE, Darbar D, Roden DM, Crawford DC, Ewart TA. Characterization of genome-wide association-identified variants for atrial fibrillation in African Americans. PLoS One. 2012;7(2):e32338. https://doi.org/10.1371/journal.pone.0032338.
99. Bress A, Han J, Patel SR, Desai AA, Mansour I, Groo V, Progar K, Shah E, Stamos TD, Wing C, Garcia JGN, Kittles R, Cavallari LH. Association of aldosterone synthase polymorphism (CYP11B2 -344T>C) and genetic ancestry with atrial fibrillation and serum aldosterone in African Americans with heart failure. PLoS ONE. 2013;8(7):e71268. https://doi.org/10.1371/journal.pone.0071268.
100. Marcus GM, Alonso A, Peralta CA, Lettre G, Vittinghoff E, Lubitz SA, Fox ER, Levitzky YS, Mehra R, Kerr KF, Deo R, Sotoodehnia N, Akylbekova M, Ellinor PT, Paltoo DN, Soliman EZ, Benjamin EJ, Heckbert SR. European ancestry as a risk factor for atrial fibrillation in African Americans. Circulation. 2010;122(20):2009–15. https://doi.org/10.1161/CIRCULATIONAHA.110.958306.
101. Meschia J, Soliman M, Soliman E, et al. Racial disparities in awareness and treatment of atrial fibrillation: the reasons for geographic and racial differences in stroke (REGARDS) study. Stroke. 2010;41(4):581–7.
102. Essien UR, Holmes DJN, Jackson LR 2nd, Fonarow GC, Mahaffey KW, Reiffel JA, Steinberg BA, Allen LA, Chan PS, Freeman JV, Blanco RG, Pieper KS, Piccini JP, Peterson ED, Singer DE. Association of race/ethnicity with oral anticoagulant use in patients with atrial fibrillation. JAMA Cardiol. 2018;3(12):1174. https://doi.org/10.1001/jamacardio.2018.3945.
103. Essien UR, Kim N, Hausmann LRM, Washington DL, Mor MK, Gellad WF, Fine MJ. Facility-level variation in racial disparities in anticoagulation for atrial fibrillation: the REACH-AF study. J Gen Intern Med. 2024;39(7):1122–6. https://doi.org/10.1007/s11606-024-08643-8.
104. Essien UR, Kim N, Magnani JW, Good CB, Litam TMA, Hausmann LRM, Mor MK, Gellad WF, Fine MJ. Association of race and ethnicity and anticoagulation in patients with atrial fibrillation dually enrolled in veterans health administration and medicare: effects of medicare part D on prescribing disparities. Circ Cardiovasc Qual Outcomes. 2022;15(2):e008389. https://doi.org/10.1161/CIRCOUTCOMES.121.008389.
105. Marini C, De Santis F, Sacco S, et al. Contribution of atrial fibrillation to incidence and outcome of ischemic stroke. Stroke. 2005;36:1115–9.
106. Roger V, Go A, Lloyd-Jones D, et al. Heart disease and stroke statistics—2012 update. Circulation. 2012;125(1):e2–e220.
107. Benjamin E, Blaha M, Chiuve S, et al. Heart disease and stroke statistics-2017 update: a report from the American Heart Association. Circulation. 2017;135(10):e146–603.
108. Akinyemi R, Tiwari HK, Arnett DK, Ovbiagele B, Irvin MR, Wahab K, Sarfo F, Srinivasasainagendra V, Adeoye A, Perry RT, Akpalu A, Jenkins C, Arulogun O, Gebregziabher M, Owolabi L, Obiako R, Sanya E, Komolafe M, Fawale M, Adebayo P, Osaigbovo G, Sunmonu T, Olowoyo P, Chukwuonye I, Obiabo Y, Onoja A, Akinyemi J, Ogbole G, Melikam S, Saulson R, Owolabi M. APOL1 CDKN2A/CDKN2B and HDAC9 polymorphisms and small vessel ischemic stroke. Acta Neurol Scand. 2018;137(1):133–41. https://doi.org/10.1111/ane.12847.

109. Kohsaka S, Volcik KA, Folsom AR, Wu KK, Ballantyne CM, Willerson JT, Boerwinkle E. Increased risk of incident stroke associated with the cyclooxygenase 2 (COX-2) G−765C polymorphism in African-Americans: the Atherosclerosis Risk in Communities Study. Atherosclerosis. 2008;196(2):926–30. https://doi.org/10.1016/j.atherosclerosis.2007.02.010.
110. Robinson DJ, Ding L, Howard G, Stanton RJ, Khoury J, Sucharew H, Haverbusch M, Nobel L, Khatri P, Adeoye O, Broderick JP, Ferioli S, Mackey J, Woo D, De Los Rios La Rosa F, Flaherty M, Slavin S, Star M, Martini SR, Demel S, Walsh KB, Coleman E, Jasne AS, Mistry EA, Kleindorfer D, Kissela B. Temporal trends and racial disparities in long-term survival after stroke. Neurology. 2024;103(3):e209653. https://doi.org/10.1212/WNL.0000000000209653.
111. Morgenstern LB, Springer MV, Porter NC, Kwicklis M, Carrera JF, Sozener CB, Campbell MS, Hijazi I, Lisabeth LD. Black Americans have worse stroke outcome compared with non-Hispanic whites. J Natl Med Assoc. 2023;115(5):509–15. https://doi.org/10.1016/j.jnma.2023.08.003.
112. Yuqi W, Xirasagar S, Nan Z, Heidari K, Sen S. Racial disparities in utilization of emergency medical services and related impact on poststroke disability. Med Care. 2023;61(11):796–804. https://doi.org/10.1097/MLR.0000000000001926.
113. Metcalf D, Zhang D. Racial and ethnic disparities in the usage and outcomes of ischemic stroke treatment in the United States. J Stroke Cerebrovasc Dis. 2023;32(12):107393. https://doi.org/10.1016/j.jstrokecerebrovasdis.2023.107393.
114. Qian F, Fonarow G, Smith E, et al. Racial and ethnic differences in outcomes in older patients with acute ischemic stroke. Circ Cardiovasc Qual Outcomes. 2013;6(3):284–92.
115. Chiou-Tan F, Keng M, Graves D, Chan K, Rintala D. Racial/ethnic differences in FIM scores and length of stay for underinsured patients undergoing stroke inpatient rehabilitation. Am J Phys Med Rehabil. 2006;85(5):415–23.
116. Mehta AM, Fifi JT, Shoirah H, Shigematsu T, Oxley TJ, Kellner CP, De LR, Mocco J, Majidi S. Racial and socioeconomic disparities in the use and outcomes of endovascular Thrombectomy for acute ischemic stroke. Am J Neuroradiol. 2021;42(9):1576–83. https://doi.org/10.3174/ajnr.A7217.
117. Gorelick PB, Leurgans S, Richardson D, Harris Y, Billingsley M, AAASPS Investigators. African American antiplatelet stroke prevention study: Clinical trial design. J Stroke Cerebrovasc Dis. 1998;7(6):426–34. https://doi.org/10.1016/S1052-3057(98)80127-4.
118. Glasser SP, Hovater MK, Lackland DT, Cushman M, Howard G, Howard VJ. Primary prophylactic aspirin use and incident stroke: reasons for geographic and racial differences in stroke study. J Stroke Cerebrovasc Dis. 2013;22(4):500–7. https://doi.org/10.1016/j.jstrokecerebrovasdis.2013.03.004.
119. Meschia JF, Bushnell C, Boden-Albala B, Braun LT, Bravata DM, Chaturvedi S, Creager MA, Eckel RH, Elkind MS, Fornage M, Goldstein LB, Greenberg SM, Horvath SE, Iadecola C, Jauch EC, Moore WS, Wilson JA, American Heart Association Stroke Council, Council on Cardiovascular and Stroke Nursing, Council on Clinical Cardiology, Council on Functional Genomics and Translational Biology, Council on Hypertension. Guidelines for the primary prevention of stroke: a statement for healthcare professionals from the American Heart Association/American Stroke Association. Stroke. 2014;45(12):3754–832. https://doi.org/10.1161/STR.0000000000000046.
120. U.S. Preventive Services Task Force. https://www.uspreventiveservicestaskforce.org/Page/Name/uspstf-a-and-b-recommendations/.
121. African American Health. Vital signs. Centers for Disease Control and Prevention. 2017. Accessed 9 May 2019.
122. Gornik HL, Aronow HD, Goodney PP, Arya S, Brewster LP, Byrd L, Chandra V, Drachman DE, Eaves JM, Ehrman JK, Evans JN, Getchius TSD, Gutiérrez JA, Hawkins BM, Hess CN, Ho KJ, Jones WS, Kim ESH, Kinlay S, Kirksey L, Kohlman-Trigoboff D, Long CA, Pollak AW, Sabri SS, Sadwin LB, Secemsky EA, Serhal M, Shishehbor MH, Treat-Jacobson D, Wilkins LR. ACC/AHA/AACVPR/APMA/ABC/SCAI/SVM/SVN/SVS/SIR/VESS guideline for the management of lower extremity peripheral artery disease: a report of the American College

of Cardiology/American Heart Association Joint Committee on clinical practice guidelines. Circulation. 2024;149(24):e1313. https://doi.org/10.1161/CIR.0000000000001251.
123. Krawisz AK, Natesan S, Wadhera RK, Chen S, Song Y, Yeh RW, Jaff MR, Giri J, Julien H, Secemsky EA. Differences in comorbidities explain black–white disparities in outcomes after femoropopliteal endovascular intervention. Circulation. 2022;146(3):191–200. https://doi.org/10.1161/CIRCULATIONAHA.122.058998.
124. Scherer ML, Nalls MA, Pawlikowska L, Ziv E, Mitchell G, Huntsman S, Hu D, Sutton-Tyrrell K, Lakatta EG, Hsueh W-C, Newman AB, Tandon A, Kim L, Kwok P-Y, Sung A, Li R, Psaty B, Reiner AP, Harris T. Admixture mapping of ankle-arm index: identification of a candidate locus associated with peripheral arterial disease. J Med Genet. 2010;47(1):1–7. https://doi.org/10.1136/jmg.2008.064808.
125. Bick AG, Akwo E, Robinson-Cohen C, Lee K, Lynch J, Assimes TL, DuVall S, Edwards T, Fang H, Freiberg SM, Giri A, Huffman JE, Huang J, Hull L, Kember RL, Klarin D, Lee JS, Levin M, Miller DR, Natarajan P, Saleheen D, Shao Q, Sun YV, Tang H, Wilson O, Chang K-M, Cho K, Concato J, Gaziano JM, Kathiresan S, O'Donnell CJ, Rader DJ, Tsao PS, Wilson PW, Hung AM, Damrauer SM. Association of APOL1 risk alleles with cardiovascular disease in blacks in the million veteran program. Circulation. 2019;140(12):1031–40. https://doi.org/10.1161/CIRCULATIONAHA.118.036589.
126. Biagetti G, Thompson E, O'Brien C, Damrauer S. The role of genetics in managing peripheral arterial disease. Ann Vasc Surg. 2024;108:279–86. https://doi.org/10.1016/j.avsg.2024.04.022.
127. Pike MM, Larson NB, Wassel CL, Cohoon KP, Tsai MY, Pankow JS, Hanson NQ, Decker PA, Berardi C, Alexander KS, Cushman M, Zakai NA, Bielinski SJ. ABO blood group is associated with peripheral arterial disease in African Americans: the multi-ethnic study of atherosclerosis (MESA). Thromb Res. 2017;153:1–6. https://doi.org/10.1016/j.thromres.2017.02.018.
128. McDermott MM, Ho KJ, Alabi O, Criqui MH, Goodney P, Hamburg N, McNeal DM, Pollak A, Smolderen KG, Bonaca M. Disparities in diagnosis treatment and outcomes of peripheral artery disease. J Am Coll Cardiol. 2023;82(24):2312–28. https://doi.org/10.1016/j.jacc.2023.09.830.
129. Ferdinand KC, Sadik K, Browne R, Desai U, Lefebvre P, Lejeune D, Mahendran M, Laliberté F, Matay L, Armstrong DG. Real-world racial variation in treatment and outcomes among patients with peripheral artery disease. Adv Ther. 2023;40(4):1850–66. https://doi.org/10.1007/s12325-023-02465-6.
130. Kalbaugh CA, Witrick B, Sivaraj LB, McGinigle KL, Lesko CR, Cykert S, Robinson WP. Non-hispanic black and hispanic patients have worse outcomes than white patients within similar stages of peripheral artery disease. J Am Heart Assoc. 2022;11(1):e023396. https://doi.org/10.1161/JAHA.121.023396.
131. Thomas VE, Beckman JA. Racial and socioeconomic health disparities in peripheral artery disease. J Am Heart Assoc. 2024;13:e031446. https://doi.org/10.1161/JAHA.123.031446.
132. Alhuneafat L, Omar YA, Naser A, Jagdish B, Alameh A, Al-Ahmad M, Al Abdouh A, Mhanna M, Hammad N, Khalid U, Yousaf A, Madanat L, Al-Amer M, Gharaibeh A, Siraj A, Nasser F, Jabri A. Racial and ethnic disparities in peripheral vascular disease admissions using a nationally representative sample. Am J Cardiol. 2023;202:74–80. https://doi.org/10.1016/j.amjcard.2023.06.055.
133. Soden PA, Zettervall SL, Deery SE, Hughes K, Stoner MC, Goodney PP, Vouyouka AG, Schermerhorn ML. Black patients present with more severe vascular disease and a greater burden of risk factors than white patients at time of major vascular intervention. J Vasc Surg. 2017;67(2):549–556.e3. https://doi.org/10.1016/j.jvs.2017.06.089.
134. Bell E, Lutsey P, Basu S, et al. Lifetime risk of venous thromboembolism in two cohort studies. Am J Med. 2016;129(3):339.e19–26.
135. Rowe VL, Weaver FA, Lane JS, Etzioni DA. Racial and ethnic differences in patterns of treatment for acute peripheral arterial disease in the United States, 1998–2006. J Vasc Surg. 2010;51:21S–6S.

136. Durazzo TS, Frencher S, Gusberg R. Influence of race on the management of lower extremity ischemia: revascularization vs amputation. JAMA Surg. 2013;148:617–23. https://doi.org/10.1001/jamasurg.2013.1436.
137. Mustapha J, Fisher B, Rizzo J, et al. Explaining racial disparities in amputation rates for the treatment of peripheral artery disease (PAD) using decomposition methods. J Racial Ethn Health Disparities. 2017;4(5):784–95.
138. Clark D, Cain L, Blaha M, et al. Cigarette smoking and subclinical peripheral arterial disease in blacks of the Jackson heart study. J Am Heart Assoc. 2019;8:e010674.
139. Ribieras AJ, Kang N, Shao T, Kenel-Pierre S, Rey J, Velazquez OC, Bornak A. Racial disparities in presentation and outcomes for endovascular abdominal aortic aneurysm repair. J Vasc Surg. 2023;77(1):69–77. https://doi.org/10.1016/j.jvs.2022.06.094.
140. Deery SE, O'Donnell TFX, Shean KE, Darling JD, Soden PA, Hughes K, Wang GJ, Schermerhorn ML. Racial disparities in outcomes after intact abdominal aortic aneurysm repair. J Vasc Surg. 2018;67(4):1059–67. https://doi.org/10.1016/j.jvs.2017.07.138.
141. Li B, Ayoo K, Eisenberg N, Lindsay TF, Roche-Nagle G. The impact of race on outcomes following ruptured abdominal aortic aneurysm repair. J Vasc Surg. 2023;77(5):1413–23. https://doi.org/10.1016/j.jvs.2023.01.181.
142. Marcaccio CL, Patel PB, de Guerre LEVM, Wade JE, Rastogi V, Anjorin A, Soden PA, Hughes K, Scali ST, Sedrakyan A, Schermerhorn ML. Disparities in 5-year outcomes and imaging surveillance following elective endovascular repair of abdominal aortic aneurysm by sex race and ethnicity. J Vas Surg. 2022;76(5):1205–1215.e4. https://doi.org/10.1016/j.jvs.2022.03.886.
143. Steffen BT, Pankow JS, Norby FL, Lutsey PL, Demmer RT, Guan W, Pankratz N, Li A, Liu G, Matsushita K, Tin A, Tang W. Proteomics analysis of genetic liability of abdominal aortic aneurysm identifies plasma neogenin and kit ligand: the ARIC study. Arterioscler Thromb Vasc Biol. 2022;43(2):367–78. https://doi.org/10.1161/ATVBAHA.122.317984.
144. Gebreab SY, Riestra P, Khan RJ, Ruihua X, Musani SK, Tekola-Ayele F, Correa A, Wilson JG, Rotimi CN, Davis SK. Genetic ancestry is associated with measures of subclinical atherosclerosis in African Americans. Arterioscler Thromb Vasc Biol. 2015;35(5):1271–8. https://doi.org/10.1161/ATVBAHA.114.304855.
145. Yang Y, Lehman EB, Aziz F. African Americans are less likely to have elective endovascular repair of abdominal aortic aneurysms. J Vasc Surg. 2019;70(2):462–70. https://doi.org/10.1016/j.jvs.2018.10.107.
146. O'Donnell TFX, Dansey KD, Marcaccio CL, Patel PB, Hughes K, Soden P, Zettervall SL, Schermerhorn ML. Racial disparities in treatment of ruptured abdominal aortic aneurysms. J Vasc Surg. 2023;77(2):406–14. https://doi.org/10.1016/j.jvs.2022.08.009.
147. Hernandez W, Gamazon ER, Smithberger E, O'Brien TJ, Harralson AF, Tuck M, Barbour A, Kittles RA, Cavallari LH, Perera MA. Novel genetic predictors of venous thromboembolism risk in African Americans. Blood. 2016;127(15):1923–9. https://doi.org/10.1182/blood-2015-09-668525.
148. Heit JA, Beckman MG, Bockenstedt PL, Grant AM, Key NS, Kulkarni R, Manco-Johnson MJ, Moll S, Ortel TL, Philipp CS. Comparison of characteristics from White- and Black-Americans with venous thromboembolism: a cross-sectional study. Am J Hematol. 2010;85(7):467–71. https://doi.org/10.1002/ajh.21735.
149. White RH, Keenan CR. Effects of race and ethnicity on the incidence of venous thromboembolism. Thromb Res. 2009;123:S11–7. https://doi.org/10.1016/S0049-3848(09)70136-7.
150. Key NS, Reiner AP. Genetic basis of ethnic disparities in VTE risk. Blood. 2016;127(15):1844–5. https://doi.org/10.1182/blood-2016-03-701698.
151. Heit JA, Armasu SM, McCauley BM, Kullo IJ, Sicotte H, Pathak J, Chute CG, Gottesman O, Bottinger EP, Denny JC, Roden DM, Li R, Ritchie MD, de Andrade M. Identification of unique venous thromboembolism-susceptibility variants in African-Americans. Thromb Haemost. 2017;117(04):758–68. https://doi.org/10.1160/TH16-08-0652.

152. Bean CJ, Boulet SL, Ellingsen D, Trau H, Ghaji N, Hooper WC, Austin H. Increased risk of venous thromboembolism is associated with genetic variation in heme oxygenase-1 in Blacks. Thromb Res. 2012;130(6):942–7. https://doi.org/10.1016/j.thromres.2012.08.300.
153. Dilley A, Austin H, Hooper WC, Lally C, Ribeiro JA, Wenger NK, Rawlins P, Evatt B. Relation of three genetic traits to venous thrombosis in an African-American population. Am J Epidemiol. 1998;147(1):30–5. https://doi.org/10.1093/oxfordjournals.aje.a009363.
154. Payne A, Miller C, Hooper W, Lally C, Austin H. High factor VIII, von Willebrand factor, and fibrinogen levels and risk of venous thromboembolism in blacks and whites. Ethn Dis. 2014;24(2):169–74.
155. Rietveld IM, Lijfering WM, le Cessie S, Bos MHA, Rosendaal FR, Reitsma PH, Cannegieter SC. High levels of coagulation factors and venous thrombosis risk: strongest association for factor VIII and von Willebrand factor. J Thromb Haemost. 2019;17(1):99–109. https://doi.org/10.1111/jth.14343.
156. Drozda K, Wong S, Patel SR, Bress AP, Nutescu EA, Kittles RA, Cavallari LH. Poor warfarin dose prediction with pharmacogenetic algorithms that exclude genotypes important for African Americans. Pharmacogenet Genomics. 2015;25(2):73–81. https://doi.org/10.1097/FPC.0000000000000108.
157. Hernandez W, Gamazon ER, Aquino-Michaels K, Patel S, O'Brien TJ, Harralson AF, Kittles RA, Barbour A, Tuck M, McIntosh SD, Douglas JN, Nicolae D, Cavallari LH, Perera MA. Ethnicity-specific pharmacogenetics: the case of warfarin in African Americans. Pharmacogenomics J. 2014;14(3):223–8. https://doi.org/10.1038/tpj.2013.34.
158. Zhang H, Alarcon C, Cavallari LH, Nutescu E, Carvill GL, Perera MA, Hernandez W. Clin Pharmacol Ther. 2023;113(3):624–33. https://doi.org/10.1002/cpt.2820.
159. Ohara M, Suzuki Y, Shinohara S, Gong IY, Schmerk CL, Tirona RG, Schwarz UI, Wen M-S, Lee MTM, Mihara K, Nutescu EA, Perera MA, Cavallari LH, Kim RB, Takahashi H. Differences in warfarin pharmacodynamics and predictors of response among three racial populations. Clin Pharmacokinet. 2019;58(8):1077–89. https://doi.org/10.1007/s40262-019-00745-5.
160. Ndadza A, Muyambo S, Mntla P, Wonkam A, Chimusa E, Kengne AP, Ntsekhe M, Dandara C. Profiling of warfarin pharmacokinetics-associated genetic variants: Black Africans portray unique genetic markers important for an African specific warfarin pharmacogenetics-dosing algorithm. J Thromb Haemost. 2021;19(12):2957–73. https://doi.org/10.1111/jth.15494.
161. Limdi NA, Brown TM, Yan Q, Thigpen JL, Shendre A, Liu N, Hill CE, Arnett DK, Beasley TM. Race influences warfarin dose changes associated with genetic factors. Blood. 2015;126(4):539–45. https://doi.org/10.1182/blood-2015-02-627042.
162. Perera MA, Cavallari LH, Limdi NA, Gamazon ER, Konkashbaev A, Daneshjou R, Pluzhnikov A, Crawford DC, Wang J, Liu N, Tatonetti N, Bourgeois S, Takahashi H, Bradford Y, Burkley BM, Desnick RJ, Halperin JL, Khalifa SI, Langaee TY, Lubitz SA, Nutescu EA, Oetjens M, Shahin MH, Patel SR, Sagreiya H, Tector M, Weck KE, Rieder MJ, Scott SA, Wu AH, Burmester JK, Wadelius M, Deloukas P, Wagner MJ, Mushiroda T, Kubo M, Roden DM, Cox NJ, Altman RB, Klein TE, Nakamura Y, Johnson JA. Genetic variants associated with warfarin dose in African-American individuals: a genome-wide association study. Lancet. 2013;382(9894):790–6. https://doi.org/10.1016/S0140-6736(13)60681-9.
163. Asiimwe IG, Blockman M, Cavallari LH, Cohen K, Cupido C, Dandara C, Davis BH, Jacobson B, Johnson JA, Lamorde M, Limdi NA, Morgan J, Mouton JP, Muyambo S, Nakagaayi D, Ndadza A, Okello E, Perera MA, Schapkaitz E, Sekaggya-Wiltshire C, Semakula JR, Tatz G, Waitt C, Yang G, Zhang EJ, Jorgensen AL, Pirmohamed M. Meta-analysis of genome-wide association studies of stable warfarin dose in patients of African ancestry. Blood Adv. 2024;8(20):5248–61. https://doi.org/10.1182/bloodadvances.2024014227.
164. Chehal PK, Uppal TS, Ng BP, Alva M, Ali MK. Trends and race/ethnic disparities in diabetes-related hospital use in medicaid enrollees: analyses of serial cross-sectional state data 2008–2017. J Gen Intern Med. 2023;38(10):2279–88. https://doi.org/10.1007/s11606-022-07842-5.

Chapter 5
A Precision Medicine Approach to the Care of Diabetes and Obesity in African Americans

Contents

5.1	Obesity...	81
5.2	Type 2 Diabetes...	86
	5.2.1 Smoking Drives Up Diabetes Risk......................................	89
	5.2.2 HbA1c Differences...	90
	5.2.3 Diabetes Treatment Approaches..	91
5.3	Diabetes Type 1...	94
5.4	Diet Management Approaches..	95
5.5	Marketing Competition...	97
References..		98

5.1 Obesity

Disparities in obesity and diabetes foreshadow important differences in health outcomes including long-term disability, cardiovascular disease, some cancers, and premature mortality. African Americans have a significantly increased rate of obesity, even starting in the school-age populations and before [1, 2]:

> Between the ages of 2 and 5 years, the proportion of (African American) children with a body mass index (BMI) at or above the 95th percentile is 11.3%, twice the proportion for (European American) children, and these differences persist through development (3.5%). Such findings suggest obesity-related risk factors present during early childhood may give rise to the differences observed through development. [3]

The widespread prevalence of obesity is best represented by the following map of the United States, showing almost nationwide obesity rates higher than 35% in the vast majority of states (Fig. 5.1).

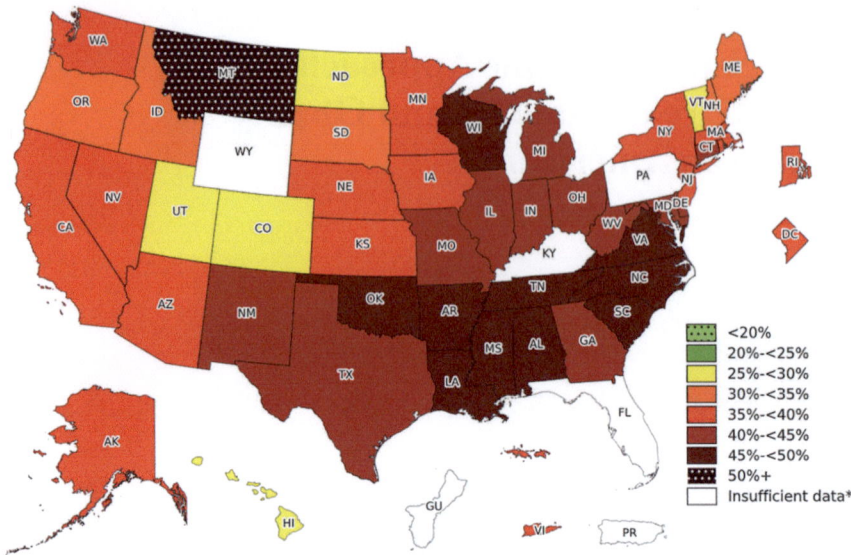

Fig. 5.1 Prevalence of self-reported obesity among African American adults by state and territory. (BRFSS, 2023. Centers for Disease Control and Prevention. *Adult Obesity Prevalence Maps*. U.S. Department of Health and Human Services)

Figure 5.2 shows the obesity rate among adults by race/ethnicity. Because the increased obesity rate leads to elevated diabetes diagnosis, we find that African Americans have an across-the-board increased rate of diabetes as compared to European Americans for all education levels. From the much earlier diagnosis of type 2 diabetes in younger African Americans to the increased occurrence of diabetes-induced heart failure and other related hospitalizations, the burden of obesity in African Americans is heavy and starts very early in life [3].

Researchers are looking into how genetics plays a role in obesity in African Americans. Any genetic influences interact with social, cultural, and environmental dynamics driven by structural racism, socioeconomic factors, perceived discrimination, stress, cardiometabolic risks, residential segregation, and cultural and behavioral factors.

Several studies have identified genetic variants associated with obesity in African Americans. For instance, copy number variations (CNVs) in genes such as PARK2, GYPA, and SGCZ have been linked to obesity-related traits in this population [4]. Additionally, renal risk variants in the APOL1 gene have been associated with higher BMI and increased odds of obesity, suggesting a genetic predisposition that may interact with environmental factors [5]. Genome-wide association studies (GWAS) have also identified loci associated with obesity in African Americans. For example, loci on chromosomes 5 and X have been implicated in obesity susceptibility [6]. Furthermore, common genetic variants in genes such as FTO and TUB have been associated with obesity in African Americans, although these associations

5.1 Obesity

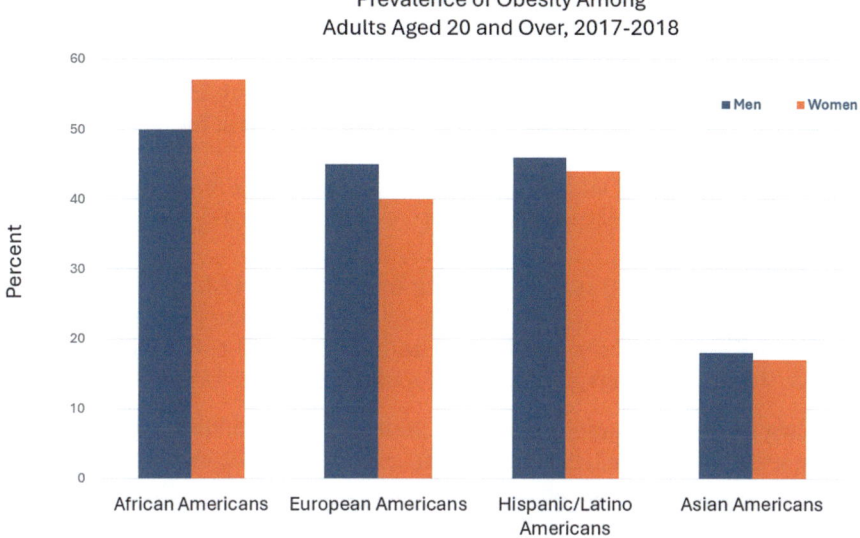

Fig. 5.2 Prevalence of obesity among adults aged 20 and over, 2017–2018 (https://www.cdc.gov/obesity/adult-obesity-facts/index.html)

often require further validation [6, 7]. These findings underscore the complex interplay between genetic and environmental factors in obesity among African Americans. Understanding these genetic predispositions can inform targeted interventions and policies to address health disparities in this population.

Environmental factors contributing to obesity in African Americans include limited access to healthy foods, which is often a result of living in food deserts where fresh produce and nutritious options are scarce. Additionally, socioeconomic constraints can lead to higher consumption of inexpensive, calorie-dense processed foods. Urban environments with fewer safe spaces for physical activity also contribute to sedentary lifestyles, further exacerbating obesity rates. Education plays a crucial role in mitigating obesity by empowering your patients with information about nutrition, healthy lifestyle choices, and the long-term health consequences of obesity. Many understand the diabetes and arthritis (wear-and-tear) connections to obesity, but few appreciate the increased risk for cancer, including:

- *Breast Cancer:* Obesity is associated with an increased risk of breast cancer, particularly postmenopausal breast cancer. African American women are more likely to be diagnosed with aggressive subtypes such as triple-negative breast cancer (TNBC), which has been linked to obesity [8–10].
- *Colorectal Cancer:* Obesity is a significant risk factor for colorectal cancer. African Americans have higher incidence and mortality rates for colorectal cancer compared to other racial groups, partly due to higher obesity rates [11].

- *Pancreatic Cancer:* Obesity increases the risk of pancreatic cancer, and African Americans have higher rates of both obesity and pancreatic cancer mortality [12, 13].
- *Endometrial Cancer:* Obesity is strongly associated with endometrial cancer. African American women with obesity are at a higher risk for this type of cancer [11].
- *Multiple Myeloma:* Obesity is linked to an increased risk of multiple myeloma, and African Americans have higher incidence and mortality rates for this cancer [14].
- *Liver Cancer:* Obesity is a risk factor for liver cancer, and African Americans are disproportionately affected by both obesity and liver cancer [11].
- *Kidney Cancer:* Obesity is associated with an increased risk of kidney cancer, and African Americans have higher rates of obesity-related kidney cancer [11].

When mentioning these connections, taking an informational approach rather than a scare tactic is vital. Scare tactics are generally not effective when educating African American patients about health risks, including obesity risks. Research indicates that African American patients often have a variable response to scare tactics, and these approaches can sometimes be counterproductive. For instance, a study by Ward et al. found that African American patients disliked the use of the word "obese" and emphasized the importance of the clinician's manner and timing when discussing weight management issues [15]. They also highlighted the necessity of a personalized approach and noted that scare tactics could hinder weight loss attempts. Additionally, Lucas et al. demonstrated that African Americans were more receptive to gain-framed messages rather than loss-framed (scare) messages when it came to educational encounters. Loss-framed messages increased perceived racism and reduced receptivity to the message [16]. This suggests that scare tactics may inadvertently increase mistrust and reduce the effectiveness of health communication.

One of the most impactful risk factors for obesity is having obese parents. Children with obese parents are ten times more likely to be obese. Through example, obese parents pass on unhealthy eating habits like increased intake of sugary beverages, higher fast food consumption, and diets that contain higher starch-content foods. Obese parents also have a more sedentary lifestyle with significantly less exercise and more watching television than their European American counterparts. Because early childhood is a critical period for habit-forming and body fat distribution formation, these environmental influences have lifelong consequences [17]. Figure 5.3 below shows the childhood obesity prevalence.

In general, African American women have a higher prevalence of obesity and are at a greater risk for weight management problems [18]. This increased propensity for obesity is directly correlated with increased chronic illnesses. Providers struggle with approaches to obese African American women given social norms that may encourage some degree of higher weight acceptance. Studies have consistently found that self-size satisfaction occurs at a higher weight among African Americans than matched European Americans. While 77% of African Americans have a BMI

5.1 Obesity

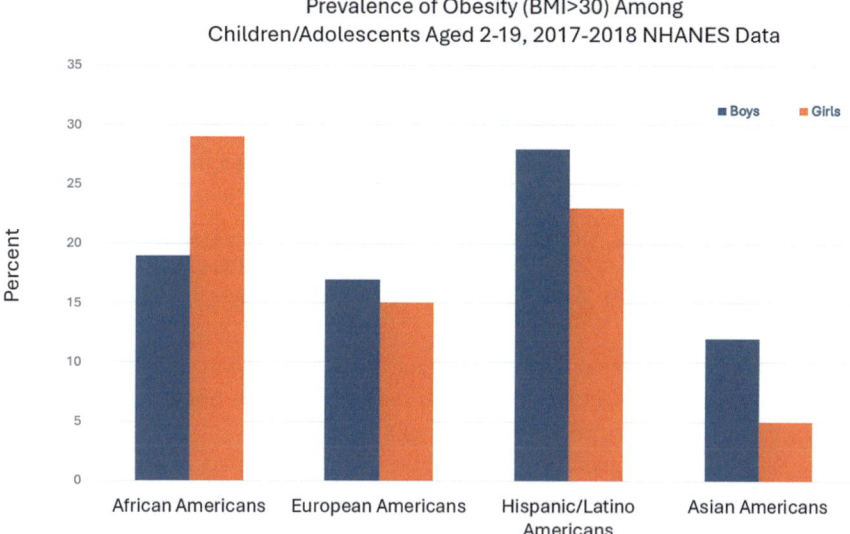

Fig. 5.3 Prevalence of obesity (BMI > 30) among children/adolescents aged 2–19, 2017–2018 NHANES Data (https://www.cdc.gov/obesity/childhood-obesity-facts/childhood-obesity-facts.html)

greater than 25, compared to 63% of European Americans, the percentage that are unhappy with their weight is significantly lower [19, 20]. Patients seeking bariatric consultation show a disproportionally lower number of African Americans "interested" in surgery. Even weight loss after bariatric surgery is more modest for African Americans due to the more tempered weight-loss goals [21]. Christina Wee and colleagues at the Beth Israel Deaconess Medical Center looked at obese patients considering bariatric surgery:

> [M]en were less likely than women and African Americans were less likely than (European American) primary care patients to have seriously considered bariatric surgery after accounting for sociodemographic factors and comorbid conditions. Much of the observed differences by race, however, appeared to be explained by higher QOL (quality of life) scores among African American relative to (European American) patients with obesity. [21]

This increased quality of life score shows the greater acceptance of some degree of obesity in African Americans and is reflected in their more conservative targets for ideal body weight. Multiple studies show that African Americans have a higher "ideal" body weight than other races, and this increased comfort at a higher weight drives down their desire for dramatic weight loss [21, 22]. These attenuated goals for weight loss are reflected even after bariatric surgery such that there are conflicting reports as to whether bariatric surgery is less effective in African Americans [23], with a number of studies showing a comparatively less overall weight loss [24–27]. Although weight loss is greater in European Americans, significant weight loss still occurs in African Americans having gastric bypass surgery. If your patient would benefit from bariatric surgery, studies have shown that having the primary care provider suggest the procedure rather than waiting for patient self-directed referrals has shown increased success [28–30].

As a disproportional number of African Americans live in higher-violence neighborhoods, there has been growing evidence of a link between increased stress from growing up in violent areas and subsequent obesity [31]. A study by Assari and others at the University of Michigan found a direct link between increased adolescent fear of violence and subsequent obesity in adulthood.

> Fear of violence in the neighborhood at age 15 is predictive of an increase in BMI from age 21 to 32 among female but not male African American youth. Thus for female African American youth who live in disadvantaged areas, fear of violence in the neighborhood is one of the contributing factors of their increased risk of obesity. [31]

It has long been accepted that psychogenic stress can lead to excess body fat and obesity, although the exact mechanism has remained elusive. Some suggest cortisol as a mediator and others put forth other hypotheses [32].

Be aware that the increased obesity we see in inner-city African American women (and men) is not completely self-induced, and approaching the patient with an accusatory tone and simple instructions to "lose weight" ignores the laundry list of contributing causes, with some of them starting before birth.

5.2 Type 2 Diabetes

Diabetes occurs at a disproportional rate in African Americans and they are 80% more likely to be diagnosed than European Americans, and the occurrence is slightly higher in women [33, 34]. Of those with diabetes, there is a higher propensity for related end-organ damage than European Americans. The prevalence of visual impairment, end-stage renal disease, wound-related leg amputations, and overall hospitalizations are dramatically higher in African Americans with diabetes [33]. The CDC reports that African American men die at over twice the rate of any other race or gender group from hyperglycemic crises [35].

Figure 5.4 also demonstrates the increased occurrence of diabetes in Native Americans and Alaskan Natives, which is dramatically higher than in the African American community. Researchers find similar drivers, including genetic factors associated with insulin resistance and beta-cell dysfunction, lower socioeconomic status, chronic stress, diet, lifestyle, and increased metabolic syndrome in those communities [36–38].

Genetic factors significantly contribute to the higher prevalence of type 2 diabetes and its complications, including increased hospital admissions and kidney failure among African Americans. Several genetic loci have been identified that are associated with type 2 diabetes in African Americans. Notably, variants in the TCF7L2 gene have shown a strong association with type 2 diabetes in this population, with the SNP rs7903146 being particularly significant [39, 40]. This gene plays a crucial role in glucose metabolism and insulin secretion. Additionally, the

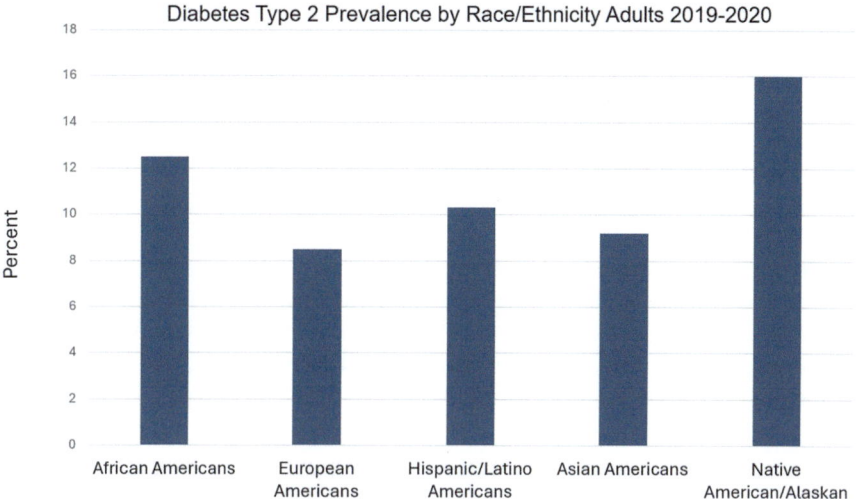

Fig. 5.4 Prevalence of diagnosed diabetes by detailed race and ethnicity among adults aged 18 years or older, United States, 2019–2021 (https://www.cdc.gov/obesity/data-and-statistics/adult-obesity-prevalence-maps.html)

KCNQ1 and HMGA2 loci have been implicated in type 2 diabetes susceptibility among African Americans [40]. These loci are involved in pancreatic beta-cell function and insulin regulation. Genetic studies have also identified novel loci specific to African Americans. For instance, the HLA-B and INS-IGF2 loci were found to be associated with type 2 diabetes in African Americans, highlighting the unique genetic architecture of diabetes in this population [40]. Regarding diabetic kidney disease, genetic variants in kidney structure-related genes such as APOL1 and MYH9 have been linked to an increased risk of end-stage kidney disease in African Americans with type 2 diabetes. These genes are involved in maintaining kidney function and structure, and their variants contribute to the higher susceptibility to kidney failure in this population [41, 42].

Several other factors contribute to the disproportionate burden of diabetes on African Americans:

- *Socioeconomic Status (SES):* Lower SES is associated with higher diabetes prevalence. African Americans often live in economically disadvantaged neighborhoods, which are linked to higher diabetes incidence due to limited access to healthy foods and safe spaces for physical activity [43, 44].
- *Perceived Racism and Discrimination:* Chronic stress from perceived racism and discrimination is linked to higher diabetes risk. African American women exposed to high levels of racism have a significantly increased risk of developing diabetes, partly mediated by higher BMI [45, 46].

- *Cultural and Behavioral Factors:* Cultural beliefs and personal experiences influence diabetes management. African Americans often perceive diabetes as a consequence of historical and ongoing racial discrimination, affecting their engagement with healthcare providers and adherence to treatment [47].
- *Social Determinants of Health (SDOH):* The American Diabetes Association emphasizes that SDOH, including food insecurity, housing instability, and limited access to healthcare, significantly impact diabetes prevalence and outcomes [48, 49].
- *Obesity and Cardiometabolic Risks:* High rates of obesity and related cardiometabolic risks, such as hypertension and insulin resistance, are prevalent [50].
- *Healthcare Access and Quality:* Disparities in healthcare access and quality, including lower rates of diabetes education and specialty care, further exacerbate the diabetes burden among African Americans [51].

Addressing these disparities requires a multifaceted approach that includes improving access to healthcare, addressing social determinants of health, and mitigating the effects of perceived racism and discrimination.

Diabetes is diagnosed at an earlier age on average (5.5–8.4 years earlier than European Americans), and this earlier age is significant because the development of diabetes complications is directly related to both glycemic control and the overall duration of the disease [52, 53].

Diabetes remains the most common cause of kidney failure across all races and is an important contributory factor among African Americans. Kidney disease is already more prevalent in African Americans due to hypertension-related causes [35]. Keeping blood sugars in the normal range and using renal-protective medications in patients with diabetes has been shown to slow the occurrence and progression of renal disease. Just in a 10-year span, significant progress has been made in decreasing new cases of renal disease, but unfortunately, significant disparities persist.

Several diabetes medications have shown renal protection, which is particularly important for African Americans, who are generally more likely to suffer from early-onset diabetes and kidney impairment. These medications can help slow the progression of kidney disease, reducing the risk of dialysis and kidney transplants. Consequently, they offer a significant advantage in managing diabetes-related complications in this high-risk population. SGLT2 inhibitors such as empagliflozin, canagliflozin, and dapagliflozin have significantly slowed chronic kidney disease (CKD) progression and improved cardiovascular outcomes. The American Diabetes Association (ADA) recommends these medications for individuals with T2D and CKD, as they reduce renal tubular glucose reabsorption, lower systemic blood pressure, reduce albuminuria, and slow the decline in glomerular filtration rate (GFR) through mechanisms independent of glycemia [54, 55]. The CREDENCE trial demonstrated a 30% relative risk reduction in the primary composite endpoint of end-stage kidney disease, doubling of serum creatinine, or renal or cardiovascular death with canagliflozin [56]. GLP-1 receptor agonists (GLP-1 RAs) such as liraglutide, semaglutide, and dulaglutide also offer renal protective effects. These medications improve kidney outcomes by reducing albuminuria and slowing GFR decline. The ADA highlights that GLP-1 RAs effectively lower glucose levels and benefit cardiovascular and kidney outcomes, making them suitable for patients with CKD [54, 55]. Semaglutide, in particular, has shown beneficial effects on cardiovascular disease, mortality, and kidney outcomes [54]. Despite these benefits, a systematic review and metaanalysis indicated that the cardiorenal protective effects of SGLT2 inhibitors and GLP-1 RAs are less pronounced in African Americans compared to European and Asian American populations, potentially due to underrepresentation in clinical trials and variations in pharmacokinetics and pharmacodynamics [57]. This underscores the necessity for a precision medicine approach, which tailors healthcare treatments to the individual's genetic, environmental, and lifestyle factors. For diverse populations, such as African Americans, personalized approaches can ensure that therapies are more effective and safer by considering unique genetic and physiological differences. Healthcare providers can optimize treatment outcomes and reduce health disparities among different demographic groups by addressing these variations.

Most research pertaining to African Americans and diabetes points to increased insulin resistance and upregulated beta cell function when compared to European Americans. To some extent, African Americans are more prone to develop diabetes genetically, but external factors like obesity, poor diet, and smoking contribute much more.

5.2.1 Smoking Drives Up Diabetes Risk

High-intensity cigarette smoking is associated with a 79% higher incidence of diabetes mellitus in African Americans compared to those who have never smoked. This increased risk is attributed to the effects of smoking on insulin resistance and beta-cell dysfunction. Smoking induces chronic inflammation and oxidative stress, which impair insulin signaling and glucose metabolism, leading to the development of type 2 diabetes [58]. Additionally, smoking interacts with genetic factors to exacerbate diabetes risk. For example, specific genetic variants, such as those in the FBN1 gene, show significant main effects only among smokers. This indicates a gene-environment interaction that heightens diabetes susceptibility in African Americans [59]. The Jackson Heart Study highlights that smoking intensity and cumulative exposure (pack-years) are critical factors in the increased diabetes risk among African Americans [58].

> Although smoking cessation should be encouraged for everyone, certain high-risk groups such as (African Americans) who are disproportionately affected by diabetes mellitus should be targeted for cessation strategies. [58]

There is fairly consistent evidence that smoking leads to increased diabetes in other racial populations as well including the "Nurses' Health Study" [60] and the "Insulin Resistance Atherosclerosis Study" [61]. Both of these large studies showed substantially increased diabetes in current smokers. The American Diabetes Association recommends routine assessment of tobacco use and combination treatment with smoking cessation counseling and pharmacologic therapy to reduce the risk of diabetes and its complications [62].

5.2.2 HbA1c Differences

Hemoglobin A1c (HbA1c) at diagnosis is generally a point higher in African Americans (8.9 in European Americans and 9.8 in African Americans), and when controlling for socioeconomic status, quality of care, self-management behaviors, and access, African Americans still have higher HbA1c levels [63]. A study by Saaddine et al. looked at NHANES data for participants aged 5–24 years and found that African American youths consistently had higher HbA1c levels [64]. Another researcher found the same persistently high HbA1c levels even "after controlling for age, sex, BMI, maternal BMI, and poverty-income ratio" [65].

Studies have consistently shown that African Americans tend to have higher HbA1c levels compared to European Americans at the same levels of glycemia [66–69]. For example, the GRADE sub-study found that HbA1c levels were 0.2–0.6 percentage points higher in African Americans compared to the majority population for average glucose levels ranging from 100 to 250 mg/dL [66]. This difference persisted even after adjusting for demographics and other factors. The American Diabetes Association (ADA) guidelines also acknowledge that HbA1c levels are generally higher in African Americans than European Americans, which may reflect higher glycemic exposure and potential genetic differences in hemoglobin glycation [67]. Genetic factors such as hemoglobinopathies (sickle cell trait) can also contribute to these differences [67, 68].

In all, HbA1c value differences in African Americans essentially equate to a 0.4% difference (higher) for glucose-matched European American patients. An HbA1c of 7.5% should be interpreted as 7.1% in African Americans, and an HbA1c of 6.5% should raise concerns for a higher risk of hypoglycemia, particularly in the elderly. This difference across a population could change the threshold for diabetes diagnosis and for targeted control in African Americans. Thus, the accepted relationship between HbA1c and the "mean blood glucose" used by clinicians and laboratories is different for African Americans:

> The relationship between mean blood glucose and HbA1c may not be the same in all people. Indeed, the published regression line from the "A1c-Derived Average Glucose" (ADAG) Study demonstrated a wide range of average glucose levels for individuals with the same HbA1c levels. [63]

Given the additional "wiggle-room" implicit in the across-the-board elevations in HbA1c levels in African Americans, some have suggested a wider "rule-in and rule-out" range in African Americans with levels lower than 5.5% representing the absence of diabetes and levels higher than 7% clearly confirming the diagnosis.

Levels within the "wiggle-room" should be further investigated with glucose plasma testing or glucose tolerance measurements. Because of the limitations of HbA1c measurements in some clinical pictures (uremia and hemolytic anemia, for example) and the racial differences discussed above, some of the patients with an HbA1c level between 5.5% and 7% will clearly have diabetes, and others will not [70]. To assume that those African Americans in that range are now "borderline" and to withhold treatment would also be a great mistake. The simple fact is the HbA1c is less accurate and dependable at "near-normal" levels and any result in this range should prompt additional confirmatory studies [65].

The American Diabetes Association (ADA) guidelines also acknowledge that HbA1c levels are generally higher in African Americans than European Americans, which may reflect higher glycemic exposure and potential genetic differences in hemoglobin glycation [62]. Hemoglobinopathies, such as sickle cell trait and glucose-6-phosphate dehydrogenase (G6PD) deficiency, significantly affect HbA1c levels in African Americans, who have a higher prevalence of early-onset diabetes and related health disparities [71]. Sickle cell trait (SCT) is prevalent in approximately 8% of African Americans. Studies have shown that individuals with SCT have lower HbA1c levels for a given glucose concentration compared to those without SCT. For example, Lacy et al. found that HbA1c values were 0.29% lower in African Americans with SCT compared to those without SCT, even after adjusting for fasting and 2-h glucose levels [72]. This suggests that HbA1c may systematically underestimate past glycemia in African Americans with SCT. Similarly, G6PD deficiency, which affects about 11% of African American males, also leads to lower HbA1c levels. Sarnowski et al. identified that the G6PD variant rs1050828-T was associated with a significant reduction in HbA1c levels, lowering HbA1c by 0.88% in hemizygous males and 0.34% in heterozygous females [71]. This genetic variant can cause underdiagnosis of diabetes when HbA1c is used as the sole diagnostic criterion. These findings suggest that HbA1c may overestimate glycemic control in African Americans, potentially leading to premature diabetes diagnoses or overtreatment. Therefore, it is essential to consider these racial differences when setting treatment goals and interpreting HbA1c levels in African American patients.

5.2.3 Diabetes Treatment Approaches

The mainstay of the initial treatment of type 2 diabetes is metformin. African Americans exhibit a better glycemic response to metformin compared to other racial-ethnic groups. A study by Williams et al. found that metformin use was associated with a 0.90% reduction in HbA1c levels among African Americans, compared to a 0.42% reduction in European Americans [73]. This suggests that African Americans may experience more significant improvements in glycemic control with metformin. Additionally, genetic factors play a role in the response to metformin. A genome-wide association study identified a variant, rs143276236, in the gene ARFGEF3, which was associated with changes in HbA1c levels among African

American patients on metformin monotherapy [74]. In the prediabetic population, African Americans also showed a more pronounced reduction in fasting plasma glucose levels with metformin treatment compared to European Americans, further supporting the enhanced glycemic response in this group [75]. Still, studies show increased side effects and fear in African Americans. Some studies suggest that African Americans may experience higher rates of gastrointestinal side effects when taking metformin [54, 74]. Additionally, there is concern about the medication's efficacy and safety due to historical disparities in healthcare [76]. To improve metformin's efficacy and safety perception among African Americans, healthcare providers should focus on personalized medicine approaches that consider genetic differences. Discuss the increased efficacy and side effects in African Americans and stress starting at a low dose and gradually titrating as tolerance improves [77]. Increased patient education about potential side effects and providing clear communication about the benefits and risks can help alleviate concerns.

The effectiveness and safety of newer diabetes medications that also result in significant weight loss have drawn considerable interest in African Americans, considering the higher prevalence of obesity, early-onset diabetes, and related health problems. When choosing one of these medications for diabetes treatment, consider the weight loss benefits as an added plus. Unlike traditional diabetes treatments that primarily focus on controlling blood sugar levels, these newer medications offer the dual benefit of aiding in weight loss. This is particularly advantageous for African Americans, who face a higher risk of obesity-related complications. By addressing both diabetes management and weight reduction, these medications provide a more comprehensive approach to improving overall health outcomes.

- *Empagliflozin:* The ongoing study designed to assess the safety and efficacy of empagliflozin in African Americans with type 2 diabetes and hypertension aims to provide further insights. Preliminary data suggest that empagliflozin is associated with significant improvements in glucose control and reductions in blood pressure. These improvements are crucial for managing diabetes and its complications in this population [78].
- *Pramlintide:* A pooled post-hoc analysis of two randomized, double-blind, placebo-controlled trials showed that pramlintide, an analog of the human beta-cell hormone amylin, significantly reduces HbA1c and body weight in insulin-treated African Americans with type 2 diabetes. The glycemic improvement and weight loss were most pronounced in African Americans, with a placebo-corrected treatment effect of −0.7% for HbA1c and −9 pounds for body weight. Hypoglycemia incidence was low, and nausea was the most common adverse event, primarily occurring in the first 4 weeks of therapy [79].

Incretin-based therapies have shown significant effectiveness and safety for diabetes and weight loss in African Americans as well.

- *Liraglutide:* A post-hoc analysis of pooled data from five double-blind randomized, placebo-controlled trials demonstrated that liraglutide 3.0 mg is effective for weight management across racial subgroups, including African Americans.

African Americans achieved a statistically significant mean weight loss of 6.3% with liraglutide compared to 1.4% with placebo. The safety profile was consistent across racial subgroups, with similar adverse events reported. Additionally, a meta-analysis of seven phase III trials confirmed that liraglutide is well tolerated and efficacious for treating type 2 diabetes in African Americans, with significant reductions in HbA1c and fasting plasma glucose levels [80, 81].
- *Semaglutide:* A post-hoc analysis of the SUSTAIN trials indicated that semaglutide was associated with consistent and clinically relevant reductions in HbA1c and body weight across race and ethnicity subgroups, including African Americans. The most commonly reported adverse events were gastrointestinal disorders, which were generally mild to moderate in severity [82].
- *Tirzepatide:* In the SURPASS clinical trial program, tirzepatide demonstrated substantial improvements in glycemic control and body weight reduction among participants with early-onset type 2 diabetes, which includes a significant proportion of African Americans. The post-hoc analysis from the SURPASS trials indicated that tirzepatide led to similar improvements in HbA1c, body weight, and cardiometabolic markers in both early-onset and later-onset type 2 diabetes groups, suggesting its efficacy across different age groups at diagnosis [80].

Once diabetes has been confirmed, studies show about a third to half of your African American patients will be nonadherent with whatever treatment you prescribe [83, 84]. Adherence to prescribed medications varies according to a number of confounding and compounding variables including access, trust in provider, medication cost, health literacy, psychological barriers, insulin preconceptions, and regime complexity.

A study of focus groups of African Americans found a high degree of skepticism regarding their own diabetes diagnosis "*as if somehow ... a mistake in diagnosis had been made*" [85]. Taking the time to explain how the diabetes diagnosis was made incorporating their presenting symptoms with an explanation of what the elevated glucose does to the body over time should help proactively convince the certainty of the diagnosis. That same focus group study found a significant number of the participants felt personally responsible for their diabetes and that "responsibility" was out of proportion to factors actually in their control. Many participants felt that if they could have adequately controlled their diet, they never would have gotten the disease ... and if they could control their diet going forward, the diabetes would go away.

Fatalism in African Americans with diabetes is common, and this attitude of hopelessness as it relates to diabetes control is "significantly associated with poor medication adherence and self-care" as found by Walker and colleagues at the Medical University of South Carolina [86].

> After adjustment for pertinent covariates, the relationship remained statistically significant for the association between increased diabetes fatalism, decreased medication adherence, and decreased levels of three self-care behaviors (diet, exercise, and blood sugar testing). [86]

Clarifying the misconceptions regarding the patient's ability to control their diabetes without medications will allow the patient to progress beyond this barrier to accepting medications as a viable option for care. While diet, exercise, and proper medications are central to diabetes care, they are not mutually exclusive in most African American patients, or anyone else for that matter. Diabetes education with every new patient with diabetes is essential to dispelling false impressions and preconceptions regarding the cause and ultimate control of the disease.

Studies have repeatedly shown that increased diabetes knowledge and understanding have been positively associated with better glycemic control and increased education leads to elevated confidence in the patient's ability to achieve control [87]. This increased confidence, also referred to as "self-efficacy," has also been associated with better "glycemic control, medication adherence, self-care, and mental health-related quality of life". Demystifying diabetes through education individually and in small groups has been shown to improve overall diabetes care [86].

> Health care providers are urged to explore the person's knowledge about the diagnosis, ask about past experiences with others who have diabetes, and inquire as to their feelings and beliefs about the purpose of prescribed medication and dispel any myths. [85]

Researchers have also found a propensity among clinicians to be slow when advancing or intensifying diabetic therapy. Having a *clinician care flow sheet* that anticipates the progression of medications typically used to achieve control will remove mental barriers clinicians may subconsciously erect that prevent the acceleration of care. Sometimes providers "stall" adding additional medications (or increasing a dose). This *slow-to-prescribe* behavior is sometimes referred to as "clinical inertia" and mimics the added energy needed to set an object in motion. By knowing what medication or next dose choice well in advance of its need, clinicians will simplify their thought process and expedite ultimate glycemic control.

5.3 Diabetes Type 1

The incidence of type 1 diabetes in African Americans is lower than in those of European descent and is 15.7 per 100,000 for both the 0–9 years and 10–19 years age groups. This incidence rate is lower compared to youth of European descent, who have the highest rates of type 1 diabetes. For example, the incidence rates for European American youth are approximately 18.6 per 100,000 for ages 0–4 years, 28.1 per 100,000 for ages 5–9 years, and 32.9 per 100,000 for ages 10–14 years [88, 89]. In comparison, Hispanic/Latino youth have an incidence rate of around 15.5 per 100,000, which is similar to African Americans, while Asian/Pacific Islanders and Native Americans have lower incidence rates [88, 89]. Genetic factors may play a significant role, as certain genetic markers associated with type 1 diabetes are more prevalent in European populations. Environmental factors, such as diet and lifestyle, could also contribute to these differences, as they can influence the development of autoimmune diseases. African Americans with early-onset type 1 diabetes mellitus are at high risk for severe diabetic nephropathy and end-stage renal disease. While type 1 diabetes typically develops from the autoimmune destruction of pancreatic beta cells, there is a subset of African American individuals who are phenotypically type 1 (thin and insulin-dependent) but do not have the immunologic markers indicative of an autoimmune destruction process. These patients have insulin deficiency but not from an immune process, and their diabetes is ketosis-prone. This nonimmune type 1 diabetes is more prevalent in African Americans [90].

5.4 Diet Management Approaches

Type 2 diabetes is a complicated disease with variable presentations and idiosyncratic causes that vary from patient to patient. As their clinician, we have the unique opportunity to personalize the explanation of their diabetes diagnosis and tailor the approach to care in a very specific manner. Obtaining a diet history from the patient with analysis of calories from foods and beverages with specific stepwise recommendations will allow for a graduated, and better tolerated, change [91]. If, for example, your patient drinks a 2-L bottle of their favorite soda on a daily basis (not an unusual example), they consume almost 1000 calories through that source alone. Cutting 1000 calories from anyone's diet is a major accomplishment and certainly a significant step in the right direction. Many African American patients will appreciate sequential and specific recommendations that target easily identifiable foods, and only represent a slight change in their overall diet (at first). For our example, an easy, impactful, and significant initial diet modification could be:

- Stop all sugary beverages.

This clear instruction would impact dietary calories, be relatively easy to accomplish, and provide a positive outcome in glycemic control. It will not achieve full control of the diabetes but will be a great first step.

It has also been clearly proven that telling patients *what not to eat* leads to more confusion about what is allowable and worse outcomes with compliance [91]. Dariush Mozaffarian looked at dietary trends and priorities for patients at risk for, or already diagnosed with, diabetes, obesity, and cardiovascular diseases. Quite simply, he affirmed what nutritionists are now emphasizing:

> [E]vidence-informed dietary priorities include increased fruits, non-starchy vegetables, nuts, legumes, fish, vegetable oils, yogurt, and minimally processed whole grains; and fewer red meats, processed (e.g., sodium-preserved) meats, and foods rich in refined grains, starch, added sugars, salt, and trans fat. [92]

Nutrition recommendations are also moving away from banning specific foods and moving toward looking at the combinations of foods in a diet that work synergistically toward better health. And better emphasizing healthy patterns in a diet versus its calorie composition:

> These lines of evidence indicate that an "energy imbalance" concept of obesity is oversimplified. Whereas short-term weight loss can be achieved by any type of calorie-reduced diet, in the long-term, counting calories may not be biologically nor behaviorally relevant. Rather, the quality and types of foods consumed influence diverse pathways related to weight homeostasis, such as satiety, hunger, brain reward, glucose-insulin responses, hepatic *de novo* lipogenesis, adipocyte function, metabolic expenditure, and the microbiome. Thus, all calories are not equal for long-term adiposity: certain foods impair pathways of weight homeostasis, others have relatively neutral effects, and others promote the integrity of weight regulation. [92]

By giving one or two specific dietary category instructions per visit, adjustments in the overall diet seem less radical to the patient and more easy to follow. At a subsequent office visit, and after success with curtailing the soda pop consumption, suggestions for increasing fruit or nut consumption can be initiated. This is framed with the patient's preferences in fruit (or nuts) elucidated, and then eliciting their agreement to the plan. It is critical to get the patient's endorsement of the diet recommendation during the visit. Simply telling the patient to start eating an orange every day, and then leaving the exam room defeats the purpose. Getting a diet history of likes and dislikes, aligning their diet plan with proven recommendations, and then gradually moving their habits to better alignment are the best approaches to sustained diet modification. The clinician will also need to stress that follow-up recommendations will be forthcoming regarding other aspects of their diet, but for now, the prime directive is whatever they have indicated, and be as helpful with specifics as needed.

For example, when preparing meals, a modest change in the quality of oils used for food preparation can have a great impact on the overall health content of a meal (Fig. 5.5). With the goal to decrease the saturated fats in a diet, talk about the different compositions of oils, their experiences with them and some practical applications with food they already eat.

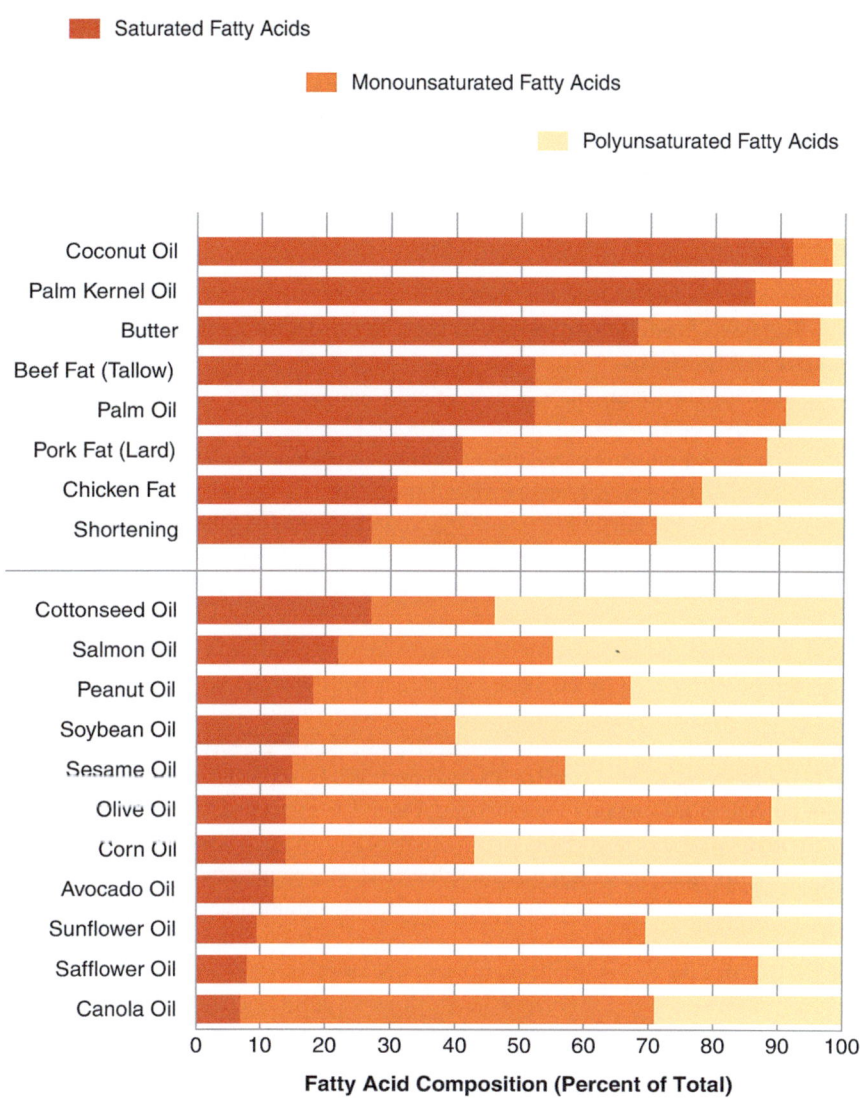

Fig. 5.5 Comparison of fats and oils. (The Dietary Guidelines for Americans 2015–2020. National Diabetes Education Program. https://health.gov/dietaryguidelines/2015/guidelines/chapter-1/a-closer-look-inside-healthy-eating-patterns/#callout-dietaryfats)

5.5 Marketing Competition

Products associated with significant population-wide morbidity in diabetes (sodas, candy, and alcoholic beverages) are advertised disproportionately in magazines, billboards, and television advertisements targeting African Americans when compared with any other racial audience [93]. Advertisements for "healthier food and beverage products" (fruits, vegetables, low-fat meats, soy, and dairy products) are disproportionately underrepresented in African American communities [91–94].

Trying to have an impact on the dietary wants of a patient with that kind of marketing barrage is like trying to explain to your children that an amusement park is not as fun as the television commercials make it seem. The important take-home message is ... your message(s) will need reinforcement and repetition, and the trust of the conveyor of the message will absolutely impact its acceptance.

> **A Precision Medicine Approach to the Care of Diabetes and Obesity in African Americans**
> - African Americans have a significantly increased rate of obesity, which directly correlates to an increased risk for chronic illnesses.
> - African American women have a higher prevalence of obesity and are at a greater risk for weight management problems.
> - African American children with obese parents are ten times more likely to be obese.
> - African Americans are more than 80% more likely to be diagnosed with type 2 diabetes than European Americans and are also diagnosed at an earlier age.
> - Ensuring optimal blood sugar control, as well as utilizing renal-protective medications, has been shown to slow the progression of renal disease.
> - HbA1c value differences in African Americans essentially equate to a 0.4% difference (higher) for glucose-matched European American patients.
> - HbA1c is less accurate and dependable at "near-normal" levels in African Americans.
> - Patients with sickle cell trait have lower HbA_{1c} at any given level.
> - HbA1c is not reliable in patients with hemoglobinopathies.
> - African Americans should be encouraged to stop smoking as smoking increases the risk of diabetes in this population.
> - Adequate diabetes education, both in small groups and individually, has been shown to improve overall diabetes care.
> - Advising patients on food and beverage use using a stepwise recommendation will allow for a graduated, better-tolerated, and accepted change.

References

1. Guerrero A, Mao C, Fuller B, Bridges M, Franke T, Kuo A. Racial and ethnic disciplines in early childhood obesity: growth trajectories in body mass index. J Racial Ethn Health Disparities. 2016;3(1):129–37.
2. Abraham P, Kazman J, Zeno S, Deuster P. Obesity and African Americans: physiologic and behavioral pathways. ISRN Obes. 2013;2013:314295.

3. Fuemmeler B, Stroo M, Lee C, Bazemore S, Blocker B, Ostbye T. Racial differences in obesity-related risk factors between 2-year-old children born of overweight mothers. J Pediatr Psychol. 2015;40(7):649–56.
4. Wei Z, Wineinger Nathan E, Tiwari Hemant K, Mosley Thomas H, Ulrich B, Arnett Donna K, Kardia Sharon LR, Kabagambe Edmond K, Sun Yan V. Copy number variations associated with obesity-related traits in African Americans: a joint analysis between GENOA and HyperGEN. Obesity. 20(12):2431–7. https://doi.org/10.1038/oby.2012.162.
5. Nadkarni Girish N, Kezhen F, Genevieve G, Yan G, Wilson James G, Richard C, Madden Ebony B, Denny Joshua C, Richardson Lynne D, Martin P, Loos Ruth JF, Horowitz Carol R. APOL1 renal risk variants are associated with obesity and body composition in African ancestry adults. Medicine. 2021;100(45):e27785. https://doi.org/10.1097/MD.0000000000027785.
6. Cheng C-Y, Linda KWH, Nick P, Arti T, Haiman Christopher A, Harris Tamara B, Chao X, John Esther M, Ambrosone Christine B, Brancati Frederick L, Josef C, Press Michael F, Parekh Rulan S, Klag Michael J, Meoni Lucy A, Wen-Chi H, Laura F, Ludmila P, Freedman Matthew L, Jandorf Lina H, Bandera Elisa V, Ciupak Gregory L, Nalls Michael A, Akylbekova Ermeg L, Orwoll Eric S, Leak Tennille S, Iva M, Rongling L, Giske U, Leslie B, Kristin A, Taylor Herman A, Eric B, Zmuda Joseph M, Henderson Brian E, Wilson James G, David R, McCarthy Mark I. Admixture mapping of 15280 African Americans identifies obesity susceptibility loci on chromosomes 5 and X. PLoS Genet. 2009;5(5):e1000490. https://doi.org/10.1371/journal.pgen.1000490.
7. Brandon C, Denada P, Arvind S, Christina L, Maria A, Martha D, Jalees R, Sreenivas K, Dawood D, Joseph D. Common genetic variants associated with obesity in an African-American and Hispanic/Latino population. PLoS One. 2021;16(5):e0250697. https://doi.org/10.1371/journal.pone.0250697.
8. Dietze Eric C, Chavez Tanya A, Seewaldt Victoria L. Obesity and triple-negative breast cancer. Am J Pathol. 188(2):280–90. https://doi.org/10.1016/j.ajpath.2017.09.018.
9. Kour SS, Amod S, Somesh VK, Wade D, Deshmukh Sachin K, Teja P, Holliday Nicolette P, Pranitha P, Cindy N, Singh Karan P, Singh Ajay P, Seema S. Obesity and early-onset breast cancer and specific molecular subtype diagnosis in black and white women. JAMA Netw Open. 7(7):e2421846. https://doi.org/10.1001/jamanetworkopen.2024.21846.
10. Rose David P, Haffner Steven M, Jacques B. Adiposity the metabolic syndrome and breast cancer in African-American and white American Women. Endocr Rev. 28(7):763–77. https://doi.org/10.1210/er.2006-0019.
11. Brooke SC, Thomas Cheryll C, Jane HS, Massetti Greta M, Galuska Deborah A, Tanya A-C, Mary P, Richardson Lisa C. MMWR Morb Mortal Wkly Rep. 2017;66(39):1052–8. https://doi.org/10.15585/mmwr.mm6639e1.
12. Twohig Patrick A, Butt Muhammad U, Gardner Timothy B, Prabhleen C, Sandhu Dalbir S. Racial and gender disparities among obese patients with pancreatic cancer. J Clin Gastroenterol. 2023;57(4):410–6. https://doi.org/10.1097/MCG.0000000000001688.
13. Bethea Traci N, Kitahara Cari M, Jennifer S, Patel Alpa V, Chinonye H, Knutsen Synnøve F, Yikyung P, Yi PS, Fraser Gary E, Jacobs Eric J, Purdue Mark P, Stolzenberg-Solomon RZ, Gillanders Elizabeth M, Blot William J, Palmer Julie R, Kolonel Laurence N. A pooled analysis of body mass index and pancreatic cancer mortality in African Americans. Cancer Epidemiol Biomarkers Prev. 2014;23(10):2119–25. https://doi.org/10.1158/1055-9965.EPI-14-0422.
14. Sonderman Jennifer S, Bethea Traci N, Kitahara Cari M, Patel Alpa V, Chinonye H, Knutsen Synnøve F, Yikyung P, Song-Yi P, Fraser Gary E, Teras LR, Purdue Mark P, Stolzenberg-Solomon Rachael Z, Gillanders Elizabeth M, Palmer Julie R, Kolonel Laurence N, Blot William J. Multiple myeloma mortality in relation to obesity among African Americans. J Natl Cancer Inst. 2016;108(10):djw120. https://doi.org/10.1093/jnci/djw120.
15. Ward Stephanie H, Gray Anastasia M, Anuradha P. African Americans' perceptions of physician attempts to address obesity in the primary care setting. J Gen Intern Med. 24(5):579–84. https://doi.org/10.1007/s11606-009-0922-z.

16. Todd L, Hayman Lenwood W, Blessman James E, Kanzoni A, Novak Julie M. Gain versus loss-framed messaging and colorectal cancer screening among African Americans: a preliminary examination of perceived racism and culturally targeted dual messaging. Br J Health Psychol. 21(2):249–67. https://doi.org/10.1111/bjhp.12160.
17. Taveras E, Gillman M, Kleinman K, Rich-Edwards J, Rifas-Shinman S. Racial/ethnic differences in early life risk factors for childhood obesity. Pediatrics. 2010;125(4):686. https://doi.org/10.1542/peds.2009-2100.
18. Bruce M, Sims M, Miller S, Elliott V, Ladipo M. One size fits all? Race, gender and body mass index among US adults. J Natl Med Assoc. 2007;99(10):1152–8.
19. Leilani D, Emily S-A. Beyond body mass index: are weight-loss programs the best way to improve the health of African American women? Prev Chronic Dis. 2017;14 https://doi.org/10.5888/pcd14.160573.
20. Sivalingam SK, Javed A, Neelima V, Jennifer F, James C, Rothberg Michael B. Ethnic differences in the self-recognition of obesity and obesity-related comorbidities: a cross-sectional analysis. J Gen Intern Med. 26(6):616–20. https://doi.org/10.1007/s11606-010-1623-3.
21. Wee C, Davis R, Jones D, et al. Sex, race, and the quality of life factors most important to patients' well-being among those seeking bariatric surgery. Obes Surg. 2016;26(6):1308–16.
22. Lori C-E, Bastian Lori A, Jessica R, Holiday D, Yuliya L, Ahinee AM, Truls O. Body Image and body satisfaction differ by race in overweight postpartum mothers. J Women's Health. 19(2):305–11. https://doi.org/10.1089/jwh.2008.1238.
23. Anderson W, Greene G, Forse R, Apovian C, Istfan N. Weight loss and health outcomes in African Americans and whites after gastric bypass surgery. Obesity (Silver Spring). 2007;15(6):1455–63.
24. Buffington C, Marema R. Ethnic differences in obesity and surgical weight loss between African Americans and Caucasian females. Obes Surg. 2006;16(2):159–65.
25. Samaan Jamil S, Yazan A, Liyun Y, Omar T, James M, Elaine Q, Nayun L, Chaitra S, Kamran S. Racial disparities in bariatric surgery postoperative weight loss and patient satisfaction. Am J Surg. 223(5):969–74. https://doi.org/10.1016/j.amjsurg.2021.09.011.
26. Wood Michael H, Carlin Arthur M, Ghaferi Amir A, Varban Oliver A, Abdelkader H, Bonham Aaron J, Birkmeyer Nancy J, Finks Jonathan F. Association of race with bariatric surgery outcomes. JAMA Surg. 154(5):e190029. https://doi.org/10.1001/jamasurg.2019.0029.
27. Jasmine Z, Samaan Jamil S, Yazan A, Kamran S. Racial disparities in bariatric surgery postoperative weight loss and co-morbidity resolution: a systematic review. Surg Obes Relat Dis. 17(10):1799–823. https://doi.org/10.1016/j.soard.2021.06.001.
28. Wee Christina C, Huskey Karen W, Dragana B-J, Ellen CM, Davis Roger B, MaryBeth H. Sex race and consideration of bariatric surgery among primary care patients with moderate to severe obesity. J Gen Intern Med. 29(1):68–75. https://doi.org/10.1007/s11606-013-2603-1.
29. Ashley O, Juang K, Quiera B, Benjamin S, Carrie MA, Messiah Sarah E. Socioecological factors associated with ethnic disparities in metabolic and bariatric surgery utilization: a qualitative study. Surg Obes Relat Dis. 16(6):786–95. https://doi.org/10.1016/j.soard.2020.01.031.
30. Lee-Shing C, Shervin M, Naoshi H, Huabing Z, Justin BC, Lei Victor J, Alexa R, Clara T, Kimhouy T, Maria S, Alexander T. Patient-provider discussions of bariatric surgery and subsequent weight changes and receipt of bariatric surgery. Obesity. 29(8):1338–46. https://doi.org/10.1002/oby.23183.
31. Assari S, Lankarani M, Caldwell C, Zimmerman M. Fear of neighborhood violence during adolescence predicts development of obesity a decade later: gender differences among African Americans. Arch Trauma Res. 2016;5(2):e31475.
32. Bjorntorp P. Do stress reactions cause abdominal obesity and comorbidities? Obes Rev. 2001;2(2):73–86.
33. U.S. Department of Health and Human Services Office of Minority Health. Diabetes and African Americans. https://minorityhealth.hhs.gov/omh/browse.aspx?lvl=4&lvlid=18
34. Chartbook on Health Care for Blacks. Agency for Healthcare Research and Quality, Rockville. https://www.ahrq.gov/research/findings/nhqrdr/chartbooks/blackhealth/acknow.html

References

35. Becles G, Chou C. Diabetes—United States, 2006 and 2010. MMWR Morb Mortal Wkly Rep. 2013;62(03):99–104.
36. Wedekind Lauren E, Mitchell Cassie M, Andersen Coley C, Knowler William C, Hanson Robert L. Epidemiology of type 2 diabetes in Indigenous communities in the United States. Curr Diab Rep. 21(11) https://doi.org/10.1007/s11892-021-01406-3.
37. Monique A, Michelle S-R, Fang X, Teresa A-M, Michael A, Greenlund Kurt J, Barbour Kamil E. Health disparities among American Indians/Alaska natives—Arizona 2017. MMWR Morb Mortal Wkly Rep. 2018;67(47):1314–8. https://doi.org/10.15585/mmwr.mm6747a4.
38. Godfrey TM, Cordova-Marks Felina M, Desiree J, Forest M, Khadijah B. Metabolic syndrome among American Indian and Alaska native populations: implications for cardiovascular health. Curr Hypertens Rep. 24(5):107–14. https://doi.org/10.1007/s11906-022-01178-5.
39. Ng Maggie CY, Richa S, Jiang L, Palmer Nicholette D, Latchezar D, Jianzhao X, Rasmussen-Torvik Laura J, Zmuda Joseph M, Siscovick David S, Patel Sanjay R, Crook Errol D, Mario S, Chen Yii-Der I, Bertoni Alain G, Mingyao L, Grant Struan FA, Josée D, Meigs James B, Psaty Bruce M, Pankow James S, Langefeld Carl D, Freedman Barry I, Rotter Jerome I, Wilson James G, Bowden Donald W. Transferability and fine mapping of type 2 diabetes loci in African Americans. Diabetes. 2013;62(3):965–76. https://doi.org/10.2337/db12-0266.
40. Ng Maggie CY, Daniel S, Chen BH, Jiang L, Wei-Min C, Guo X, Jiankang L, Bielinski Suzette J, Yanek Lisa R, Nalls Michael A, Comeau Mary E, Rasmussen-Torvik Laura J, Jensen Richard A, Evans Daniel S, Sun Yan V, Ping A, Patel Sanjay R, Lu Y, Jirong L, Armstrong Loren L, Lynne W, Yang L, Snively Beverly M, Palmer Nicholette D, Poorva M, Langefeld Carl D, Keene Keith L, Freedman BI, Mychaleckyj Josyf C, Uma N, Raffel Leslie J, Goodarzi Mark O, Ida CY-D, Taylor Herman A, Adolfo C, Mario S, David C, Pankow James S, Eric B, Adebowale A, Ayo D, Guanjie C, Mathias Rasika A, Dhananjay V, Singleton Andrew B, Zonderman Alan B, Igo Robert P, Sedor John R, Kabagambe Edmond K, Siscovick David S, Barbara MK, Kenneth R, Yongmei L, Wen-Chi H, Wei Z, Bielak Lawrence F, Aldi K, Province Michael A, Bottinger Erwin P, Omri G, Qiuyin C, Zheng W, Blot William J, Lowe William L, Pacheco Jennifer A, Crawford Dana C, Elin G, Rich Stephen S, Geoffrey HM, Xiao-Ou S, Loos Ruth JF, Borecki Ingrid B, Peyser Patricia A, Cummings Steven R, Psaty Bruce M, Myriam F, Iyengar Sudha K, Evans MK, Becker Diane M, Linda KWH, Wilson James G, Rotter Jerome I, Sale Michèle M, Simin L, Rotimi Charles N, Bowden Donald W, Eleftheria Z. Meta-analysis of genome-wide association studies in African Americans provides insights into the genetic architecture of type 2 diabetes. PLoS Genet. 2014;10(8):e1004517. https://doi.org/10.1371/journal.pgen.1004517.
41. Palmer Nicholette D, Ng Maggie CY, Hicks Pamela J, Poorva M, Langefeld Carl D, Freedman Barry I, Bowden Donald W, Giuseppe R. Evaluation of candidate nephropathy susceptibility genes in a genome-wide association study of African American diabetic kidney disease. PLoS One. 2014;9(2):e88273. https://doi.org/10.1371/journal.pone.0088273.
42. Meijian G, Jun M, Keaton Jacob M, Latchezar D, Poorva M, Mary S, Bonomo Jason A, Hicks Pamela J, Freedman Barry I, Bowden Donald W, Ng Maggie CY. Association of kidney structure-related gene variants with type 2 diabetes-attributed end-stage kidney disease in African Americans. Hum Genet. 135(11):1251–62. https://doi.org/10.1007/s00439-016-1714-2.
43. Andy M, Sarah C, Linda G, Cowie Catherine C. Prevalence of and trends in diabetes among adults in the United States 1988–2012. JAMA. 314(10):1021. https://doi.org/10.1001/jama.2015.10029.
44. Mario S, Diez Roux Ana V, Shawn B, Daniel S, Gebreab Samson Y, Wyatt Sharon B, DeMarc H, Marinelle P, Lynette E, Taylor Herman A. The socioeconomic gradient of diabetes prevalence awareness treatment and control among African Americans in the Jackson Heart Study. Ann Epidemiol. 21(12):892–8. https://doi.org/10.1016/j.annepidem.2011.05.006.
45. Brancati FL, Linda KWH, Folsom Aaron R, Watson Robert L, Moyses S. Incident Type 2 diabetes mellitus in African American and White adults. JAMA. 283(17):2253. https://doi.org/10.1001/jama.283.17.2253.

46. Trudy G, Haiying C, Effoe Valery S, Adolfo C, Mercedes C, Kalyani Rita R, Echouffo-Tcheugui Justin B, Joseph Joshua J, Bertoni Alain G. Glucometabolic state transitions: the Jackson Heart Study. Ethn Dis. 2022;32(3):203–12. https://doi.org/10.18865/ed.32.3.203.
47. Mary M, Chrisman Matthew S, Tiffany MA, McDonald Olevia D. Fostering healthy lifestyles in the African American population. Health Educ Behav. 42(1):109–16. https://doi.org/10.1177/1090198114540465.
48. Brian L, Peng L, Crouse Andrew B, Tiffany G, Matthew M, Fernando O, Anath S. Data-driven cluster analysis reveals increased risk for severe insulin-deficient diabetes in black/African Americans. J Clin Endocrinol Metabol. 2024;110(2):387–95. https://doi.org/10.1210/clinem/dgae516.
49. David K. Special considerations of care and risk management for African American patients with type 2 diabetes mellitus. J Natl Med Assoc. 104(5–6):265–73. https://doi.org/10.1016/S0027-9684(15)30158-9.
50. Flaxel CJ, Adelman RA, Bailey ST, Amani F, Jennifer L I, Atma VG, Gui-shuang Y. Diabetic retinopathy Preferred Practice Pattern®. Ophthalmology. 127(1):P66–P145. https://doi.org/10.1016/j.ophtha.2019.09.025.
51. Chuck RS, Dunn Steven P, Flaxel Christina J, Gedde Steven J, Mah Francis S, Miller Kevin M, Wallace David K, Musch David C. Comprehensive adult medical eye evaluation Preferred Practice Pattern®. Ophthalmology. 128(1):P1–P29. https://doi.org/10.1016/j.ophtha.2020.10.024.
52. ElSayed Nuha A, McCoy Rozalina G, Grazia A, Kirthikaa B, Beverly Elizabeth A, Kathaleen BE, Dennis B, Osagie E, Echouffo-Tcheugui Justin B, Laya E, Gaglia Jason L, Rajesh G, Kamlesh K, Rayhan L, Ildiko L, Glenn M, Naushira P, Pekas Elizabeth J, Pilla Scott J, Sarit P, Segal Alissa R, Jeffrie SJ, Stanton Robert C, Bannuru Raveendhara R. 3. Prevention or delay of diabetes and associated comorbidities: standards of care in diabetes—2025. Diabetes Care. 2024;48(Supplement_1):S50–8. https://doi.org/10.2337/dc25-S003.
53. Lee DC, Ta'Loria Y, Koziatek Christian A, Shim Christopher J, Marcela O, Vinson Andrew J, Ravenell Joseph E, Wall Stephen P. Age disparities among patients with type 2 diabetes and associated rates of hospital use and diabetic complications. Prev Chronic Dis. 2019;16 https://doi.org/10.5888/pcd16.180681.
54. ElSayed Nuha A, McCoy Rozalina G, Grazia A, Mandeep B, Kirthikaa B, Beverly Elizabeth A, Kathaleen BE, Dennis B, Echouffo-Tcheugui Justin B, Laya E, Gaglia Jason L, Rajesh G, Monica G, Kamlesh K, Rayhan L, Ildiko L, Glenn M, Neumiller Joshua J, Naushira P, Pekas Elizabeth J, Pilla Scott J, Sarit P, Segal Alissa R, Jeffrie SJ, Stanton Robert C, Bannuru Raveendhara R. 9. Pharmacologic approaches to glycemic treatment: standards of care in diabetes—2025. Diabetes Care. 2024;48(Supplement_1):S181–206. https://doi.org/10.2337/dc25-S009.
55. ElSayed Nuha A, McCoy Rozalina G, Grazia A, Kirthikaa B, Beverly Elizabeth A, Kathaleen BE, Dennis B, Echouffo-Tcheugui Justin B, Laya E, Rajesh G, Kamlesh K, Rayhan L, Ildiko L, Glenn M, Naushira P, Pekas Elizabeth J, Pilla Scott J, Sarit P, Segal Alissa R, Jeffrie SJ, Stanton Robert C, Bannuru Raveendhara R. 11. Chronic kidney disease and risk management: standards of care in diabetes—2025. Diabetes Care. 2024;48(Supplement_1):S239–51. https://doi.org/10.2337/dc25-S011.
56. Das Sandeep R, Everett Brendan M, Birtcher Kim K, Brown Jenifer M, Januzzi James L, Kalyani Rita R, Mikhail K, Melissa M, Morris Pamela B, Neumiller Joshua J, Sperling Laurence S. Expert consensus decision pathway on novel therapies for cardiovascular risk reduction in patients with type 2 diabetes. J Am Coll Cardiol. 2020;76(9):1117–45. https://doi.org/10.1016/j.jacc.2020.05.037.
57. Kunutsor Setor K, Kamlesh K, Samuel S. Racial ethnic and regional differences in the effect of sodium–glucose co-transporter 2 inhibitors and glucagon-like peptide 1 receptor agonists on cardiovascular and renal outcomes: a systematic review and meta-analysis of cardiovascular outcome trials. J R Soc Med. 2025;117(8):267–83. https://doi.org/10.1177/01410768231198442.

58. White W, Cain L, Benjamin E, et al. High-intensity cigarette smoking is associated with incident diabetes mellitus in black adults: the Jackson Heart Study. J Am Heart Assoc. 2018;7(2):e007413.
59. Peitao W, Denis R, Bielak Lawrence F, Feitosa MF, Nora F, Yize L, Yingchang L, Jonathan M, Musani Solomon K, Raymond N, Sridharan R, Rose Lynda M, Karen S, Smith Albert V, Tajuddin Salman M, Dina V, Najaf A, Arnett Donna K, Bottinger Erwin P, Ayse D, Florez Jose C, Mohsen G, Harris Tamara B, Launer Lenore J, Jingmin L, Jun L, Mook-Kanamori Dennis O, Murray Alison D, Nalls Mike A, Peyser Patricia A, Uitterlinden André G, Trudy V, Claude B, Daniel C, Adolfo C, de Mutsert R, Evans Michele K, Vilmundur G, Caroline H, Linda K, Kardia Sharon LR, Charles K, Loos Ruth JF, Province Michael M, Tuomo R, Susan R, Ridker Paul M, Rotter Jerome I, David S, Smith Blair H, van Duijn C, Zonderman Alan B, Rao DC, Wilson James G, Josée D, Meigs James B, Ching-Ti L, Vassy Jason L, David M. Smoking-by-genotype interaction in type 2 diabetes risk and fasting glucose. PLoS One. 2020;15(5):e0230815. https://doi.org/10.1371/journal.pone.0230815.
60. Zhang L, Curhan G, Hu F, Rimm E, Forman J. Association between passive and active smoking and incident type 2 diabetes in women. Diabetes Care. 2011;34(4):892–7.
61. Foy C, Bell R, Farmer D, Goff D, Wagenknecht L. Smoking and incidence of diabetes among US adults. Diabetes Care. 2005;28(10):2501–7.
62. ElSayed Nuha A, McCoy RG, Grazia A, Kirthikaa B, Beverly EA, Kathaleen BE, Dennis B, Echouffo-Tcheugui JB, Barbara E, Laya E, Rajesh G, Mohamed H, Kamlesh K, Rayhan L, Ildiko L, Glenn M, Middelbeek Roeland JW, Naushira P, Pekas EJ, Pilla SJ, Sarit P, Segal AR, Jeffrie SJ, Stanton RC, Tanenbaum ML, Patti U, Bannuru RR. 5. Facilitating positive health behaviors and Well-being to improve health outcomes: standards of care in diabetes—2025. Diabetes Care. 2024;48(Supplement_1):S86–S127. https://doi.org/10.2337/dc25-S005.
63. Herman W, Cohen R. Racial and ethnic differences in the relationship between HbA1c and blood glucose: implications for the diagnosis of diabetes. J Clin Metab. 2012;97(4):1067–72.
64. Saaddine J, Fagot-Campagna A, Rolka D, et al. Distribution of HbA1c levels for children and young adults in the U.S.: third National Health and nutrition examination survey. Diabetes Care. 2002;25(8):1326–30.
65. Eldeirawi K, Lipton R. Predictors of hemoglobin A1c in a national sample of nondiabetic children: the Third National Health and Nutrition Examination Survey, 1988–1994. Am J Epidemiol. 2003;157(7):624–32.
66. Nathan DM, Herman WH, Larkin ME, Heidi K-S, Hiba AA, Ahmann AJ, Janet B-F, Hsia DS, Tasma H, Mary J, Arends VL, Butera NM, Rosin SP, Lachin JM, Naji Y, Everett BM, Abdouch I, Bahtiyar G, Brantley P, Broyles FE, Canaris G, Copeland P, Craine JJ, Fein WL, Gliwa A, Hope L, Lee MS, Meiners R, Meiners V, O'Neal H, Park JE, Sacerdote A, Sledge E, Soni L, Steppel-Reznik J, Turchin A. Relationship between average glucose levels and HbA1c differs across racial groups: a substudy of the GRADE randomized trial. Diabetes Care. 2024;47(12):2155–63. https://doi.org/10.2337/dc24-1362.
67. Sacks DB, Mark A, Bakris GL, Bruns DE, Horvath AR, Åke L, Metzger BE, Nathan DM, Sue KM. Guidelines and recommendations for laboratory analysis in the diagnosis and management of diabetes mellitus. Diabetes Care. 2023;46(10):e151–99. https://doi.org/10.2337/dci23-0036.
68. Marie-France H, Costas C, Kathleen J, Sharon E, Steven K, Hill GS, Samuel D-J, Mather Kieren J, Luchsinger José A, Enrique CA, Elizabeth B-C, Knowler William C, Florez Jose C, Herman William H. Genetic ancestry markers and difference in A1c between African-American and White in the diabetes prevention program. J Clin Endocrinol Metab. 2018;104:328. https://doi.org/10.1210/jc.2018-01416.
69. Karter AJ, Parker MM, Moffet HH, Gilliam LK. Racial and ethnic differences in the association between mean glucose and hemoglobin A1c. Diabetes Technol Ther. 25(10):697–704. https://doi.org/10.1089/dia.2023.0153.
70. Ziemer D, Kolm P, Weintraub W, et al. Glucose-independent, black-white differences in hemoglobin A1c levels: a cross-sectional analysis of 2 studies. Ann Intern Med. 2010;152(12):770–7.

71. Chloé S, Aaron L, Raffield Laura M, Peitao W, de Vries Paul S, Daniel DC, Xiuqing G, Huichun X, Yongmei L, Xiuwen Z, Yao H, Brody Jennifer A, Goodarzi Mark O, Hidalgo Bertha A, Highland Heather M, Deepti J, Ching-Ti L, Naik Rakhi P, O'Connell Jeffrey R, Perry James A, Porneala Bianca C, Elizabeth S, Jennifer W, Psaty Bruce M, Curran Joanne E, Peralta Juan M, John B, Charles K, Rasika M, Johnson Andrew D, Reiner Alexander P, Mitchell Braxton D, Adrienne CL, Vasan Ramachandran S, Adolfo C, Morrison Alanna C, Eric B, Rotter Jerome I, Rich Stephen S, Manning Alisa K, Josée D, Meigs James B. Impact of rare and common genetic variants on diabetes diagnosis by hemoglobin A1c in multi-ancestry cohorts: the trans-omics for precision medicine program. Am J Human Genet. 105(4):706–18. https://doi.org/10.1016/j.ajhg.2019.08.010.
72. Lacy M, Wellenius G, Sumner A, et al. Association of sickle cell trait with hemoglobin A1c in African Americans. JAMA. 2017;217(5):507–15.
73. Keoki WL, Badri P, Ahmedani Brian K, Peterson Edward L, Wells Karen E, Esteban GB, Lanfear David E. Differing effects of metformin on glycemic control by race-ethnicity. J Clin Endocrinol Metab. 99(9):3160–8. https://doi.org/10.1210/jc.2014-1539.
74. Baojun W, Wah YS, Shujie X, Fei X, Sridhar Sneha B, Mao Y, Samantha H, Whitney C, Lanfear David E, Hedderson Monique M, Giacomini Kathleen M, Keoki WL. Genome-wide association study identifies pharmacogenomic variants associated with metformin glycemic response in African American patients with type 2 diabetes. Diabetes Care. 2023;47(2):208–15. https://doi.org/10.2337/dc22-2494.
75. Zhang C, Zhang R. More effective glycaemic control by metformin in African Americans than in Whites in the prediabetic population. Diabetes Metab. 41(2):173–5. https://doi.org/10.1016/j.diabet.2015.01.003.
76. Huang Elbert S, Brown Sydney ES, Nidhi T, Lisabeth C, Edward F, Bernard E, Meltzer David O. Racial/ethnic differences in concerns about current and future medications among patients with type 2 diabetes. Diabetes Care. 32(2):311–6. https://doi.org/10.2337/dc08-1307.
77. Giovanni Antonio S. Optimizing metformin therapy in practice: tailoring therapy in specific patient groups to improve tolerability efficacy and outcomes. Diabetes Obes Metab. 26(S3):42–54. https://doi.org/10.1111/dom.15749.
78. Ferdinand KC, Leo S, Afshin S. Design of a 24-week trial of empagliflozin once daily in hypertensive black/African American patients with type 2 diabetes mellitus. Curr Med Res Opin. 34(2):361–7. https://doi.org/10.1080/03007995.2017.1405800.
79. Maggs D, Shen L, Strobel S, Brown D, Kolterman O, Weyer C. Effect of pramlintide on A1C and body weight in insulin-treated African Americans and Hispanics with type 2 diabetes: a pooled post hoc analysis. Metabolism. 52(12):1638–42. https://doi.org/10.1016/j.metabol.2003.06.003.
80. Ard J, Cannon A, Lewis CE, Lofton H, Vang Skjøth T, Stevenin B, Pi-Sunyer X. Diabetes Obes Metab. 18(4):430–5. https://doi.org/10.1111/dom.12632.
81. Shomali ME, Ørsted DD, Cannon AJ. Efficacy and safety of liraglutide a once-daily human glucagon-like peptide-1 receptor agonist in African-American people with type 2 diabetes: a meta-analysis of sub-population data from seven phase III trials. Diabetic Med. 34(2):197–203. https://doi.org/10.1111/dme.13185.
82. Cyrus DS, Bertrand C, Satish G, Nanna L, Andrea N, Vivian F. Efficacy and safety of Semaglutide for type 2 diabetes by race and ethnicity: a post hoc analysis of the SUSTAIN trials. J Clin Endocrinol Metabol. 2019;105(2):543–56. https://doi.org/10.1210/clinem/dgz072.
83. Shenolikar R, Balkrishnan R, Camacho F, Whitmire J, Anderson R. Race and medication adherence in medicaid enrollees with type 2 diabetes. J Natl Med Assoc. 2006;98(7):1071–7.
84. Kyanko K, Franklin R, Angell S. Adherence to chronic disease medications among New York City medicaid participants. J Urban Health. 2013;90(2):323–8.
85. Bockwoldt D, Staffileno B, Coke L, et al. Understanding experiences of diabetes medications among African Americans living with type 2 diabetes. J Transcult Nurs. 2017;28(4):363–71.

References

86. Walker R, Smalls B, Hernandez-Tejada M, Campbell J, Davis K, Egede L. Effect of diabetes fatalism on medicaition adherence and self-care behaviors in adults with diabetes. Gen Hosp Psychiatry. 2012;34(6):598–603.
87. Bains S, Egede L. Associations between health literacy, diabetes knowledge, self-care behaviors, and glycemic control in a low income population with type 2 diabetes. Diabetes Technol Ther. 2011;13(3):335–41.
88. Wagenknecht Lynne E, Lawrence Jean M, Scott I, Jensen Elizabeth T, Dana D, Liese Angela D, Dolan Lawrence M, Shah Amy S, Anna B, Katherine S, Santica M, Kristi R, Catherine P, Giuseppina I, Jasmin D. Trends in incidence of youth-onset type 1 and type 2 diabetes in the USA 2002–18: results from the population-based SEARCH for Diabetes in Youth study. Lancet Diabetes Endocrinol. 2025;11(4):242–50. https://doi.org/10.1016/S2213-8587(23)00025-6.
89. The Writing Group for the SEARCH for Diabetes in Youth Study Group. Incidence of diabetes in youth in the United States. JAMA. 297(24):2716. https://doi.org/10.1001/jama.297.24.2716.
90. Shivani A, Kanapka Lauren G, Raymond Jennifer K, Ashby W, Andrea G-G, Davida K, Redondo Maria J, Rickels Michael R, Shah Viral N, Ashley B, Jeffrey G, Verdejo Alandra S, Gal Robin L, Steven W, Long Judith A. Racial-ethnic inequity in young adults with type 1 diabetes. J Clin Endocrinol Metab. 2020;105(8):e2960–9. https://doi.org/10.1210/clinem/dgaa236.
91. The Dietary Guidelines for Americans 2015–2020. National Diabetes Education Program. https://www.cdc.gov/diabetes/ndep/pdfs/dietary_guidelines_slides.pdf. Accessed 9 May 2019.
92. Mozaffarian D. Dietary and policy priorities for cardiovascular disease, diabetes, and obesity. A comprehensive review. Circulation. 2016;133:187–225.
93. Yancey A, Cole B, Brown R, et al. A cross-sectional prevalence study of ethnically targeted and general audience outdoor obesity-related advertising. Milibank Q. 2009;87(1):155–84.
94. Outley CW, Taddese A. A content analysis of health and physical activity messages marketed to African American children during after-school television programming. Arch Pediatr Adolesc Med. 2006;160(4):432–5.

Chapter 6
A Precision Medicine Approach to Cancer in African Americans

Contents

6.1	Breast Cancer	109
6.2	Colon Cancer	112
6.3	Prostate Cancer	115
6.4	Lung Cancer	117
	6.4.1 Equitable Tobacco Cessation Advice	119
	6.4.2 African American Smoking Paradox	120
6.5	Multiple Myeloma	121
6.6	"Chemotherapy"	123
References		125

African Americans have the highest death rates and shortest survival rates of any racial/ethnic group in the US for most cancers (see Fig. 6.1). Several factors contribute to these disparities, including socioeconomic differences, limited access to healthcare, and a higher prevalence of risk factors, including diet, smoking, and higher obesity rates. A precision medicine approach that "considers the genetics, environment, and lifestyle" [1] to cancer prevention, diagnosis, and treatment can potentially eliminate many gaps. Genetics is frequently ignored in deference to "race being a social construct," but validated research continues to show that African Americans are more likely to have specific genetic differences and mutations that increase their risk of certain types of cancer. Additionally, African Americans often face barriers to early detection and treatment, leading to later-stage diagnoses. Tailored and nuanced cancer screening recommendations are frequently advanced for African Americans, but in-the-trenches clinicians rarely get clear directives. Finally, African Americans are more likely to receive inadequate cancer treatment, leading to poorer overall outcomes. Figure 6.1 shows the latest cancer mortality differences by race and/or ethnicity.

Compared to European American men, African American men had a 6% higher cancer incidence rate but a 19% higher mortality rate [2]. Multiple myeloma,

© The Author(s), under exclusive license to Springer Nature Switzerland AG 2025
G. L. Hall, *Precision Medicine for African Americans*,
https://doi.org/10.1007/978-3-031-95774-1_6

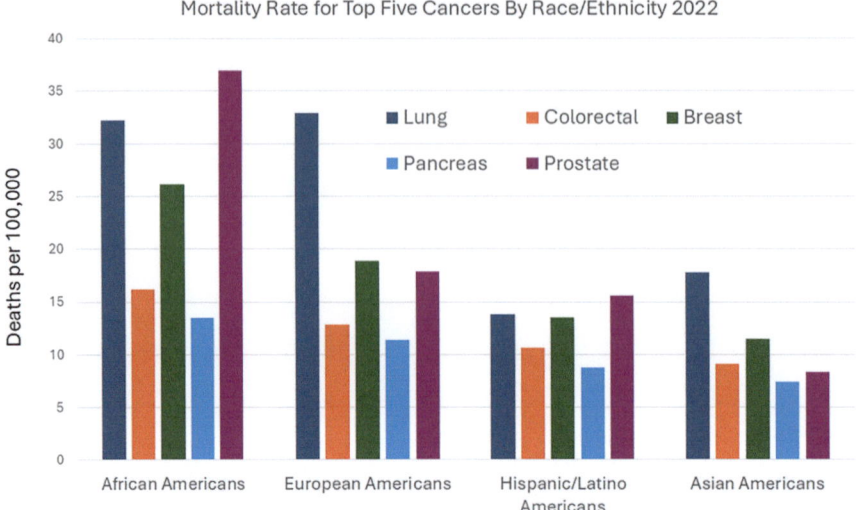

Fig. 6.1 U.S. Cancer Statistics Working Group. U.S. Cancer Statistics Data Visualizations Tool. (U.S. Department of Health and Human Services, Centers for Disease Control and Prevention and National Cancer Institute; https://www.cdc.gov/cancer/dataviz, released in June 2024)

stomach cancer, and prostate cancer had twofold higher mortality rates [2]. The overall cancer mortality disparity is narrowing between African American and European American men because of a more dramatic drop in African American men for lung and prostate cancers. However, the decline in prostate cancer mortality in African American men slowed after recommendations from multiple sources suggested that screening for prostate cancer was more harmful due to prostate cancer's indolent nature in the majority population [2]. Prostate cancer deaths declined 5% annually from 2010 through 2014 and then slowed to 1.3% from 2015 through 2019, likely reflecting the 5% annual increase in advanced-stage diagnoses since 2012 [2] when clinicians stopped or slowed their screening for prostate cancer. This change in screening reflected a "best practice" recommendation for the overall US population, but African American men suffered disproportionately from the more advanced prostate cancer disease at diagnosis and the ensuing higher mortality.

The incidence rate of cancer in African American women is 8% lower than in European American women, but the mortality rate is 12% higher; in addition, mortality rates are twofold higher for endometrial cancer and 41% higher for breast cancer despite similar or lower incidence rates. As a result of later diagnosis (57% localized stage vs. 67% in European American women) and lower 5-year survival (82% vs. 92%, respectively), breast cancer disparities are significant across all stage categories [2]. As of 2019, breast cancer surpassed lung cancer as the leading cause of cancer death among African American women [2].

Genetic predispositions can play a significant role in increasing cancer risk as certain inherited mutations can make individuals more susceptible to developing specific types of cancer. For example, mutations in genes such as BRCA1 and

BRCA2, which occur at a higher rate in African American women, have been linked to higher risks of breast and ovarian cancers [3]. Hereditary nonpolyposis colorectal cancer (HNPCC or Lynch syndrome) is another example of a significant genetic cancer predisposition. It is caused by mutations in certain genes that increase the risk of colon and rectal cancers. HNPCC is most commonly associated with people of Eastern European descent, occurring in 1 in 518 people, but a recent study found the highest prevalence of genetic risk in African Americans (1 in 299), and the vast majority had no idea they were at increased risk and had never previously been tested [4].

Familial, or inherited, prostate cancer has been recognized for decades, but a lack of specific predisposition genes has historically limited the use of genetic testing for this condition. However, in recent years, progress has been made in identifying genetic risk factors for familial prostate cancer. One study found an increased occurrence of prostate cancer-related "variants of uncertain significance" in African Americans (7.3%) compared to European Americans (2.2%) [5]. These and other discoveries will further enable the development of genetic tests to identify those at risk for developing an array of cancers. The persistent disparity of research on genetic predispositions, particularly in African Americans, has been a disadvantage in terms of timely diagnosis, prevention, and treatment. There is also a substantial gap in clinician-generated referrals for genetic testing [3], even among patients with strong family histories of cancer or who have had cancer themselves. Clinicians are generally aware of African Americans' increased risk for cancer, but that should not preclude an investigation into genetic drivers of these risks. This lack of access to genetic testing can lead to delays in diagnosis and treatment, which logically can have a significant negative impact on patient outcomes. Additionally, the documented gap in genetic testing referrals [6–8] can lead to a lack of access to preventive care, and health education within impacted families.

6.1 Breast Cancer

The incidence of breast cancer is highest in European American women at 139 per 100,000, while the African American rate is slightly lower at 132 per 100,000 (see Fig. 6.2). In sharp contrast, the breast cancer mortality for African American women is 26 deaths per 100,000 women, while European American women have 19 deaths per 100,000 women. Nationally, African American women were 43% more likely to die from breast cancer than their European American counterparts, yet the disease occurs less [9].

Yang and colleagues at Emory University suggested that the poor clinical outcomes in African American women with breast cancer can be associated with the abnormal elevation of individual gene expression. They proposed that this abnormal expression could be due to genetic factors, epigenetic modifications, or environmental factors [10].

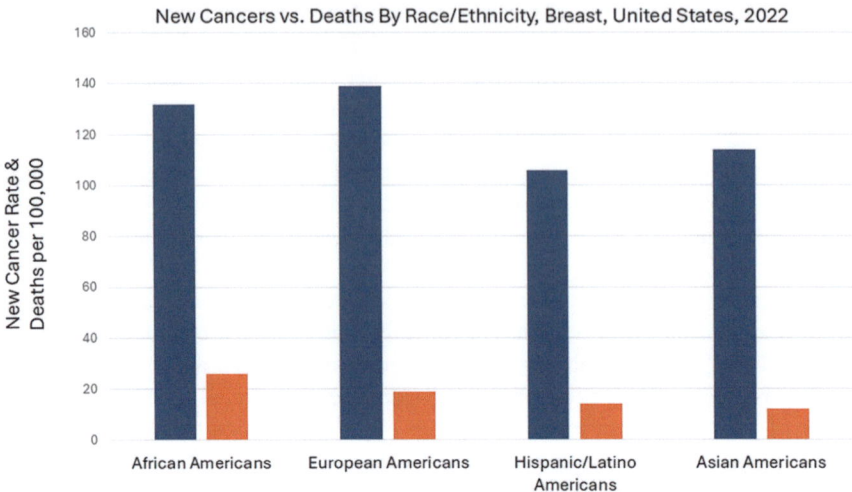

Fig. 6.2 New breast cancer and deaths by race/ethnicity, Breast Cancer U.S. Cancer Statistics Working Group. U.S. Cancer Statistics Data Visualizations Tool. (U.S. Department of Health and Human Services, Centers for Disease Control and Prevention and National Cancer Institute; https://www.cdc.gov/cancer/dataviz, released in June 2024)

We found that more than 30% of all protein-coding genes are differentially expressed in White and African American breast cancer patients. We have determined a set of 32 genes whose overexpression in African American patients strongly correlates with decreased survival of African American but not White breast cancer patients. Among those genes, the overexpression of mitogen-activated protein kinase kinase 3 (MKK3) has one of the most dramatic and race-specific negative impacts on the survival of African American patients, specifically with triple-negative breast cancer. We found that MKK3 can promote the TNBC tumorigenesis in African American patients in part by activating the epithelial-to-mesenchymal transition induced by master regulator MYC. [10]

Triple-negative breast cancers (TNBCs) are a breast cancer subgroup characterized by their lack of expression of estrogen receptor (ER), progesterone receptor (PR), and human epidermal growth factor receptor 2 (HER2). TNBC is unique in that its lack of receptor expression coincides with a poor prognosis related to chemotherapy resistance, aggressive behavior, and more frequent cancer recurrences. African American women are disproportionately affected by triple-negative breast cancer compared to other races or ethnicities. They tend to have a higher incidence of TNBC and are often diagnosed at a younger age with more aggressive forms of the disease. This disparity is likely influenced by a combination of genetic, socioeconomic, and healthcare access factors. Recent research suggests that genetic factors, such as mutations in the BRCA1 and BRCA2 genes, may contribute to the higher incidence of TNBC in African American women. Additionally, variations in other genes associated with breast cancer risk, like PALB2 and TP53, could also play a role.

African American women are also more likely to have a family history of breast cancer, which may also contribute to the increased risk of TNBC in this population.

Additionally, environmental factors, such as diet and lifestyle, may also play a role in the increased risk of TNBC in African American women. Focusing on prevention strategies for TNBC could involve increasing awareness and education about genetic testing for high-risk genes like BRCA1 and BRCA2 [11]. Early detection programs and regular screenings tailored to African American women may help identify TNBC at an earlier, more treatable stage. Additionally, lifestyle interventions, such as promoting a healthy diet and regular physical activity, could reduce risk factors associated with the development of TNBC.

A study of almost 20,000 cancer patients of the Southwest Oncology Statistical Center found results that "when controlled for uniform stage, treatment, and follow up, African American sex-specific cancers (breast, ovarian, and prostate) still did worse" [12]. The startling nature of this outcome might initially suggest that clinicians are powerless to have an impact on these cancers, but in reality, more vigorous surveillance and research, coupled with more aggressive therapy, is the simple answer. For breast cancer, most studies verify that increased mammography, chemotherapy, and hormone therapy (if indicated) will lead to decreased mortality.

There is almost uniform consensus that obesity adds to all-cause mortality in patients with breast cancer [13, 14], and given the increased obesity in African American women, the worsened outcomes in this population may, at least partially, be explained by this. Add the increased mortality and morbidity of breast cancer to the long list of reasons for weight loss in your obese African American patients.

The American College of Radiology recently recommended that African American and Ashkenazi Jewish women have a breast cancer "risk assessment by age 25 to determine if screening earlier than age 40 is needed" [15]. The presence of the BRCA gene, a history of any breast cancer, ductal carcinoma in situ (DCIS) or lobular carcinoma in situ (LCIS), or previous radiation therapy to the chest for treatment of Hodgkin lymphoma dramatically increases the risk. The screening begins with the demographics of age and race/ethnicity (older age and African American race conveying higher risk). Other factors in the risk assessment include age at first menstrual period (age 11 or earlier conveying increased risk), age at birth of first child (older age conveying higher risk), and the number of first-degree relatives with breast cancer [15]. It has been well established that African American women have on average a younger age of first menses [16], so documenting this historical risk factor as well as parity details (with age) and breast-feeding history (breast-feeding is protective) [17] should all be documented in their record.

A team of researchers at Stanford looked at over 2700 women with breast cancer and examined their reproductive characteristics and breast cancer risk [18]. They confirmed the risks listed above, as well as a curious association of increased parity, which is usually protective, coupled with lower breast-feeding rates in African Americans, resulting in an increased breast cancer risk. African American women historically have the lowest breast-feeding rates and duration [19].

> Breast-feeding is likely the only reproductive risk factor for breast cancer that is potentially modifiable. Efforts focused on improving knowledge on the benefits of breast-feeding and creating a more supportive environment that facilitates breast-feeding could have major impact on lowering breast cancer risk for all subtypes, particularly among premenopausal

African American women who are at higher risk. Breast-feeding disparities are tied at multiple levels to social determinants of health that impose barriers to breast-feeding, particularly among African American women (e.g., shorter parental leave; differential access to breast-feeding programs and lactation support; limited accommodations for pumping and storing breast milk at work; and historical and cultural factors. Effective primary breast cancer prevention efforts focused on increasing breast-feeding need to address these barriers among African American women and implement tailored approaches that overcome them. [18]

Among African American women, increased knowledge of the precise benefits and detriments of seemingly innocuous life decisions (like personal size, breast-feeding, or the age of child-bearing) can have ramifications down the road, particularly if a family history of breast cancer exists. In these cases, early detection with screening earlier than age 40 can lead to improved outcomes.

False perceptions of the diagnosis of "cancer" can negatively impact outcomes and decrease engagement of African American women. A study from Drew University of Medicine and Science looked at perceptions about cancer and early detection in African American women.

> Given that 5-year survival rates range from 84% to 93% for all three cancers (breast, cervical, and colorectal) if detected early, our data suggest that a substantial proportion of African American women in South Los Angeles are not aware of the benefits of early detection, particularly for colorectal and cervical cancers. For these two types of cancers, almost one out of two African American women in our study believed that chances of survival are fair or poor, even if the cancer was detected early. Our findings confirm results from previous studies that have identified fatalistic attitudes towards cancer outcomes among African American women and the attitude that cancer is a death sentence. [20]

Patient education involving the specifics of why a screening test is done and what advantage is gleaned is essential when ordering a test. Frequently, African Americans are not aware of the true value of finding a cancer early versus just "finding a cancer." Many have the (perfectly understandable) perspective that they "do not want to find a cancer in them" and the benefit of finding the cancer early is lost on many because of the fatalistic misconceptions they hold. Explain the benefits and what is avoided by having a mammogram, Pap test, or colonoscopy early and the dramatic differences in survival from finding localized cancer versus one that has spread. These conversations, although time-consuming, can also be life-saving down the road.

6.2 Colon Cancer

African American men and women continue to have higher colorectal cancer incidence and mortality rates and are diagnosed at more advanced stages than European Americans (see Fig. 6.3). Even when adjustments are made for socioeconomic status, African Americans still have significantly lower screening [21]. The colon cancer incidence and death rate is so high in the African American community that the American College of Gastroenterology recommended 20 years ago that screening in

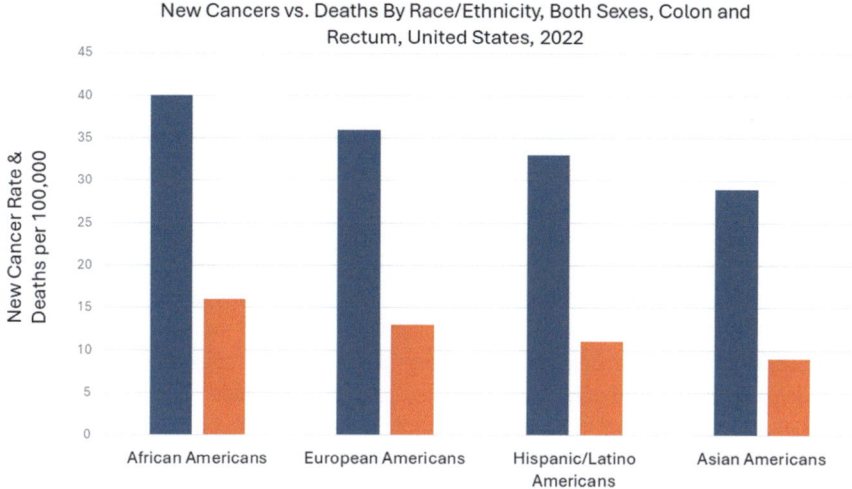

Fig. 6.3 U.S. Cancer Statistics Working Group. U.S. Cancer Statistics Data Visualizations Tool. (U.S. Department of Health and Human Services, Centers for Disease Control and Prevention and National Cancer Institute; https://www.cdc.gov/cancer/dataviz, released in June 2024)

African Americans begin at age 45 rather than age 50, which in the past had been the recommendation for the rest of the US population [22]. Updated recommendations now include universally starting colorectal cancer screening at 45, which will inadvertently also help African Americans [23].

This recommendation was confirmed by Paquette et al., who did a retrospective database review of all patients with colon cancer from 2000 through 2011, and given the cancer stage at discovery, he concluded that African Americans would benefit significantly from earlier surveillance [24]. The lower screening rate in African Americans has also been postulated as a cause for finding more advanced cancers upon diagnosis, but researchers are also looking into other causes for these more aggressive cancers. Studies also showed an increased occurrence in African Americans for right-sided colon cancer tumors, prompting recommendations against sigmoidoscopy in these patients because a significant number of tumors would be missed [25]. That recommendation, which was ratified by the American College of Gastroenterology, was issued in 2005:

> The committee recommends colonoscopy as a "first line" screening procedure for colorectal cancer for African Americans rather than the flexible sigmoidoscopy because of the high overall risk and as well as some evidence that African Americans have more right-sided cancers and polyps. March 21, 2005 American College of Gastroenterology. [22]

Because most colorectal cancers progressed from colorectal adenomas, screening has continued to save lives. A recent study showed that concerted efforts have nearly erased colon cancer screening disparities in African Americans [26, 27], and the addition of alternative means of screening beyond colonoscopy has helped greatly. Multitarget stool DNA testing (DNA-FIT), marketed as Cologuard®, was approved for use in the US in 2014 as an equitable alternative to colonoscopy [28], and blood testing for colon cancer was approved in July 2024 but has not been widely adopted by insurance companies [29, 30]. As primary care clinicians and insurances shift their attention from treatment to prevention, the potential impact financially, in terms of lives saved, and suffering prevented, becomes palpable.

A large study looking at over 60,000 Medicare recipients found that interval colorectal cancer after a screening colonoscopy was more common in African American patients and it occurred more frequently with gastroenterologists with high polyp detection rates [31]. The assumption is gastroenterologists with lower polyp detection rates could have missed precancerous lesions at the original colonoscopy and are the reason for some of these new cancers being found. Another contributing factor is faster-growing interval cancers that aggressively grew in between procedures and presumably needed sooner surveillance than occurred. The study also suggested that screening parameters may need to be adjusted based on race in order to minimize the added cancer risk.

Spending the time to plan for follow-up colonoscopies in African Americans more critically may show benefit mainly when a procedure found numerous polyps; the more polyps that were found, the more that may have been missed.

Studies have found that trained patient navigators (tailored navigation) help patients with cancer screening options and increase adherence particularly well with African Americans [32]. In addition, leaving the options freely open for the patients to choose (colonoscopy, CT colonography, or FIT DNA, etc.) versus strongly stressing one particular option improved completion with African Americans [33].

Computer-delivered tailored interventions with African Americans have also been reviewed in a number of studies, and most have shown a significant positive impact in changed perception of colorectal screening or actual screening behavior [34, 35]. As discussed later in the book, presentations that are delivered in the form of stories connect better, are easier to remember, and tend to more positively impact behavior. With more use of electronic medical records, having a computer screen in the exam room on which to present an educational video is becoming less of a barrier. Tailoring the video, as much as possible, to the specifics of the patients' history also helps ultimate success. Showing a video tailored to address known African American preconceptions and discussing the various screening options and outcomes provide another objective source of useful information that the patient can add to your thoughtful advice.

When talking about colon cancer screening, it is prudent practice to also talk about preventive diet measures. A diet that lowers colon cancer risk typically includes high-fiber foods such as fruits, vegetables, whole grains, and beans. Reducing red and processed meat intake, maintaining a healthy weight, and incorporating plenty of antioxidants from sources like berries and nuts can also be beneficial. Additionally, staying hydrated and limiting alcohol consumption are significant dietary considerations.

6.3 Prostate Cancer

Prostate cancer is notably prevalent among African American men, who have a 70% higher incidence rate compared to European American men (see Fig. 6.4). This demographic also experiences a mortality rate that is approximately double that of other racial groups [36]. Despite the higher incidence and mortality rates, African American men are less likely to receive definitive treatments such as radical prostatectomy or radiation therapy compared to their European American counterparts [37, 38]. This disparity persists even in equal-access healthcare settings, although the gap is somewhat reduced [39]. Overall, the 5-year survival rate for prostate cancer in the United States is nearly 98%, indicating that most men diagnosed with the disease survive at least 5 years after diagnosis [36]. However, survival rates can vary significantly based on factors such as diagnosis stage and healthcare access. Early detection and effective treatment are crucial in improving these outcomes for all men.

Several studies have identified specific genetic variants that contribute to prostate cancer risk and aggressiveness in this population. For instance, a meta-analysis of genome-wide association studies (GWAS) identified nine novel susceptibility loci for prostate cancer, seven of which were either unique to or more common in men of African ancestry. These include an African-specific stop-gain variant in the prostate-specific gene anoctamin 7 (ANO7) [40]. Another study found novel risk-associated alleles on chromosomes 13q34 and 22q12, which are specific to men of African ancestry. These alleles were associated with a significantly increased

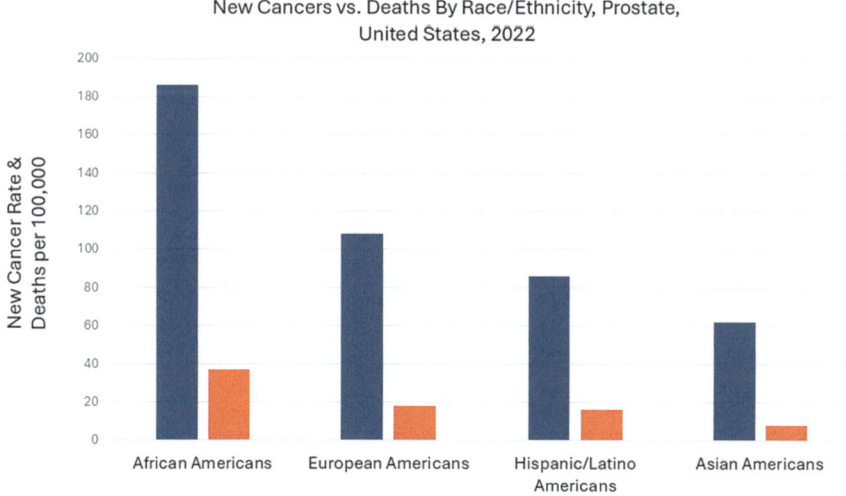

Fig. 6.4 Prostate cancer new and deaths by race/ethnicity. U.S. Cancer Statistics Working Group. U.S. Cancer Statistics Data Visualizations Tool. (U.S. Department of Health and Human Services, Centers for Disease Control and Prevention and National Cancer Institute; https://www.cdc.gov/cancer/dataviz, released in June 2024)

prostate cancer risk [41]. Additionally, "genetic hitchhiking" and "population bottlenecks" have been suggested to contribute to the elevated prostate cancer risks in men of African descent, with certain single nucleotide polymorphisms (SNPs) driving these disparities [42]. Moreover, a germline variant at 8q24 has been shown to contribute to familial clustering of prostate cancer in men of African ancestry, with significant associations with earlier age at diagnosis and more aggressive disease [43]. Certain genetic variations, such as mutations in the BRCA1 and BRCA2 genes, are more prevalent in African Americans and can also increase the risk of prostate cancer [44].

Financially, finding an aggressive cancer later in stage is costlier to society than finding it earlier. Advanced cancers put a serious strain on our medical system and our ability to distribute limited healthcare dollars. So what is the sense in screening these high-risk, high-cost diseases less? A commonly held perception is that prostate cancer is an indolent disease and most that get it die from other unrelated causes. While this may be the case across multiple populations, prostate cancer occurs earlier, is more aggressive, and ultimately kills African American men at a much higher rate.

In a stunning move, the United States Preventive Services Task Force (USPSTF) issued guidelines recommending that all male patients, irrespective of race, no longer be routinely screened for prostate cancer with a prostate-specific antigen (PSA) test [45]. An amended guideline issued in May 2018 suggests that men age 55–69 engage in an individualized decision-making process with their physician. At the time of this writing, the USPSTF was in the final stages of reviewing its recommendations yet again, and given multiple other urology organizations having specific recommendations for African American men, more personalized guidelines should be forthcoming [46].

The course of prostate cancer has been shown to be different in African American men; prostate cancer volume is greater in African American men, and advanced metastatic prostate cancer occurs at a stunning 4:1 ratio when compared to European American men [47]. The more aggressive nature of prostate cancer in African American men has prompted some to think the cancer has an augmented growth rate. Because of this increased growth rate, African American men present at a later stage of disease than age-matched European American patients. African American men also have higher PSA values and higher PSA density when compared to European Americans, and some have suggested this is linked to a higher tumor burden [48].

The American Urological Association has listed African American race as a risk factor for prostate cancer:

> The Panel recognizes that certain subgroups of men age 40 to 54 years may realize added benefit from earlier screening. For example, men at increased risk for prostate cancer, such as those with a strong family history or those of African-American race, may benefit from earlier detection, given their higher incidence of disease. [49]

Statements such as these are found within urologic guideline summaries that essentially advise against widespread PSA screening, but if your patient population is African American, an entirely different screening approach is "assumed" due to your knowledge of the prostate cancer difference in African Americans.

By not acknowledging that different populations require different approaches in America, well-meaning initiatives may actually cause more suffering. The overarching message in most urological guidelines is to decrease PSA screening, and the parenthetical exception is … but not in African Americans and people with strong family histories. Unfortunately, these parenthetical exceptions are frequently lost to most readers, and the overarching message (stop PSA measurements) is reported in media and summary statements for wide distribution.

Several lifestyle suggestions can lower your patient's risk for prostate cancer. Regular exercise, maintaining a healthy weight, and consuming a diet rich in fruits, vegetables, and whole grains can help reduce the risk of prostate cancer. Additionally, quitting smoking and limiting alcohol intake are crucial lifestyle changes that can contribute to overall health and lower cancer risk. Limiting red meat and processed foods can also lower prostate cancer risk [50]. Vitamin D deficiency has been hypothesized to contribute to higher prostate cancer risk in African American men [50]. Due to higher levels of melanin, individuals with darker skin have a reduced capacity to synthesize vitamin D from sunlight, potentially leading to lower vitamin D levels. Some studies suggest that adequate vitamin D levels may offer a protective effect against prostate cancer, highlighting the importance of addressing vitamin D deficiency as part of prostate cancer prevention strategies in this population. Encouraging patients to adopt these healthy habits can significantly improve their overall well-being and reduce their risk of developing prostate cancer.

Prostate cancer in African American men is the most prevalent cancer and the second most common cause of overall cancer deaths. When compared to other racial/ethnic groups, we see an entirely different prevalence and mortality rate. Given that there is no cure for metastatic prostate cancer, finding it sooner in populations at risk for early metastasis is the only logical course.

Screen for prostate cancer annually starting at age 40 with a prostate-specific antigen (PSA) lab test in your African American male population.

6.4 Lung Cancer

While the rate of lung cancer in African Americans looks comparable to European Americans at first glance, with African American and European American men having an identical 1 in 13 probability of diagnosis (and European women having higher incidence of 1 in 15 versus 1 in 19 for African American women), the age-adjusted lung cancer incidence is 32% higher in African Americans (see Fig. 6.5) [51]. Fundamentally, lung cancer is diagnosed 3 years earlier in African Americans [52]. In addition, African Americans are diagnosed more often with lung cancer in intermittent and light smokers when compared to European Americans despite the fact that, on average, they start smoking later in life.

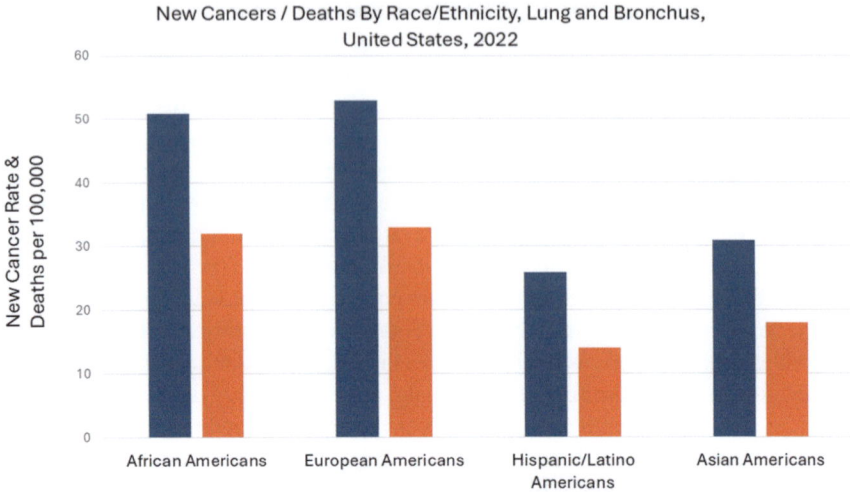

Fig. 6.5 New cancers/deaths by race/ethnicity, lung, and bronchus, United States, 2022

African Americans exhibit distinct lung cancer genetic mutational profiles. For instance, mutations in genes such as STK11 and RB1 are more prevalent in African American lung adenocarcinoma tumors than in European American tumors [53]. Additionally, dysregulation of long noncoding RNAs (lncRNAs) like MALAT1 has been implicated in modulating the tumor immune microenvironment, contributing to lung cancer aggressiveness in African Americans [54]. Genome-wide association studies have confirmed that loci near CHRNA5 on chromosome 15q25.1 and TERT on chromosome 5p15.33 are significantly associated with lung cancer risk in African Americans [55, 56]. These loci are linked to increased lung cancer risk and smoking dependence. Elevated levels of MALAT1 in African American lung cancer patients modulate the tumor immune microenvironment, enhancing tumor growth and invasiveness through interactions with miR-206 and monocyte chemoattractant protein-1 (MCP-1) [56]. Socioeconomic factors, including lower rates of lung cancer screening and limited access to high-quality treatment, exacerbate these disparities. African Americans are less likely to receive timely and appropriate treatments, such as surgery and biomarker testing, which are critical for improving outcomes [57, 58]. The American College of Chest Physicians highlights that the later stage of diagnosis and lack of access to evidence-based treatments are significant contributors to poorer survival rates in African Americans [59].

While smoking is the main driver of lung cancer, there are other causes including alcohol consumption, decreasing BMI, radon exposure, geography, and more. Interestingly, a Kaiser Permanente Medical Care Cohort found that while drinking three glasses of alcohol a day was associated with an increased risk for lung cancer in European Americans, it was not associated with increased risk in African Americans [60]. Living near industrial sources of pollution is associated with increased lung cancer mortality, and African Americans disproportionately fit this demographic. Additionally, industrial exposure is associated with even higher rates of lung cancer in African Americans than would be predicted, essentially showing the same potentiated effect tobacco exposure has in the otherwise less-exposed African American population [61, 62].

In terms of lung cancer subtypes, non-small cell cancers still compose the majority of lung cancers in African Americans, but there is a 30% increased risk for adenocarcinoma and a 70% increased risk for squamous cell carcinoma within that category. Overall the incidence of small cell carcinoma tends to be lower in African Americans [61].

With the acceptance of low-dose computed tomography (LDCT) as a reimbursed annual screening for the early detection of lung cancer in adults 50–80 years with a 20-pack-year history (and currently smoke or have quit within the last 15 years), we can expect a significant reduction in lung cancer mortality overall simply due to early detection [63]. But with African Americans starting smoking later in life, smoking fewer cigarettes, having more advanced tumors at diagnosis, and living more in industry-dense locations, many with substantially increased lung cancer risk will more likely be deemed screening ineligible. Research has shown that African Americans are less likely to meet these criteria despite having a higher risk of lung cancer. A study by Gudina et al. proposed tailored eligibility criteria for African Americans, suggesting a reduction in the minimum age to 43 years and a decrease in the cumulative number of cigarettes smoked to 15 pack-years. This adjustment aims to equalize the odds of eligibility for lung cancer screening between African Americans and the majority population [64].

6.4.1 Equitable Tobacco Cessation Advice

Studies have shown that smoking cessation improves when providers discuss the topic at clinical encounters [65, 66]. That discussion, and its focus and intensity, varies across clinicians. Only half (48%) of African American smokers reported receiving advice to quit from physician providers (2010 National Health Interview Survey), and the rate for advising European Americans was better, but not by much (52%) [67, 68]. With the widespread health impact and societal cost of tobacco use and abuse, advising only half of smokers to stop smoking is a missed clinical opportunity of monumental proportions. Julia Soulakova found African Americans are twice as likely to profess an intention to quit smoking after getting advice to quit than European Americans [69]. Another study by Kulak and others found distinct racial differences in smoking cessation, with African Americans having more attempts to quit and European Americans being significantly more successful in quitting [70]. Making the time to discuss the merits of quitting and reviewing the various strategies available for African Americans takes full synergistic advantage of their increased motivation to attempt to quit.

6.4.2 African American Smoking Paradox

Among African Americans, there is a curious and deadly paradox that has confounded researchers. Alexander and colleagues comment:

> Despite their social disadvantage, African American youth have lower smoking prevalence rates, initiate smoking at older ages, and during adulthood, smoking rates are comparable to (European Americans). Smoking frequency and intensity among African American youth and adults are lower compared to (European Americans) and American Indian and Alaska Natives, but tobacco-caused morbidity and mortality rates are disproportionately higher. Disease prediction models have not explained disease causal pathways in African Americans. [71]

European American male smokers consume 30–40% more cigarettes than their African American counterparts, but African American male smokers are 34% more likely to develop lung cancer. This higher incidence based on lower exposure highlights the imperative of smoking cessation campaigns. An equitable approach would dictate that clinicians spend a disproportionately high amount of time on smoking cessation in African Americans because preventing the initiation of smoking and promoting complete cessation can have a dynamic impact on a patient population.

Studies have also shown a higher propensity among African Americans to smoke mentholated cigarettes (80%) and a higher risk of stroke in that subpopulation [72]. Smoking cessation, for unknown reasons, among menthol cigarette smokers is worse in both African American and Hispanic/Latino smokers, and for those who stopped, fewer were able to remain abstinent [73, 74]. Studies also suggest that it is easier to start smoking a menthol cigarette and there is a higher rate of progression to an established smoker. Menthol cigarettes are more heavily marketed in younger, poorer, and more African American or Hispanic/Latino communities [75, 76].

African Americans tend to have higher levels of total nicotine equivalents (TNE) and the tobacco-specific lung carcinogen 4-(methylnitrosamino)-1-(3-pyridyl)-1-butanol (NNAL) per cigarette smoked [77, 78]. This indicates greater toxicant uptake per cigarette, which contributes to increased lung cancer risk. Genetic variations, such as those found on chromosomes 5p15 and 15q25, are associated with higher lung cancer susceptibility in African Americans [55]. These loci are linked to genes involved in nicotine addiction and carcinogen metabolism, further elevating their risk despite lower cigarette consumption. African Americans may smoke cigarettes differently, such as taking deeper puffs or smoking more of each cigarette, leading to a higher intake of nicotine and carcinogens per cigarette. This behavior results in an increased exposure to harmful substances even with fewer cigarettes smoked [79].

With 80% of deaths from lung cancer deemed smoking-related, and half of all deaths from cancers of the mouth, esophagus, and urinary bladder caused by smoking, and worse cessation rates among African Americans, a deliberate clinical plan needs to be organized to better educate African Americans that smoke. A start in the discussion is to assess what baseline knowledge exists related to lung cancer and the other risks. Studies have shown that "low income and limited education adversely affect cessation attempts and that often (African American) smokers underestimate the link between cancer and tobacco smoking compared with (European American) smokers" [60]. Successful smoking cessation processes include:

- Clinician-led discussions
- Pertinent educational videos for the patient to see while waiting for their visit
- Patient navigator educational support and discussions

On average, male smokers die 13 years earlier than male nonsmokers, and female smokers die 14 years earlier than female nonsmokers. Saving those years represents an indelible impact on someone's life. What else in medicine can we affect so significantly?

6.5 Multiple Myeloma

Multiple myeloma (MM), a neoplasm of plasma cells, is the most common hematologic malignancy in African Americans, with two to three times the incidence of European Americans (see Fig. 6.6). The overall incidence rates of multiple myeloma increase with age, particularly after age 40, and are higher in men, particularly African American men [80]. Family history, radiation exposure, workplace exposure, and Agent Orange exposure all place an increased risk for multiple myeloma [81]. A National Cancer Institute study also found that the age of onset of multiple myeloma occurred at significantly younger ages in African Americans [82]. African Americans have a higher incidence of multiple myeloma compared to other racial groups, with rates approximately twice that of the majority population. This

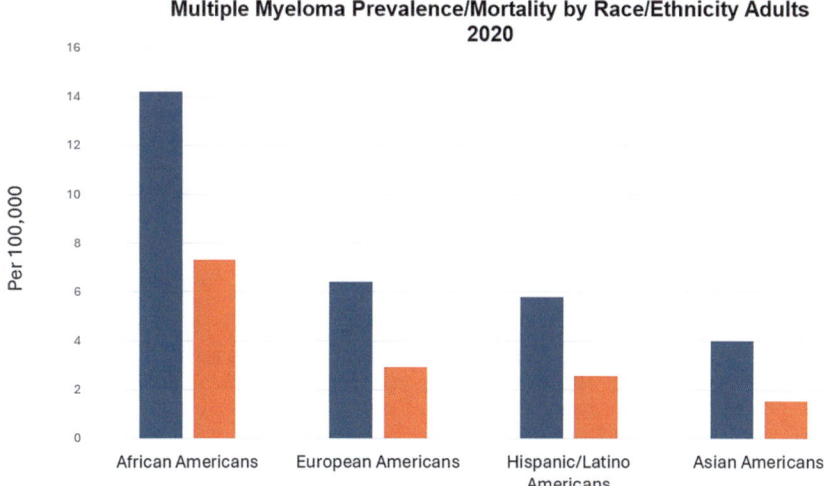

Fig. 6.6 Multiple myeloma, incidence/mortality by race/ethnicity, 2020

increased incidence is partly attributed to a higher prevalence of monoclonal gammopathy of undetermined significance (MGUS), a precursor condition to MM, in African Americans [83, 84].

Despite the higher incidence, African Americans often experience delays in diagnosis and disparities in treatment access and outcomes. They are less likely to receive autologous stem cell transplantation and other advanced therapies compared to majority populations, which contributes to poorer outcomes. Additionally, African Americans with multiple myeloma tend to be diagnosed at a younger age and have a higher burden of disease at presentation. Genetic factors also play a role in these disparities. African Americans have different genetic profiles, including a lower frequency of certain high-risk cytogenetic abnormalities, which may influence disease progression and response to treatment. However, the underrepresentation of African Americans in clinical trials limits the understanding of these genetic differences and their impact on treatment outcomes.

Because of the stark racial differences in the age of onset and the prevalence of multiple myeloma in African Americans, geneticists began to look for trends and dissimilarities. What they found were specific differences in the genetics of the myeloma cells that varied by race [85]. Overall, African Americans had a genetic version of multiple myeloma that occurred more often but also was consistent with better susceptibility to current therapeutic modalities and, therefore, improved outcomes [85]. The increased mortality of multiple myeloma in African Americans is related to the pure increased occurrence, whereas the improved survival is within the entire population with multiple myeloma. More African Americans with multiple myeloma lead to higher mortality, even in the presence of better survival outcomes.

Monoclonal gammopathy of undetermined significance (MGUS) is a precursor to multiple myeloma and is one of the most common premalignant plasma cell disorders. MGUS indicates the presence of a monoclonal immunoglobulin called an M-protein at a level of less than 10% clonal bone marrow plasma cells. Greater than 10% of these cells (and associated symptoms) confirm the diagnosis of multiple myeloma. MGUS occurs at a threefold higher rate in African Americans compared to European Americans, but the rate of progression to multiple myeloma is equal [86]. In other words, all racial groups progress from MGUS to multiple myeloma at the same rate, but African Americans have a significantly increased risk to develop MGUS. The racial disparity in the occurrence of MGUS is present even after adjusting for socioeconomic status [87].

The overall conclusion regarding the "racial disparities" in multiple myeloma rests in a theory best summarized by Greenberg et al.:

> Although MM is clinically considered as a unique disease, it is likely a collection of several cytogenetically unique malignancies that are considered together as one entity solely, because they arise from plasma cells and have roughly similar clinical features. As the racial disparity in the incidence of MM is marked (relative risk of ≥2 in African Americans), it is unlikely that the increase in risk is shared by all cytogenetic subtypes of the disease. Our hypothesis is that the racial predisposition in MM is driven largely by an excess risk of one or more specific cytogenetic subtypes of MM. [86]

The classic clinical manifestations of multiple myeloma include hypercalcemia (>11 mg/dL), renal failure, anemia, and lytic bone lesions as well as greater than 10% clonal bone marrow plasma cells. Patients frequently present with bone pain, pathologic fractures, and recurrent bacterial infections.

After diagnosis, patients are risk stratified and are begun on chemotherapy and/or bone marrow transplantation. Unfortunately, African Americans are less likely to receive adequate treatment for multiple myeloma including getting newer medications or bone marrow transplants [88–91]. Drs. Mark Fiala and Tanya Wildes looked at racial disparities in patient choice and utilization for multiple myeloma and found that African Americans were 37% less likely to choose stem cell transplantation and 21% less likely to utilize bortezomib (a newer, more targeted MM medication) than European Americans after controlling for access barriers and overall health status [92]. This difference in patient decision-making as it relates to treatment options impacts cancer outcomes overall.

6.6 "Chemotherapy"

Chemotherapy as a treatment option is a scary word for any patient to hear. Multiple studies have demonstrated significant delays in the initiation and completion of chemotherapy predict inferior outcomes [93–97]. African Americans may have a cultural aversion to the word "chemotherapy" that makes them less likely to agree to this potentially life-saving treatment. Because of a history of seeing their African American family and friends "get cancer" and then "get chemotherapy" and then lose weight and hair and then die, an unfortunate direct association of chemotherapy with death ensues. The specifics of the cancer and the chemotherapy are frequently lost on many patients.

As providers, it is our responsibility to explain the vast differences in cancers and why and how they occur, as well as clarify that all chemotherapies are not equal nor equivalent in effectiveness or side effects. In fact, all of the medications that a patient takes, from over-the-counter to prescriptions, are a form of "chemotherapy." Encourage the patient to ask questions about their options and ways to minimize adverse reactions. Too many African Americans are saying "no to chemotherapy" before getting the information they need. As the cancer progresses, many change their minds, but worse outcomes can now be predicted because of a potentially avoidable delay.

> **A Precision Medicine Approach to Cancer in African Americans**
> - Breast cancer incidence is lower in African American women, while the mortality is significantly higher.
> - African Americans tend to have breast cancer tumors with worse prognostic factors.

(continued)

- African Americans have a lower frequency of hormone receptor-positive tumors in breast cancer.
- Increased knowledge of the benefits of early detection of breast cancers leads to improved outcomes among African American women.
- African American women tend to believe their prognosis when cancer is detected is much worse than reality.
- The American College of Gastroenterology recommends colorectal screening in African Americans to begin at age 45.
- Sigmoidoscopy is contraindicated in African Americans due to a propensity to have more right-sided polyps.
- In African Americans, prostate cancer occurs earlier, is more aggressive, and has a higher mortality rate.
- The PSA (prostate-specific antigen) is a more sensitive and specific test for prostate cancer in African Americans.
- African Americans are more likely to smoke menthol cigarettes and therefore inhale more deeply and absorb more nicotine, making it harder to quit.
- African Americans are more likely to develop lung cancer if they smoke; therefore, it is imperative that clinicians spend more time discussing smoking cessation.
- Lung cancer is diagnosed at younger ages, is more advanced, and occurs in lighter smokers in African Americans.
- Living near industrial sources of pollution is associated with increased lung cancer mortality, stressing the importance of a more detailed history in regard to geography.
- African Americans have a 30% increased risk for adenocarcinoma and a 70% increase in squamous cell carcinoma of the lung compared to European Americans.
- The US Preventive Services Task Force (USPSTF) recommends annual screening for lung cancer with low-dose computed tomography in adults aged 55–80 years who have a 30-pack-year smoking history and currently smoke or have quit within the past 15 years.
- Multiple myeloma, a neoplasm of plasma cells, is the most common blood-based malignancy in African Americans, with two to three times the incidence of European Americans.
- Age of onset of multiple myeloma is significantly younger in African Americans.
- African Americans have a genetic version of multiple myeloma that occurs more often but also is consistent with better susceptibility to current therapeutic modalities and, therefore, improved outcomes.
- MGUS occurs at a threefold higher rate in African Americans compared to European Americans, but the rate of progression to multiple myeloma is equal.
- African Americans may have a cultural aversion to the word "chemotherapy" that makes them less likely to agree to this potentially life-saving treatment in a timely manner.

References

1. The Promise of Precision Medicine. National Institute of Health. https://www.nih.gov/about-nih/what-we-do/nih-turning-discovery-into-health/promise-precision-medicine. Accessed 4 Dec 2024.
2. Giaquinto AN, Miller KD, Tossas KY, Winn RA, Ahmedin J, Siegel RL. Cancer statistics for African American/Black people 2022. CA Cancer J Clin. 72(3):202–29. https://doi.org/10.3322/caac.21718.
3. Ambreen K, Rogers Charles R, Kennedy Carson D, AnaMaria L, Joanne J. Genetic evaluation for hereditary cancer syndromes among African Americans: a critical review. Oncologist. 2022;27(4):285–91. https://doi.org/10.1093/oncolo/oyab082.
4. Rosenblum RE, Celina A, Suckiel SA, Soper ER, Sigireddi MR, Sinead C, Belbin GM, Lucas AL, Kenny EE, Abul-Husn NS. Lynch syndrome–associated variants and cancer rates in an ancestrally diverse biobank. JCO Precis Oncol. 4:1429–44. https://doi.org/10.1200/PO.20.00290.
5. Giri VN, Knudsen KE, Kelly WK, Wassim A, Andriole GL, Bangma CH, Bekelman JE, Benson MC, Amie B, Arthur B, Catalona WJ, Cooney KA, Matthew C, Crawford DE, Den Robert B, Dicker AP, Scott E, Neil F, Freedman ML, Hamdy FC, Jean H-C, Hurwitz MD, Colette H, Isaacs WB, Kane CJ, Philip K, Jeffrey KR, Karsh LI, Klein EA, Lin DW, Loughlin KR, Grace L-Y, Bruce MS, Mann MJ, Mark JR, McCue PA, Miner MM, Todd M, Moul JW, Myers RE, Nielsen SM, Elias O, Pavlovich CP, Peiper SC, Penson DF, Daniel P, Pettaway CA, Robert P, Pinto PA, Wendy P, Raj GV, Rebbeck TR, Robson ME, Rosenberg MT, Howard S, Oliver S, Edward S, Schwartz GF, Shahin MS, Shore ND, Brian S, Soule Howard R, Tomlins Scott A, Trabulsi Edouard J, Robert U, Vander Griend Donald J, Walsh Patrick C, Weil Carol J, Richard W, Gomella Leonard G. Role of genetic testing for inherited prostate cancer risk: Philadelphia Prostate Cancer Consensus Conference 2017. J Clin Oncol. 36(4):414–24. https://doi.org/10.1200/JCO.2017.74.1173.
6. Siegel JB, Melanie B, Rupak M, Kiersten M, Hughes KS, Abbott AM. Racial disparities in breast cancer genetic testing may be mitigated by counseling. Ann Surg Oncol. 31(8):5197–204. https://doi.org/10.1245/s10434-024-15434-2.
7. Walker EJ, Dena G, Gordon KM, Christina P, Julia C, Pelin C, Collisson EA, Tempero MA, Ko AH, Blanco AM, Mallika D. Oncologist. 2021;26(11):e1982–91. https://doi.org/10.1002/onco.13968.
8. Frey Melissa K., Finch Amy, Kulkarni Amita, Akbari Mohammad R., Chapman-Davis Eloise, Genetic testing for all: overcoming disparities in ovarian cancer genetic testing. Am Soc Clin Oncol Educ Book 42 471–482 https://doi.org/10.1200/EDBK_350292.
9. U.S. Cancer Statistics Working Group. U.S. Department of Health and Human Services, Centers for Disease Control and Prevention and National Cancer Institute. https://www.cdc.gov/cancer/dataviz. Released in June 2024.
10. Xuan Y, Mohamed A, Cooper Lee AD, Du Yuhong, Haian F, Ivanov Andrey A. High expression of MKK3 is associated with worse clinical outcomes in African American breast cancer patients. J Transl Med. 18(1) https://doi.org/10.1186/s12967-020-02502-w.
11. Tuya P, Devon B, Deborah C, Monteiro Alvaro NA, Catherine P, Lily S, Jongphil K, Narod SA, Akbari MR, Vadaparampil ST. Cancer. 121(23):4173–80. https://doi.org/10.1002/cncr.29645.
12. Albain K, Unger J, Crowley J, Coltman C, Hershman D. Racial disparities in cancer survival among randomized clinical trials patients of the southwest oncology group. J Natl Cancer Inst. 2009;101(14):984–92.
13. Devericks EN, Carson MS, McCullough LE, Coleman MF, Hursting SD. The obesity-breast cancer link: a multidisciplinary perspective. Cancer Metastasis Rev. 41(3):607–25. https://doi.org/10.1007/s10555-022-10043-5.
14. Manuel P-R, Cynthia M-T, Valle-Goffin JJ, Friedman ER, Slingerland JM. Obesity and adverse breast cancer risk and outcome: mechanistic insights and strategies for intervention. CA Cancer J Clin. 67(5):378–97. https://doi.org/10.3322/caac.21405.

15. Monticciolo DL, Newell MS, Linda M, Lee CS, Destounis SV. Breast cancer screening for women at higher-than-average risk: updated recommendations from the ACR. J Am Coll Radiol. 20(9):902–14. https://doi.org/10.1016/j.jacr.2023.04.002.
16. Reagan PB, Salsberry PJ, Fang MZ, Gardner WP, Kathleen P. African-American/white differences in the age of menarche: accounting for the difference. Soc Sci Med. 75(7):1263–70. https://doi.org/10.1016/j.socscimed.2012.05.018.
17. Britta S. Breastfeeding reduces the risk of breast cancer: a call for action in high-income countries with low rates of breastfeeding. Cancer Med. 12(4):4616–25. https://doi.org/10.1002/cam4.5288.
18. John EM, Jocelyn K, Phipps AI, Longacre TA, Kurian AW, Ingles SA, Wu AH, Hines LM. Reproductive characteristics menopausal status race and ethnicity and risk of breast cancer subtypes defined by ER PR and HER2 status: the breast cancer etiology in minorities study. Breast Cancer Res. 2024;26(1) https://doi.org/10.1186/s13058-024-01834-5.
19. Chiang KV, Ruowei L, Anstey EH, Perrine CG. Racial and ethnic disparities in breastfeeding initiation—United States 2019. MMWR Morb Mortal Wkly Rep. 2021;70(21):769–74. https://doi.org/10.15585/mmwr.mm7021a1.
20. Bazargan M, Lucas-Wright A, Jones L, et al. Understanding perceived benefit of early cancer detection: community-partnered research with African American women in South Los Angeles. J Womens Health (Larchmt). 2015;24(9):755–61.
21. Ananthakrishnan A, Schellhase K, Sparapani R, Laud P, Neuner J. Disparities in colon cancer screening in the Medicare population. Arch Intern Med. 2007;167(3):258–64.
22. Rex D, Johnson D, Anderson J, et al. Colorectal cancer screening. Am J Gastroenterol. 2009;104:739–50.
23. Davidson KW, Barry MJ, Mangione CM, Michael C, Caughey AB, Davis EM, Donahue KE, Doubeni CA, Krist AH, Martha K, Li L, Gbenga O, Owens DK, Lori P, Michael S, James S, Chien-Wen T, Wong JB. Screening for colorectal cancer. JAMA. 325(19):1965. https://doi.org/10.1001/jama.2021.6238.
24. Paquette I, Ying J, Shah S, Abbott D, Ho S. African Americans should be screened at an earlier age for colorectal cancer. Gastrointest Endosc. 2015;82(5):878–83.
25. Chattar-Cora D, Onime G, Valentine I, Cudjoe E, Rivera L. Colorectal cancer in a multi-ethnic urban group: its anatomical and age profile. Int Surg. 2000;85(2):137–42.
26. Hollis RH, Chu DI. Healthcare disparities and colorectal cancer. Surg Oncol Clin N Am. 31(2):157–69. https://doi.org/10.1016/j.soc.2021.11.002.
27. Castañeda-Avila MA, Mayra T, Oyinbo AG, Kate L. Racial and ethnic disparities in use of colorectal cancer screening among adults with chronic medical conditions: BRFSS 2012–2020. Prevent Chronic Dis. 2024;21 https://doi.org/10.5888/pcd21.230257.
28. Abraham S, Mehmood SS. Reducing disparities and achieving health equity in colorectal cancer screening. Tech Innov Gastrointest Endosc. 25(3):284–96. https://doi.org/10.1016/j.tige.2023.02.007.
29. Colorectal cancer screening: where does the shield liquid biopsy fit in? National Cancer Institute. https://www.cancer.gov/news-events/cancer-currents-blog/2024/shield-blood-test-colorectal-cancer-screening. 11 Oct 2024.
30. Chung DC, Gray DM, Harminder S, Issaka RB, Raymond VM, Craig E, Sylvia H, Chudova Darya I, AmirAli T, Greenson Joel K, Sinicrope Frank A, Samir G, Grady William M. A cell-free DNA blood-based test for colorectal cancer screening. New Engl J Med. 390(11):973–83. https://doi.org/10.1056/NEJMoa2304714.
31. Fedewa S, Flanders W, Ward K, et al. Racial and ethnic disparities in interval colorectal cancer incidence: a population-based cohort study. Ann Intern Med. 2017;166(12):857–66.
32. Myers R, Sifri R, Daskalakis C, et al. Increasing colon cancer screening in primary care among African Americans. J Natl Cancer Inst. 2014;106(12):dju344.
33. Myers R, Bittner-Fagan H, Daskalakis C, et al. A randomized controlled trial of a tailored navigation and a standard intervention in colorectal cancer screening. Cancer Epidemiol Biomarkers Prev. 2013;22(1):109–17.

34. Rawl S, Skinner C, Perkins S, et al. Computer-delivered tailored intervention improves colon cancer screening knowledge and health beliefs of African Americans. Health Educ Res. 2012;27(5):868–85.
35. Jerant A, Sohler N, Fiscella K, et al. Tailored interactive multimedia computer programs to reduce health disparities: opportunities and challenges. Patient Educ Couns. 2011;85:323–30.
36. William L, Robert D, Jarrard DF, Scarpato KR, Kim SK, Erin K, Buckley DI, Griffin JC, Cookson MS. Updates to advanced prostate cancer: AUA/SUO guideline (2023). J Urol. 209(6):1082–90. https://doi.org/10.1097/JU.0000000000003452.
37. Mahal BA, Aizer AA, Ziehr DR, Hyatt AS, Sammon JD, Marianne S, Choueiri TK, Hu JC, Sweeney CJ, Beard CJ, D'Amico AV, Martin NE, Kim SP, Quoc-Dien T, Nguyen PL. Trends in disparate treatment of African American men with localized prostate cancer across national comprehensive cancer network risk groups. Urology. 84(2):386–92. https://doi.org/10.1016/j.urology.2014.05.009.
38. Nnenaya A-M, Yongmei Q, Samuel K, Mary O, Randy V, Danil M, Caram MV, Christina C, Joseph R, Hollenbeck BK, Skolarus TA. Understanding the role of urology practice organization and racial composition in prostate cancer treatment disparities. JCO Oncol Pract. 19(5):e763–72. https://doi.org/10.1200/OP.22.00147.
39. Kosj Y, Min LK, Shivanshu A, Alba PR, Cristina P, Anglin-Foote TR, Brian R, Anthony G, DuVall Scott L, Evangelia K, Yu-Ning W, Markt SC, Rose BS, Ryan B, Carrie W, Okoduwa A, Fink AK, Nickols NG, Lynch JA, Garraway IP. Racial and ethnic disparities in prostate cancer outcomes in the veterans affairs health care system. JAMA Netw Open. 5(1):e2144027. https://doi.org/10.1001/jamanetworkopen.2021.44027.
40. Chen Fei, Madduri Ravi K., Rodriguez Alex A., Darst Burcu F., Chou Alisha, Sheng Xin, Wang Anqi, Shen Jiayi, Saunders Edward J., Rhie Suhn K., Bensen Jeannette T., Ingles Sue A., Kittles Rick A., Strom Sara S., Rybicki Benjamin A., Nemesure Barbara, Isaacs William B., Stanford Janet L., Zheng Wei, Sanderson Maureen, John Esther M., Park Jong Y., Xu Jianfeng, Wang Ying, Berndt Sonja I., Huff Chad D., Yeboah Edward D., Tettey Yao, Lachance Joseph, Tang Wei, Rentsch Christopher T., Cho Kelly, Mcmahon Benjamin H., Biritwum Richard B., Adjei Andrew A., Tay Evelyn, Truelove Ann, Niwa Shelley, Sellers Thomas A., Yamoah Kosj, Murphy Adam B., Crawford Dana C., Patel Alpa V., Bush William S., Aldrich Melinda C., Cussenot Olivier, Petrovics Gyorgy, Cullen Jennifer, Neslund-Dudas Christine M., Stern Mariana C., Kote-Jarai Zsofia, Govindasami Koveela, Cook Michael B., Chokkalingam Anand P., Hsing Ann W., Goodman Phyllis J., Hoffmann Thomas J., Drake Bettina F., Hu Jennifer J., Keaton Jacob M., Hellwege Jacklyn N., Clark Peter E., Jalloh Mohamed, Gueye Serigne M., Niang Lamine, Ogunbiyi Olufemi, Idowu Michael O., Popoola Olufemi, Adebiyi Akindele O., Aisuodionoe-Shadrach Oseremen I., Ajibola Hafees O., Jamda Mustapha A., Oluwole Olabode P., Nwegbu Maxwell, Adusei Ben, Mante Sunny, Darkwa-Abrahams Afua, Mensah James E., Diop Halimatou, Van Den Eeden Stephen K., Blanchet Pascal, Fowke Jay H., Casey Graham, Hennis Anselm J., Lubwama Alexander, Thompson Ian M., Leach Robin, Easton Douglas F., Preuss Michael H., Loos Ruth J., Gundell Susan M., Wan Peggy, Mohler James L., Fontham Elizabeth T., Smith Gary J., Taylor Jack A., Srivastava Shiv, Eeles Rosaline A., Carpten John D., Kibel Adam S., Multigner Luc, Parent Marie-Élise, Menegaux Florence, Cancel-Tassin Geraldine, Klein Eric A., Andrews Caroline, Rebbeck Timothy R., Brureau Laurent, Ambs Stefan, Edwards Todd L., Watya Stephen, Chanock Stephen J., Witte John S., Blot William J., Michael Gaziano J., Justice Amy C., Conti David V., Haiman Christopher A., Evidence of novel susceptibility variants for prostate cancer and a multiancestry polygenic risk score associated with aggressive disease in men of african ancestry. Eur Urol 84(1) 13–21. https://doi.org/10.1016/j.eururo.2023.01.022.
41. Conti David V, Wang K, Xin S, Bensen Jeannette T, Hazelett Dennis J, Cook Michael B, Ingles Sue A, Kittles Rick A, Strom Sara S, Rybicki Benjamin A, Barbara N, Isaacs William B, Stanford Janet L, Zheng W, Maureen S, John Esther M, Park Jong Y, Xu J, Stevens Victoria L, Berndt Sonja I, Huff Chad D, Wang Z, Yeboah Edward D, Yao T, Biritwum Richard B, Adjei Andrew A, Evelyn T, Ann T, Shelley N, Sellers Thomas A, Kosj Y, Murphy Adam B, Crawford

Dana C, Gapstur Susan M, Bush William S, Aldrich Melinda C, Olivier C, Gyorgy P, Jennifer C, Christine N-D, Stern Mariana C, Zsofia-Kote J, Koveela G, Chokkalingam Anand P, Hsing Ann W, Goodman Phyllis J, Thomas H, Drake Bettina F, Hu Jennifer J, Clark Peter E, Van Den Eeden SK, Pascal B, Fowke Jay H, Graham C, Hennis Anselm JM, Ying H, Alexander L, Thompson IM, Robin L, Easton Douglas F, Fredrick S, Van den Berg DJ, Gundell Susan M, Alex S, Wan P, Lucy X, Pooler Loreall C, Mohler James L, Fontham Elizabeth TH, Smith Gary J, Taylor Jack A, Shiv S, Eeles Rosalind A, John C, Kibel Adam S, Luc M, Marie-Elise P, Florence M, Geraldine C-T, Klein Eric A, Laurent B, Stram Daniel O, Stephen W, Chanock Stephen J, Witte John S, Blot William J, Henderson Brian E, Haiman Christopher A. Two novel susceptibility loci for prostate cancer in men of African ancestry. JNCI J Natl Cancer Inst. 2017;109(8) https://doi.org/10.1093/jnci/djx084.

42. Joseph L, Berens AJ, Hansen Matthew EB, Teng AK, Tishkoff SA, Rebbeck TR. Genetic hitchhiking and population bottlenecks contribute to prostate cancer disparities in men of African descent. Cancer Res. 2018;78(9):2432–43. https://doi.org/10.1158/0008-5472.CAN-17-1550.

43. Darst Burcu F, Peggy W, Xin S, Bensen Jeannette T, Ingles Sue A, Rybicki Benjamin A, Barbara N, John Esther M, Fowke Jay H, Stevens Victoria L, Berndt Sonja I, Huff Chad D, Strom Sara S, Park Jong Y, Wei Z, Ostrander Elaine A, Walsh Patrick C, Shiv S, John C, Sellers Thomas A, Kosj Y, Murphy Adam B, Maureen S, Crawford Dana C, Gapstur Susan M, Bush William S, Aldrich Melinda C, Olivier C, Meredith Y, Gyorgy P, Jennifer C, Christine N-D, Kittles Rick A, Jianfeng X, Stern Mariana C, Zsofia K-J, Koveela G, Chokkalingam Anand P, Luc M, Marie-Elise P, Florence M, Geraldine C-T, Kibel Adam S, Klein Eric A, Goodman Phyllis J, Drake Bettina F, Hu Jennifer J, Clark Peter E, Pascal B, Graham C, Hennis Anselm JM, Alexander L, Thompson Ian M, Robin L, Gundell Susan M, Loreall P, Lucy X, Mohler James L, Fontham Elizabeth TH, Smith Gary J, Taylor Jack A, Eeles Rosalind A, Laurent B, Chanock Stephen J, Stephen W, Stanford Janet L, Diptasri M, Isaacs William B, Kathleen C, Blot William J, Conti David V, Haiman Christopher A. A germline variant at 8q24 contributes to familial clustering of prostate cancer in men of african ancestry. Eur Urol. 78(3):316–20. https://doi.org/10.1016/j.eururo.2020.04.060.

44. Indu K, Xijun Z, Shyh-Han T, Darryl N, Kevin B, Lakshmi R, Gauthaman S, Elisa M-M, John R, Camille A, Amina A, Denise Y, Yongmei C, Jennifer C, Rosner IL, Sesterhenn IA, Albert D, Gregory C, Clesson T, Clifton D, Wilkerson MD, Pollard HB, Shiv S, Gyorgy P. Germline mutation landscape of DNA damage repair genes in African Americans with prostate cancer highlights potentially targetable RAD genes. Nature. Communications. 2022;13(1) https://doi.org/10.1038/s41467-022-28945-x.

45. U.S. Preventative Services Task Force. Published final recommendations. https://www.uspreventiveservicestaskforce.org/. Accessed 9 May 2019.

46. US Preventative Services Task Force, Grossman DC, Curry SJ, et al. Screening for prostate cancer: US preventative services task force recommendation statement. JAMA. 2018;319(18):1901–13.

47. Kaushal JB, Pratima R, Sakthivel M, Siddiqui JA, Alsafwani ZW, Parthasarathy S, Nair SS, Tewari AK, Batra SK. Racial disparity in prostate cancer: an outlook in genetic and molecular landscape. Cancer Metastasis Rev. 43(4):1233–55. https://doi.org/10.1007/s10555-024-10193-8.

48. Carter H, Albertsen P, Barry M, et al. Early detection of prostate cancer: AUA guideline. J Urol. 2013;190(2):419–26.

49. Shenoy D, Packiananthan S, Chen A, Vijayakumar S. Do African American men need separate prostate cancer screening guidelines? BMC Urol. 2016;16:19.

50. Johnson JR, Nicole M, Leanne W-B, Mya W, Deyana L, Hooker SE, Dorothy G, Brian R, Kittles RA. The complex interplay of modifiable risk factors affecting prostate cancer disparities in African American men. Nat Rev Urol. 21(7):422–32. https://doi.org/10.1038/s41585-023-00849-5.

51. Lathan C, Waldman BE, Gagne J, Emmons K. Perspectives of African Americans on lung cancer: a qualitative analysis. Oncologist. 2015;20(4):393–9.

52. American Cancer Society. Cancer facts & figures for African Americans 2016–2018. Atlanta: American Cancer Society, Inc; 2016.
53. Arauz RF, Byun JS, Mayank T, Sanju S, Skyler K, Sheryse T, Adriana Z, Mitchell KA, Pine SR, Kevin G, Perez-Stable EJ, Napoles AM, Ryan BM. Whole-exome profiling of NSCLC among African Americans. J Thorac Oncol. 15(12):1880–92. https://doi.org/10.1016/j.jtho.2020.08.029.
54. Jin L, Pushpa D, Holden Van K, Ashutosh S, Todd NW, Feng J. Dysregulation of lncRNA MALAT1 contributes to lung cancer in African Americans by modulating the tumor immune microenvironment. Cancers. 2024;16(10):1876. https://doi.org/10.3390/cancers16101876.
55. Zanetti, Krista A, Zhaoming W, Melinda A, Amos Christopher I, Blot William J, Bowman Elise D, Laurie B, Qiuyin C, Neil C, Chung Charles C, Gillanders Elizabeth M, Haiman Christopher A, Hansen Helen M, Henderson Brian E, Kolonel Laurence N, Le ML, Shengchao L, Haughton MNL, Ryan Bríd M, Schwartz Ann G, Sison Jennette D, Spitz Margaret R, Margaret T, Wenzlaff Angela S, Wiencke John K, Lynne W, Wrensch Margaret R, Xifeng W, Wei Z, Weiyin Z, David C, Palmer Julie R, Penning Trevor M, Rieber Alyssa G, Lynn R, Ruiz-Narvaez Edward A, Li S, Anil V, Yongyue W, Whitehead Alexander S, Chanock Stephen J, Harris Curtis C. Genome-wide association study confirms lung cancer susceptibility loci on chromosomes 5p15 and 15q25 in an African-American population. Lung Cancer. 98:33–42. https://doi.org/10.1016/j.lungcan.2016.05.008.
56. Amos CI, Gorlov IP, Dong Qiong W, Xifeng ZH, Lu EY, Paul S, Greisinger AJ, Mills GB, Spitz MR. Nicotinic acetylcholine receptor region on chromosome 15q25 and lung cancer risk among African Americans: a case–control study. JNCI J Natl Cancer Inst. 2010;102(15):1199–205. https://doi.org/10.1093/jnci/djq232.
57. Narjust D, Nathaniel E, Edith M. Disparities in lung cancer. J Natl Med Assoc. 115(2):S46–53. https://doi.org/10.1016/j.jnma.2023.02.004.
58. Yee TNW, Carracedo UC, Andres A, Meri M, Raez LE. Diversity and disparities in lung cancer outcomes among minorities. Cancer J. 29(6):323–7. https://doi.org/10.1097/PPO.0000000000000689.
59. Alberg AJ, Brock MV, Ford JG, Samet JM, Spivack SD. Epidemiology of lung cancer. Chest. 143(5):e1S–29S. https://doi.org/10.1378/chest.12-2345.
60. Ryan B. Lung cancer health disparities. Carcinogenesis. 2018;39(6):741–51.
61. Tran H, et al. Predictors of lung cancer: noteworthy cell type differences. Penn J. 2013;17:23–9.
62. Luo J, et al. Environmental carcinogen releases and lung cancer mortality in rural-urban areas of the United States. J Rural Health. 2011;27:342–9.
63. Katki H, Kovalchik S, Berg C, Cheung L, Chaturvedi A. Development and validation of risk models to select ever-smokers for CT lung cancer screening. JAMA. 2016;315(21):2300–11.
64. Gudina AT, Charles K, Hardy SJ, Lee K, Eva C, Ana-Paula C. Revisiting the lung cancer screening eligibility criteria to promote equity for Black individuals. Lung Cancer. 191:107539. https://doi.org/10.1016/j.lungcan.2024.107539.
65. Stead L, Buitrago S, Preciado N, et al. Does advice from doctors encourage people who smoke to quit. Cochrane. https://www.cochrane.org/CD000165/TOBACCO_does-advice-from-doctors-encourage-people-who-smoke-to-quit
66. Dhumal G, Pednekar M, Gupta P, et al. Quit history, intentions to quit, and reasons for considering quitting among tobacco users in India: findings from the wave 1 TCP India survey. Indian J Cancer. 2014;51(01):S39–45.
67. Danesh D, Paskett E, Ferketich A. Disparities in receipt of advice to quit smoking from health care providers: 2010 National Health Interview Survey. Prev Chronic Dis. 2014;11:e131.
68. Hooks-Anderson Denise R, Joanne S, Scott S, Sarah S-H, Scherrer Jeffrey F. Association between race and receipt of counselling or medication for smoking cessation in primary care. Fam Pract. 2017;35(2):160–5. https://doi.org/10.1093/fampra/cmx099.
69. Soulakova J, Li J, Crockett L. Race/ethnicity and intention to quit cigarette smoking. Prev Med Rep. 2017;5:160–5.

70. Kulak J, Cornelius M, Fong G, Giovino G. Differences in quit attempts and cigarette smoking abstinence between whites and African Americans in the United States: literature review and results from the International Tobacco Control US Survey. Nicotine Tob Res. 2016;18(Suppl 1):S79–87.
71. Alexander L, Trinidad D, Sakuma K, et al. Why we must continue to investigate menthol's role in the African American smoking paradox. Nicotine Tob Res. 2016;18(Suppl 1):S91–101.
72. Gandhi K, Foulds J, Steinberg M, Lu S, Williams J. Lower quit rates among African Americans and Latino menthol cigarette smokers at a tobacco treatment clinic. Int J Clin Pract. 2009;63(3):360–7.
73. Delnevo CD, Gundersen DA, Hrywna M, et al. Smoking-cessation prevalence among U.S. smokers of menthol versus non-menthol cigarettes. Am J Prev Med. 2011;41:357–65.
74. Nonnemaker J, Hersey J, Homsi G, et al. Initiation with menthol cigarettes and youth smoking uptake. Addiction. 2013;108:171–8.
75. Henriksen L, Schleicher NC, Dauphinee AL, et al. Targeted advertising, promotion, and price for menthol cigarettes in California high school neighborhoods. Nicotine Tob Res. 2012;14:116–21.
76. Moreland-Russell S, Harris J, Snider D, et al. Disparities and menthol marketing: additional evidence in support of point of sale policies. Int J Environ Res Public Health. 2013;10:4571–83.
77. Murphy SE, Cherie G, Thomson NM, Carmella SG, Milo W, Aldrich MC, Qiuyin C, Sullivan SM, Stram DO, Loïc LM, Hecht SS, Blot WJ, Lani PS. Association of urinary biomarkers of tobacco exposure with lung cancer risk in African American and white cigarette smokers in the southern community cohort study. Cancer Epidemiol Biomarkers Prev. 2024;33(8):1073–82. https://doi.org/10.1158/1055-9965.EPI-23-1362.
78. Gideon SH, Benowitz Neal L, Jennifer K, Peyton J, Gregorich Steven E, Pérez-Stable Eliseo J, Murphy Sharon E, Hecht Stephen S, Hatsukami Dorothy K, Donny Eric C. Differences in exposure to toxic and/or carcinogenic volatile organic compounds between Black and White cigarette smokers. J Expo Sci Environ Epidemiol. 31(2):211–23. https://doi.org/10.1038/s41370-019-0159-9.
79. Benowitz NL, Dains KM, Dempsey D, Wilson M, Jacob P. Racial differences in the relationship between number of cigarettes smoked and nicotine and carcinogen exposure. Nicotine Tob Res. 2011;13(9):772–83. https://doi.org/10.1093/ntr/ntr072.
80. Zhu DT, Andrew P, Alan L, Lingxiao Z, Hiba A, Rebbeck TR. Multiple myeloma incidence and mortality trends in the United States 1999–2020. Sci Rep. 2024;14(1) https://doi.org/10.1038/s41598-024-65590-4.
81. Greenberg AJ, Vachon CM, Rajkumar SV. Disparities in the prevalence, pathogenesis and progression of monoclonal gammopathy of undetermined significance and multiple myeloma between blacks and whites. Leukemia. 2012;26(4):609–14.
82. Waxman AJ, Mink PJ, Devesa SS, et al. Racial disparities in incidence and outcome in multiple myeloma: a population-based study. Blood. 2010;116:5501–6. https://doi.org/10.1182/blood-2010-07-298760.
83. Samer AH, Deepa D, Hamisu S, Kamble RT, Lulla PD, LaQuisa H, George C, Almeida RC, Heslop HE, Zafar US. Health disparities experienced by Black Americans with multiple myeloma in the United States: a population-based study. J Clin Oncol. 39(15_suppl):e18512. https://doi.org/10.1200/JCO.2021.39.15_suppl.e18512.
84. Ashley S, Samantha S, Krishnaveni S, Tao G, Kwan-Keat A, Alyssa QM, Seth RA. Clinical characteristics treatment patterns and outcomes among African American and White patients with multiple myeloma in the United States. Leuk Lymphoma. 65(1):109–17. https://doi.org/10.1080/10428194.2023.2273746.
85. Kumar S, Fonseca R, Ketterling RP, et al. Trisomies in multiple myeloma: impact on survival in patients with high-risk cytogenetics. Blood. 2012;119(9):2100–5.
86. Greenberg AJ, Philip S, Paner A, et al. Racial differences in primary cytogenetic abnormalities in multiple myeloma: a multi-center study. Blood Cancer J. 2015;5:e271. https://doi.org/10.1038/bcj.2014.91.

References

87. Landgren O, Rajkumar SV, Pfeiffer RM, et al. Obesity is associated with an increased risk of monoclonal gammopathy of undetermined significance (MGUS) among African American and Caucasian women. Blood. 2010;116(7):1056–9.
88. Costa LJ, Huang JX, Hari PN. Disparities in utilization of autologous hematopoietic cell transplantation for treatment of multiple myeloma. Biol Blood Marrow Transplant. 2015;21(4):701–6.
89. Hari PN, Majhail NS, Zhang MJ, et al. Race and outcomes of autologous hematopoietic cell transplantation for multiple myeloma. Biol Blood Marrow Transplant. 2010;16:395–402.
90. Joshua TV, Rizzo JD, Zhang MJ, et al. Access to hematopoietic stem cell transplantation: effect of race and sex. Cancer. 2010;116:3469–76.
91. Al-Hamadani M, Hashmi SK, Go RS. Use of autologous hematopoietic cell transplantation as initial therapy in multiple myeloma and the impact of socio-geo-demographic factors in the era of novel agents. Am J Hematol. 2014;89:825.
92. Fiala MA, Wildes TM. Racial disparities in treatment use for multiple myeloma. Cancer. 2017;123:1590–6.
93. Biagi JJ, Raphael M, King WD, et al. The effect of delay in time to adjuvant chemotherapy (TTAC) on survival in breast cancer (BC): a systematic review and meta-analysis. ASCO Meet Abstr. 2011;29(15_suppl):1128.
94. Colleoni M, Bonetti M, Coates AS, The International Breast Cancer Study Group, et al. Early start of adjuvant chemotherapy may improve treatment outcome for premenopausal breast cancer patients with tumors not expressing estrogen receptors. J Clin Oncol. 2000;18(3):584–90.
95. Kim YW, Choi EH, Kim BR, et al. The impact of delayed commencement of adjuvant chemotherapy (eight or more weeks) on survival in stage II and III colon cancer: a national population-based cohort study. Oncotarget. 2017;8(45):80061–72.
96. Salazar MC, Rosen JE, Wang Z, et al. Association of delayed adjuvant chemotherapy with survival after lung cancer surgery. JAMA Oncol. 2017;3(5):610–9.
97. Petrelli F, Zaniboni A, Ghidini A, et al. Timing of adjuvant chemotherapy and survival in colorectal, gastric, and pancreatic cancer. A systemic review and meta-analysis. Cancers (Basel). 2019;11(4):E550. https://doi.org/10.3390/cancers11040550.

Chapter 7
A Precision Medicine Approach to Renal Disease in African Americans

Contents

7.1	Hypertensive Nephrosclerosis	136
7.2	Obesity and Proteinuria	136
7.3	Kidney Disease Progression	137
7.4	Treatment and Counseling	137
7.5	Kidney Transplantation	138
7.6	Kidney Stones	139
References		141

The prevalence of renal disease in African Americans is significantly higher compared with other racial groups. African Americans are approximately 3.5 times more likely to develop chronic kidney disease (CKD) and 3 times more likely to progress to end-stage renal disease (ESRD) compared to European Americans. This disparity is influenced by a combination of genetic, socioeconomic, and healthcare-related factors [1, 2].

Genetic factors include the presence of certain variants in the APOL1 gene, which are more common in individuals of African descent. These variants have been associated with an increased risk of developing kidney disease. Genetically, variants in the APOL1 gene are associated with a higher risk of CKD and progression to ESRD among African Americans. Individuals carrying two APOL1 risk alleles have a 1.49-fold increased risk of CKD and a 1.88-fold increased risk of ESRD compared with those with zero or one risk allele [3–5]. Approximately 13% of African Americans carry both high-risk APOL1 genotypes. The prevalence of high-risk APOL1 genotypes in West African populations, the ancestral origin of most African Americans, is reported to be almost 30%, which is higher than the prevalence among African Americans due to the admixture with European ancestry [5]. This increased renal-risk variant emanates from sub-Saharan African ancestors associated with a survival advantage conferred against African sleeping sickness (trypanosomiasis) [6, 7].

Socioeconomic factors play a crucial role in these disparities. African Americans often face barriers such as lower socioeconomic status, limited access to healthcare, and lower health literacy, which can delay the diagnosis and treatment of CKD. Joseph Lunyera and colleagues at Duke University found that African Americans in the lowest socioeconomic cohort had a higher rate of CKD [1]:

> [L]ow cumulative lifetime socioeconomic status was associated with increased odds of prevalent CKD at baseline both directly and indirectly *via* allostatic load. After follow-up, low cumulative lifetime socioeconomic status was only indirectly associated with increased odds of incident CKD and faster eGFR decline *via* baseline allostatic load. Thus, our data link low life course socioeconomic status with kidney outcomes in (African) Americans and allostatic load is a potential mediator of this link. [1]

Prior to 1994, hypertension was the clear most common cause of end-stage renal disease in African Americans, but with progressive obesity, diabetes has become a major contributor [6, 8]. Since hypertension frequently accompanies diabetes in African Americans, the exact driver (hypertension versus diabetes) of ESRD is complicated. The APOL1 variant strongly increases the risk for hypertensive nephropathy, and that frequently leads to ESRD.

Why Have an APOL1 Gene?
Overall, the APOL1 genetic variant (including the high-risk and low-risk variant combinations) is found in more than 30% of African Americans and largely absent in European Americans [7]. It is hypothesized that this gene offered protection from *Trypanosoma brucei* carried by the tsetse fly and was the vector for African sleeping sickness (African trypanosomiasis), an otherwise deadly disease if untreated [7, 9–11]. Through natural selection, those with APOL1 (a functional gene for apolipoprotein L1) had a trypanolytic factor in their serum that conferred natural resistance to the disease. The population with the APOL1 gene was completely immune to African sleeping sickness, while those without the gene lacked protection from the disease. In Africa the APOL1 gene modification was extremely beneficial and provided life-saving protection from a widespread insect-mediated infectious disease that was almost impossible to avoid, but now, in America, it presents a significant long-term renal disadvantage. However, once on dialysis, investigators at the Center for Kidney Disease Research and Epidemiology in California found that there was a relative survival advantage in African American dialysis patients that was also related to the APOL1 gene variation. The APOL1 gene is associated with increased kidney failure but is also associated with better outcomes once on dialysis [12].

With the increased renal disease, African Americans make up 35% of all patients on chronic dialysis [13]. The preferred options for kidney failure are home dialysis or, ideally, kidney transplantation, but the most common approach is center-based hemodialysis. Center-based hemodialysis involves traveling to a facility three times per week for the nurse-supervised multihour procedure. This approach can negatively impact the ability to keep employment as well as lower the overall quality of life. Wang and colleagues looked at racial and ethnic disparities in home dialysis access and use and found that African Americans had a consistently lower rate of home hemodialysis and peritoneal dialysis rate when compared with European Americans [14]. This analysis also demonstrated that African Americans had better mortality rates with these modes of dialysis [15].

Vascular access for hemodialysis also remains inadequate for too many African Americans. Nee and colleagues found that African Americans and Hispanics/Latinos were less likely to initiate hemodialysis with an arteriovenous fistula "independent of predialysis nephrology care, area-level income, dual-eligibility status and other insurance types" [16].

African Americans are less likely to have had a nephrology evaluation prior to kidney failure [16, 17]. An appropriate referral to a specialist can positively impact quality of care.

> The involvement of a nephrologist throughout the more advanced stages of chronic kidney disease, preferably in collaboration with a multidisciplinary team, has been strongly recommended. Earlier referral provides the nephrologist time to identify and manage reversible conditions, ensure avoidance of nephrotoxic agents, administer specific therapies, recommend dietary and lifestyle changes to slow the progression of kidney decline, manage comorbidities and complications and institute regular follow-up, education and activation of social support. Even if progression to ESRD is inevitable, earlier nephrology care can optimally prepare the patient for renal replacement therapy, both physically and mentally. [18]

Researchers suggest that 12 months of pre-ESRD care by a specialist is optimal [18, 19].

As has been covered earlier, African American patients with ESRD and on dialysis have better outcomes than matched European American groups, but Kalbfleisch and colleagues looked at racial disparities in outcomes within almost 6000 dialysis facilities [20].

> Without race adjustment, facilities with higher proportions of black patients had better survival outcomes; facilities with the highest percentage of black patients (top 10%) had overall mortality rates approximately 7% lower than expected. After adjusting for within-facility racial differences, facilities with higher proportions of black patients had poorer survival outcomes among black and non-black patients; facilities with the highest percentage of black patients (top 10%) had mortality rates approximately 6% worse than expected. [20]

Essentially, the researchers contend that the better outcomes in African American-predominant dialysis centers are misleading because they should actually be higher. It is only after adjusting for the better survival on dialysis by race do these differences become evident.

Although poor access to healthcare, the APOL1 gene, and increased diabetes and hypertension greatly contribute to added renal disease burden in African Americans, well-designed studies have still failed to fully account for all of the excess kidney disease. Despite similar dietary sodium intake, renal handling, and plasma volume regulation, renal disease burden is substantially worse in African Americans [21].

7.1 Hypertensive Nephrosclerosis

Persistent hypertension results in progressive kidney changes including arteriosclerosis, cortical fibrosis, tubular atrophy and loss, and glomerulosclerosis, which is collectively referred to as hypertensive nephrosclerosis [22]. When compared with the majority population, African Americans have more severe nephrosclerosis; it begins at a younger age, and it results in renal failure more often [22]. The increased prevalence of hypertensive nephrosclerosis is principally attributed to the risk alleles associated with APOL1 and is directly related to the increased burden of end-stage renal disease among African Americans [6, 8].

7.2 Obesity and Proteinuria

In addition to the genetic differences, researchers also suspect that obesity and its increased prevalence leading to diabetes in the African American community is driving up kidney disease [23]:

> We found that BMI was related independently to both urine total protein–creatinine and albumin-creatinine ratios, and that higher urine total protein–creatinine and urine albumin-creatinine ratios were observed in those with the highest BMI. This association was independent of traditional factors previously observed or hypothesized to be related to proteinuria, including BP, level of kidney function, glycemia, and hyperuricemia. In addition, we found that this association was particularly evident in individuals younger than 61 years. This finding raises the possibility that obesity is a risk factor for proteinuria and albuminuria in hypertensive nephrosclerosis and may have a role in the development and progression of kidney disease, particularly in younger patients. [23]

The African American Study of Kidney Disease and Hypertension (AASK) cohort study found that higher body mass index (BMI) is significantly associated with increased urine total protein and albumin excretion. Specifically, each 2-kg/m^2 increase in BMI was associated with a 3.5% increase in proteinuria and a 5.6% increase in albuminuria after adjusting for various confounders such as age, sex, systolic blood pressure, serum glucose, uric acid, and creatinine levels [24]. Additionally, the Jackson Heart Study highlighted that higher visceral adipose volume, a measure of central obesity, was independently associated with incident CKD, particularly in those with lower dietary quality [25]. This suggests that metabolic factors may be crucial in obesity-associated CKD risk. Moreover, metabolic syndrome, which often accompanies obesity, has been linked to increased levels of proteinuria in hypertensive African Americans. However, when adjusting for proteinuria, the association between metabolic syndrome and CKD progression was insignificant, indicating that proteinuria is a critical mediator in this relationship [23].

7.3 Kidney Disease Progression

In terms of tracking kidney disease progression, the African American Study of Kidney Disease and Hypertension (AASK) found that proteinuria (both baseline and follow-up) was a better predictor of subsequent kidney disease in African Americans than a baseline glomerular filtration rate (GFR) which is generally accepted as the best predictor [24, 26]. In all, it is important to remember that measuring proteinuria is the most predictive in all racial and ethnic subgroups as a marker for renal disease.

Decreased education and low socioeconomic status have been shown to contribute to excess ESRD in African Americans [27, 28]. Other risk factors include:

- Male
- Diabetes history
- Smoking
- Hypertension

Despite the high prevalence and incidence of chronic and end-stage renal disease in African Americans, among those with kidney disease, African Americans have a better-adjusted survival rate [27]. This paradox of improved survival in African Americans after initiation of dialysis has befuddled researchers given the disproportionate occurrence and increased comorbidities. Ma and colleagues at the Wake Forest School of Medicine suggest that the improved survival in nondiabetic-induced nephropathy may also be due to the very gene that causes the disparity, the APOL1 gene, but this time, it conveys protection against further advancing atherosclerosis while on dialysis [29].

Time will sort out these genetic and phenotypic peculiarities, but the overall poor outcomes in renal disease persist, and their impact on the African American population remains clear and present.

7.4 Treatment and Counseling

As far as treatment, in contrast to the contraindications for the use of ACE inhibitors as a singular first-line treatment of hypertension, the use of ACE inhibitors (and ARBs) is the mainstay of therapy for the reduction of adverse clinical outcomes for African American patients with kidney disease. Using an ACE or ARB in combination with a thiazide diuretic in African Americans with hypertensive nephrosclerosis has been shown to decrease the progression of disease [30]. Elevated blood pressure should be aggressively treated.

Thiazide-type diuretics and Calcium Channel Blockers (CCBs): These are recommended as initial antihypertensive treatments in African Americans without chronic kidney disease (CKD), as they are more effective in lowering blood pressure in this population [31]. *Renin-Angiotensin System (RAS) Blockade:* For African

Americans with CKD, the ACC/AHA guidelines recommend the use of ACE inhibitors or angiotensin receptor blockers (ARBs) to slow kidney disease progression, particularly in those with albuminuria (≥300 mg/day) [32, 33]. This recommendation ignores the increased risk for angioedema in African Americans on ACE inhibitors. ARBs are preferred in African Americans [32, 34, 35]. *Blood Pressure Targets:* The ACC/AHA guidelines recommend a blood pressure target of less than 130/80 mm Hg for adults with hypertension and CKD to reduce cardiovascular and renal outcomes [32]. *APOL1 Genotype Considerations:* Individuals with APOL1 risk variants may have differential responses to antihypertensive therapies. For example, those with APOL1 risk alleles may experience greater blood pressure and albuminuria reduction with ARBs like candesartan. Strict blood pressure control is particularly beneficial in reducing mortality risk in those with high-risk APOL1 genotypes [36, 37].

Continued cigarette smoking also negatively impacts renal function, accelerates albuminuria, and decreases the glomerular filtration rate (GFR) in African Americans [38]. A large study of over 5000 participants found a dose-dependent (cigarette-per-day dependent) direct relationship between renal function decline and smoking: the more cigarettes per day, the faster the renal function decline. The study also found that smoking was also related to elevated CRP (C-reactive protein) levels, suggesting that smoking elevates inflammation in some way [38]. The more likely explanation links smoking and progressive vascular disease and worsened blood pressure control. Most patients with chronic kidney disease die of cardiovascular disease, which speaks to the value of adequate hypertension control in patients with kidney disease, as well as persistent smoking cessation counseling [39, 40].

7.5 Kidney Transplantation

Finally, disparities also exist in kidney transplantation, with fewer African American referrals for kidney transplantation [41, 42]. Barriers to organ transplantation include African Americans being less likely than European Americans to be supportive of organ donation [42, 43], to be referred and evaluated for transplant [44], to be identified as a donor, and to consent to organ donation [42, 44].

The issues related to African Americans consenting to organ donation have been the topic of much research, and the basis for skepticism in this sometimes-life-saving process rests in cultural and experiential differences. Because African Americans have fewer transplants, the awareness in the community of successful and productive transplants remains low. It is important for many African American patients to understand that kidney donation does not require the sacrifice of life or that agreeing to other organ donations does not initiate a grand conspiracy to prematurely be declared dead for the benefit of others. The history of earned distrust of the medical community negatively impacts outcomes related to the donation and the receiving of life-saving organ transplantation. A study by Esther Brown at the

School of Nursing at Widener University found five fundamental areas of "reluctance" to transplantation [43]:

1. A lack of awareness
2. Lack of trust in the medical profession
3. Fear of premature death
4. Racial discrimination
5. Religious beliefs and misconceptions

The overall decreased organ donation in the African American population decreases the options for closer genetic matches, which can usually lead to better long-term graft survival. Another barrier is the increased comorbidities (diabetes and hypertension) in African Americans, which may disqualify a potential African American donor. Families with members who have end-stage renal disease are frequently populated with others with the same problems, thus decreasing the pool of potential high-match living donors. Breakthroughs in genomic medicine have revealed that individuals with APOL1 genetic variants are associated with significantly decreased transplant graft survival [45]. Nephrologists have long known that kidneys from African American donors had significantly shorter allograft survival no matter the race of the recipient. In fact, African American recipients of non-African American kidneys have a higher likelihood of prolonged allograft survival [45].

Other African Americans simply disqualify themselves as potential donors due to a misperception of their own health and the thought that because of a history of poor dietary habits and lifestyle decisions, no one would want their organs [46].

Once kidney transplantation is indicated, several factors increase waiting time and negatively influence graft survival after transplantation. Outside of related donors, minimizing the genetic mismatches greatly improves transplant opportunity and ultimate success but naturally will negatively impact African Americans' waiting for the reasons discussed above. Having an African American donor or recipient negatively impacts graft survival for a number of factors that are poorly understood. Taber, Egede, and Baliga found a consistently higher rate of acute rejection and delayed graft function in African Americans, with over 90% compromised after 5 years [47].

With a myriad of issues related to early diagnosis, occurrence, progression, preparation for dialysis, dialysis initiation, transplant planning, and posttransplant preservation, much work still needs to be done with African Americans and kidney disease.

7.6 Kidney Stones

Urinary tract calculi (kidney stones) are far more common in European Americans and Asians than in African Americans [48]. European American males are affected three to four times more often than African American males, though African

Americans have a higher incidence of infected ureteral calculi than European Americans. The difference in the occurrence of stones between African American men and women is small compared to the large difference based on sex in European Americans. African Americans tend to develop stones at an older age, and there is a curious but verified association with increased gallstones [49].

If an African American develops kidney stones, calcium oxalate and calcium phosphate stones are still the most common, but African Americans also have a higher propensity to form uric acid stones, have diabetes, and have a higher BMI and waist circumference. As part of the workup for kidney stone, a 24-h urine collection is a key aspect. Unfortunately, Eric Ghiraldi at the Einstein Healthcare Network found that "African American patients were half as likely to submit a 24-h urine collection than (European American) patients" [50]. Spending more time describing the process and purpose of a 24-h urine collection should improve your success with patient compliance.

A Precision Medicine Approach to Renal Disease in African Americans
- There is at least a threefold increase in occurrence of renal disease among African Americans, but African Americans have a better-adjusted survival rate.
- Diabetes and hypertension are generally the cause of ESRD in African Americans, with nephropathy caused by renal-risk variants in the apolipoprotein L1 gene (*APOL1*).
- Vascular injury caused by smoking, obesity, diabetes, hyperlipidemia, and persistent hypertension accelerates kidney injury.
- For African Americans with CKD, the use of angiotensin receptor blockers (ARBs) to slow kidney disease progression, particularly in those with albuminuria, is preferred over ACE inhibitors.
- A blood pressure target of less than 130/80 mm Hg for adults with hypertension and CKD to reduce cardiovascular and renal outcomes is essential.
- Measuring proteinuria is the best way to track kidney function in African Americans.
- African Americans should be advised of the one-to-one correlation between the amount of their cigarette smoking and their continued renal function decline.
- Kidney transplantation differences:
  – African Americans tend to be less open to donating organs for transplantation.
  – African Americans tend to be less aware of their options as related to kidney transplantation and also less aware of the specifics regarding the maintenance of a transplanted organ.

(continued)

- Kidney transplants in African Americans tend to have a shorter duration of viability.
- Allograft survival is shorter in recipients of kidneys from African American donors relative to those donated by European Americans, regardless of the race of the recipient.

• African Americans have a lower incidence of urinary tract calculi.

- When they occur, African Americans have a *higher incidence* of infected ureteral calculi than European Americans.
- When collecting a 24-h urine sample, spend more time explaining the process and purpose of the collection.

References

1. Marciana L, Shen JI, Norris KC. Kidney disease among African Americans: a population perspective. Am J Kidney Dis. 72(5):S3–7. https://doi.org/10.1053/j.ajkd.2018.06.021.
2. Friedman DJ, Pollak MR. APOL1 nephropathy: from genetics to clinical applications. Clin J Am Soc Nephrol. 16(2):294–303. https://doi.org/10.2215/CJN.15161219.
3. Ingelfinger JR, Lee CD, Asaf V. Genetics of chronic kidney disease. New Engl J Med. 391(7):627–39. https://doi.org/10.1056/NEJMra2308577.
4. Parnaz D, Kopp JB, Winkler CA, Rosenberg AZ. The evolving story of apolipoprotein L1 nephropathy: the end of the beginning. Nat Rev Nephrol. 18(5):307–20. https://doi.org/10.1038/s41581-022-00538-3.
5. Gbadegesin RA, Ifeoma U, Samuel A, Yemi R, Timothy O, Charlotte O, Ademola AD, Adanze A, Winkler CA, David B, Fatiu A, Ivy E, Jacob P-R, Manmak M, Michael M, Olukemi A, Richard C, Sampson A, Adeyemo AA, Ilori TO, Victoria A, Alexander N, Anita G, Toyin A, Adaobi S, Olugbenga A, Kimmel PL, Chip BF, Muhammad M, Uzoma O, Matthias K, Hodgin JB, Pollak MR, Vincent B, Freedman BI, Palmer ND, Bernard C, Milind P, Jill S, Agwai CI, Ogochukwu O, Aliyu A, Jillian W, Winfred W, Salako Babatunde L, Parekh Rulan S, Bamidele T, Dwomoa A, Akinlolu O. New Engl J Med. 392(3):228–38. https://doi.org/10.1056/NEJMoa2404211.
6. Sinha S, Shaheen M, Rajavashisth T, Pan D, Norris K, Nicholas S. Association of race/ethnicity, inflammation, and albuminuria in patients with diabetes and early chronic kidney disease. Diabetes Care. 2014;37(4):1060–8.
7. Parsa A, Kao W, Xie D, et al. APOL1 risk variants, race, and progression of chronic kidney disease. N Engl J Med. 2013;369(23):2183–96.
8. 2017 United States Renal Data System annual data report: executive summary. https://www.usrds.org/2017/download/2017_Volume_1_CKD_in_the_US.pdf
9. Freedman B, Limou S, Ma L, Kopp J. APOL1-associated nephropathy: a key contributor to racial disparities in CKD. Am J Kidney Dis. 72(5 Suppl 1):S8–16.
10. Kruzel-Davila E, Wasser WG, Aviram S, Skorecki K. APOL1 nephropathy: from gene to mechanisms of kidney injury. Nephrol Dial Transplant. 2016;31(3):349–58.
11. Genovese G, Friedman DJ, Ross MD, Lecordier L, Uzureau P, Freedman BI, et al. Association of trypanolytic ApoL1 variants with kidney disease in African Americans. Science. 2010;329(5993):841–5.

12. Lertdumrongluk P, Streja E, Rhee CM, et al. Survival advantage of African American dialysis patients with end-stage renal disease causes related to APOL1. Cardiorenal Med. 2019;9(4):212–21.
13. African Americans and Kidney Disease. National Kidney Foundation. https://www.kidney.org/news/newsroom/factsheets/African-Americans-and-CKD. Accessed 10 May 2019.
14. Wang V, Zepel L, Coffman CJ, Diamantidis CJ, Scholle SH, Maciejewski ML. Have racial disparities in home dialysis utilization changed over time? Am J Manag Care. 2023;29(3):152–8. https://doi.org/10.37765/ajmc.2023.89329.
15. Mehrotra R, Soohoo M, Rivara MB, Himmelfarb J, Cheung AK, Arah OA, et al. Racial and ethnic disparities in use of and outcomes with home dialysis in the United States. J Am Soc Nephrol. 2016;27(7):2123–34. Epub 2015/12/15. Eng.
16. Nee R, Moon DS, Jindal RM, et al. Impact of poverty and health care insurance on arteriovenous fistula use among incident hemodialysis patients. Am J Nephrol. 2015;42(4):328–36.
17. Kimberly H, Mersha TB, Vassalotti JA, Webb FJ, Nicholas SB. Current state and future trends to optimize the care of chronic kidney disease in African Americans. Am J Nephrol. 2017;46(2):176–86. https://doi.org/10.1159/000479481.
18. Gillespie BW, Morgenstern H, Hedgeman E, et al. Nephrology care prior to end-stage renal disease and outcomes among new ESRD patients in the USA. Clin Kidney J. 2015;8(6):772–80.
19. Norris KC, Williams SF, Rhee CM, et al. Hemodialysis disparities in African Americans: the deeply integrated concept of race in the social fabric of our society. Semin Dial. 2017;30(3):213–23.
20. Kalbfleisch J, Wolfe R, Bell S, et al. Risk adjustment and the assessment of disparities in dialysis mortality outcomes. J Am Soc Nephrol. 2015;26(11):2641–5.
21. Williams S, Ogedegbe G. Unraveling the mechanism of renin-angiotensin-aldosterone system activation and target organ damage in hypertensive blacks. Hypertension. 2011;59:10–1.
22. Hughson M, Puelles V, Hoy W, Douglas-Denton R, Mott S, Bertram J. Hypertension, glomerular hypertrophy and nephrosclerosis: the effect of race. Nephrol Dial Transplant. 2014;297(7):1399–409.
23. Lea J, Greene T, Hebert L, Lipkowitz M, Massry S, Middleton J, Rostand S, Miller E, Smith W, Bakris G. The relationship between magnitude of proteinuria reduction and risk of end-stage renal disease: results of the African American study of kidney disease and hypertension. Arch Intern Med. 2005;165(8):947–53.
24. Toto RD, Tom G, Hebert LA, Leena H, Lea JP, Lewis JB, Velvie P, Mohammed S, Xuelei W. Relationship between body mass index and proteinuria in hypertensive nephrosclerosis: results from the African American study of kidney disease and hypertension (AASK) cohort. Am J Kidney Dis. 56(5):896–906. https://doi.org/10.1053/j.ajkd.2010.05.016.
25. Olivo Robert E, Davenport Clemontina A, Diamantidis Clarissa J, Bhavsar Nrupen A, Tyson Crystal C, Rasheeda H, Aurelian B, Bessie Y, Mwasongwe Stanford E, Jane P, Ebony BL, Scialla Julia J. Obesity and synergistic risk factors for chronic kidney disease in African American adults: the Jackson heart study. Nephrol Dial Transplant. 2017;33(6):992–1001. https://doi.org/10.1093/ndt/gfx230.
26. Toto R. Lessons from the African American study of kidney disease and hypertension: an update. Curr Hypertens Rep. 2006;8(5):409–12.
27. Lipworth L, Mumma M, Cavanaugh K, Edwards T, Ikizler T, Tarone R, McLaughlin J, Blot W. Incidence and predictors of end stage renal disease among low-income blacks and whites. PLoS One. 2012;7(10):e48407.
28. Ward M. Socioeconomic status and the incidence of ESRD. Am J Kidney Dis. 2008;51(4):563–72.
29. Ma L, Langefeld C, Comeau M. APOL1 renal-risk genotypes associate with longer hemodialysis survival in prevalent nondiabetic African American patients with end-stage renal disease. Kidney Int. 2016;90(2):389–95.
30. Dirkx TC, Woodell T. Kidney disease. In: Papadakis MA, SJ MP, Rabow MW, editors. Current medical diagnosis & treatment. New York: McGraw-Hill; 2019. http://0-accessmedicine.mhmedical.com.crusher.neomed.edu/content.aspx?bookid=2449&sectionid=194574729. Accessed 11 May 2019.

31. Whelton Paul K., Carey Robert M., Aronow Wilbert S., Casey Donald E., Collins Karen J., Dennison Himmelfarb Cheryl, DePalma Sondra M., Gidding Samuel, Jamerson Kenneth A., Jones Daniel W., MacLaughlin Eric J., Muntner Paul, Ovbiagele Bruce, Smith Sidney C., Spencer Crystal C., Stafford Randall S., Taler Sandra J., Thomas Randal J., Williams Kim A., Williamson Jeff D., Wright Jackson T., 2017 ACC/AHA/AAPA/ABC/ACPM/AGS/APhA/ASH/ASPC/NMA/PCNA guideline for the prevention detection evaluation and management of high blood pressure in adults: a report of the American College of Cardiology/American Heart Association Task Force on clinical practice guidelines. Circulation 138(17) https://doi.org/10.1161/CIR.0000000000000596.
32. Whelton PK, Carey RM, Aronow WS, Casey DE, Collins KJ, Cheryl DH, DePalma Sondra M, Samuel G, Jamerson KA, Jones DW, MacLaughlin EJ, Paul M, Bruce O, Smith SC, Spencer CC, Stafford RS, Taler SJ, Thomas RJ, Williams KA, Williamson JD, Wright JT. ACC/AHA/AAPA/ABC/ACPM/AGS/APhA/ASH/ASPC/NMA/PCNA guideline for the prevention detection evaluation and management of high blood pressure in adults. J Am Coll Cardiol. 2017;71(19):e127–248. https://doi.org/10.1016/j.jacc.2017.11.006.
33. Sula Karreci Esilida, Jacas Sonako, Donovan Olivia, Pintye Diana, Wiley Nicholas, Zsengeller Zsuzsanna K., Schlondorff Johannes, Alper Seth L., Friedman David J., Pollak Martin R., Differing sensitivities to angiotensin converting enzyme inhibition of kidney disease mediated by APOL1 high-risk variants G1 and G2. Kidney Int 106(6) 1072–1085 https://doi.org/10.1016/j.kint.2024.07.026.
34. Zuraw BL, Bernstein JA, Lang DM, Timothy C, David D, Fred H, David K, Javed S, David W, Bernstein DI, Joann B-M, Linda C, Nicklas RA, John O, Portnoy JM, Randolph CR, Schuller DE, Spector SL, Tilles SA, Dana W. A focused parameter update: hereditary angioedema acquired C1 inhibitor deficiency and angiotensin-converting enzyme inhibitor–associated angioedema. J Allergy Clin Immunol. 131(6):1491–3.e25. https://doi.org/10.1016/j.jaci.2013.03.034.
35. Vincenzo M, Marco C. ACE inhibitor-mediated angioedema. Int Immunopharmacol. 78:106081. https://doi.org/10.1016/j.intimp.2019.106081.
36. Cunningham PN, Zhiying W, Grove ML, Cooper-DeHoff RM, Beitelshees AL, Yan G, Gums JG, Johnson JA, Turner ST, Eric B, Chapman AB, Tatsuo S. Hypertensive APOL1 risk allele carriers demonstrate greater blood pressure reduction with angiotensin receptor blockade compared to low risk carriers. PLoS One. 2019;14(9):e0221957. https://doi.org/10.1371/journal.pone.0221957.
37. Elaine K, Lipkowitz MS, Appel LJ, Afshin P, Jennifer G, Glidden DV, Miroslaw S, Chi-yuan H. Strict blood pressure control associates with decreased mortality risk by APOL1 genotype. Kidney Int. 91(2):443–50. https://doi.org/10.1016/j.kint.2016.09.033.
38. Hall M, Wang W, Okhomina V, Agarwal M, Hall J, Dreisbach A, Juncos L, Winniford M, Payne T, Robertson R, Bhatnagar A, Young B. Cigarette smoking and chronic kidney disease in African Americans in the Jackson heart study. J Am Heart Assoc. 2016;5(6):e003280.
39. Rahman M, Pressel S, Davis B. Cardiovascular outcomes in high-risk hypertensive patients stratified by baseline glomerular filtration rate (GFR). Report from the antihypertensive and lipid-lowering treatment to prevent heart trial (ALLHAT). Ann Intern Med. 2006;144(3):172–80.
40. Cheung A, Rahman M, Reboussin D, for the SPRINT Research Group. Effects of intensive blood-pressure control in CKD. J Am Soc Nephrol. 2017;28:2812–23. ISSN: 1046-6673/2809.
41. Kumar K, Holscher C, Luo X, Wang J, Anjum S, King E, Massie A, Tonascia J, Purnell T, Segev D. Persistent regional and racial disparities in nondirected living kidney donation. Clin Transpl. 2017;31(12):e13135.
42. Hannah W, Graham FC, Yuridia L, Xingyuan L, Chang C-CH, Amanda DM, Kellee K, Emilee C, Pleis JR, Harn NY, Unruh ML, Ron S, Larissa M. Social determinants of health and race disparities in kidney transplant. Clin J Am Soc Nephrol. 16(2):262–74. https://doi.org/10.2215/CJN.04860420.
43. Brown E. African American present perceptions of organ donation: a pilot study. ABNF J. 2012;23(2):29–33.

44. Sieverdes J, Nemeth L, Magwood G, Baliga P, Chavin K, Ruggiero K, Treiber F. African American kidney transplant patients' perspective on challenges in the living donation process. Prog Transplant. 2015;25(2):164–75.
45. Freedman B, Julian B. Should kidney donors be genotyped for APOL1 risk alleles? Kidney Int. 2015;87(4):671–3.
46. DuBay D, Ivankova N, Herby I, Wynn T, Kohler C, Berry B, Foushee H, Carson A, Redden D, Holt C, Siminoff L, Fouad M, Martin M. African American organ donor registration: a mixed methods design using the theory of planned behavior. Prog Transplant. 2014;24(3):273–83.
47. Taber D, Egede L, Baliga P. Outcome disparities between African Americans and Caucasians in contemporary kidney transplant recipients. Am J Surg. 2017;213(4):666–72.
48. Akoudad S, Szklo M, McAdams M, Fulop T, Anderson C, Coresh J, Kottgen A. Correlates of kidney stone disease differ by race in a multi-ethnic middle aged population: the ARIC study. Prev Med. 2010;51(5):416–20.
49. Ahmed M, Barakat S, Almobarak A. The association between renal stone disease and cholesterol gallstones: the easy to believe and not hard to retrieve theory of the metabolic syndrome. Ren Fail. 2014;36(6):957–62.
50. Ghiraldi E, Reddy M, Li T, Lawler A, Friedlander J. Factors associated with compliance in submitting 24-hour urine collections in an underserved community. J Endourol. 2017;31(S1):S64–8.

Chapter 8
A Precision Medicine Approach to Rheumatic Diseases in African Americans

Contents

8.1	Osteoarthritis	147
8.2	Rheumatoid Arthritis	148
8.3	Systemic Lupus Erythematosus	149
8.4	Ankylosing Spondylitis	152
8.5	Primary Sjögren's Syndrome	152
8.6	Scleroderma (Systemic Sclerosis)	153
8.7	Polymyalgia Rheumatica and Giant Cell Arteritis	154
8.8	Gout	154
References		157

Rheumatic diseases encompass a wide range of conditions affecting the joints, muscles, and connective tissues. These diseases can lead to chronic pain, inflammation, and varying degrees of disability. African Americans are disproportionately affected by several rheumatic diseases. Studies indicate that African Americans experience higher rates of rheumatic diseases compared to other racial groups. For instance, conditions like rheumatoid arthritis (RA), systemic lupus erythematosus (SLE), and osteoarthritis (OA) are more prevalent in this population [1]. African American women are particularly susceptible to SLE. The prevalence is estimated to be two to three times higher in African American women compared with European American women. They also tend to experience more severe manifestations of the disease [2]. African Americans are diagnosed with rheumatoid arthritis at a younger age and experience more severe symptoms throughout the disease course [3]. Socioeconomic factors, including lower household income and education levels, are associated with worse disease activity and health outcomes in African Americans [4]. Genetic factors play a significant role in the higher prevalence and severity of SLE and RA in African Americans. For SLE, several studies have identified specific genetic loci that contribute to the increased risk and severity in African Americans. The *APOL1* gene, which has nephropathy risk alleles G1 and G2, is strongly associated with

© The Author(s), under exclusive license to Springer Nature
Switzerland AG 2025
G. L. Hall, *Precision Medicine for African Americans*,
https://doi.org/10.1007/978-3-031-95774-1_8

lupus nephritis and progression to end-stage renal disease in African Americans. Genetic variations within the major histocompatibility complex (MHC), particularly HLA alleles such as HLA-DRB1*15:03, are more prevalent in African Americans and contribute to the increased risk of SLE. Transancestral studies have also highlighted unique genetic drivers in African Americans, such as those related to B cell activity and metabolic dysfunction, which are less prominent in European populations [5–8]. For rheumatoid arthritis, genetic studies have identified loci that are specific to African Americans, such as GPC5 and RBFOX1, which are not commonly seen in European or Asian populations. These loci, along with other immune-related genes, contribute to the susceptibility and severity of RA in African Americans [9]. The unique linkage disequilibrium patterns in African Americans have also helped identify novel candidate variants that may influence disease expression and severity [10]. Overall, the genetic predisposition in African Americans for these rheumatic diseases involves a complex interplay of ancestry-specific and shared genetic factors, which contribute to the observed disparities in disease prevalence and severity.

Mobility disability manifested as arthritis and other rheumatic disorders are the leading causes of physical disability in the United States. The proportion impacted increases as poverty increases with African Americans disproportionately comprising this group. There are important considerations when treating African American patients with rheumatic diseases in particular, and some can make a significant impact in terms of early diagnosis and morbidity aversion [11].

In contrast to osteoarthritis, which is conventionally viewed as a result of "wear and tear," rheumatic disorders comprise an array of autoimmune-mediated diseases including:

- Rheumatoid arthritis
- Systemic lupus erythematosus
- Ankylosing spondylitis and psoriatic arthritis
- Sjögren syndrome
- Scleroderma
- Polymyalgia rheumatica and giant cell arteritis

There has been a significant debate regarding whether African Americans express autoimmune diseases differently than other racial/ethnic groups and whether these differences are genetically mediated or related to the social determinants of health. Does the disproportionate occurrence of systemic lupus erythematosus in African American women, in particular a greater risk of progression to end-stage renal disease and dialysis, relate somehow to their innate immune function? Or is the immune response related to the stresses of living a life of poverty, social pressure, and racism? The outcomes are clear: African Americans have more severe cases of immune-mediated diseases overall. The exact causes of these adverse outcomes are still being investigated.

Early-life socioeconomic disadvantage has become increasingly targeted as a lasting social determinant of health [12]. Data in rheumatologic studies across the spectrum of diseases suggest that childhood low socioeconomic status increases the risk of later disease [13–16].

While the mystery of increased autoimmune disorders in African Americans will remain essentially a modern-day "nature versus nurture" debate, clinicians have to treat the patients in front of them including their social determinants, and African Americans with immune-mediated diseases will require specialized attention.

8.1 Osteoarthritis

Osteoarthritis (OA) is a multifactorial joint disease characterized by cartilage degradation and structural changes in the subchondral bone, which often leads to joint pain, activity limitations, and physical disability. Middle-aged and older African Americans experience disproportionate rates of functional limitations and disabilities from osteoarthritis when compared with other racial/ethnic groups [17–21]. Specifically, African Americans report greater pain and activity limitation than European Americans. Although researchers have suggested that these disproportionate rates of functional limitations in African Americans may be due to increased obesity rates, poor physical activity, and decreased tolerance of pain in general, it remains unclear what other factors may be related to this disparity [22, 23].

Jordan and colleagues at the Thurston Arthritis Research Center at the University of North Carolina found that "African Americans had a slightly higher prevalence of knee symptoms, radiographic knee OA, and symptomatic knee OA, but a significantly higher prevalence of severe radiographic knee OA compared with (European Americans)" [24].

The Johnston County Osteoarthritis Project in Durham, North Carolina, looked at knee, hip, and multiple joint outcomes and found that "African Americans and (European Americans) with only hip OA or both hip and knee OA did not differ in self-reported pain or function." But the study did find differences in patients with only knee OA and attributed the difference to increased BMI (obesity) and the presence of depression. The authors suggested improving the management of obesity and depressive symptoms as key avenues to successful management of osteoarthritis pain [25]. This Project also found distinct differences in common foot disorders with flat feet (pes planus) being three times more common in African Americans and high arches (pes cavus) being five times less common [26]. African Americans were also more likely to have bunions (hallux valgus), hammer toes, and overlapping toes [26].

Vaughn et al. did a meta-analysis comparing pain from osteoarthritis in European Americans and African Americans, and their review confirmed differences in clinical pain severity, functional limitations, and poor performance between African Americans and European Americans with osteoarthritis [27, 28].

Burns et al. added another confounding layer to the OA debate by reporting that frequently African American and European Americans "with radiographically documented knee OA reported equivalent functional ability and pain severity. However, both (African Americans)'s OA severity rating and tested performance were significantly worse than those of (European Americans)" [29].

Wu and colleagues found significant disparities in management:

> We found racial/ethnic disparities in the utilization of imaging, intra-articular injections, and total joint arthroplasty (TJA) for the diagnosis and treatment of hip and knee OA. Specifically, Asian patients had lower odds of receiving knee intra-articular injections and hip radiographs, and African American (AA) patients had lower odds of receiving knee injections and MRI compared to (European American) patients. Additionally, AA, Hispanic, and Asian patients all had lower odds of undergoing total hip arthroplasty (THA) and total knee arthroplasty (TKA) compared to (European American) patients after controlling several baseline demographic and socioeconomic factors. We also found that higher income quartiles had greater odds of undergoing MRI and TJA, males had lower odds of receiving injections, and greater odds of undergoing TJA, and Medicaid and self-pay patients had lower odds of undergoing TJA. These findings highlight sociodemographic inequities that exist in the management of hip and knee OA [30].

In addition to lower odds of arthritis interventions mentioned above, researchers also found lower referrals for education, weight management, and physical therapy in racial and ethnic minorities when compared with the majority population [23]. These differences are most frequently clinician-driven and we should be more deliberate about balancing our interventions across our patient population.

Liu and colleagues at the University of North Carolina revealed a genome-wide association study (GWAS) in African Americans that identified a significant variant in the LINC01006 gene associated with radiographic knee OA, which is less common in European populations. This variant has a minor allele frequency of 12% in African Americans, compared with less than 3% in European American populations, highlighting its unique relevance in this group [31].

Additionally, pathway analyses have identified significant associations with dorsal/ventral neural tube patterning and iron ion transport pathways. These pathways were significantly associated with knee OA in African Americans [31]. These genetic findings suggest that there may be underlying biological differences in the pathogenesis of knee OA among different racial/ethnic groups. Understanding these differences can help tailor more effective treatment strategies and lead to the development of targeted therapies. Furthermore, acknowledging these genetic variations emphasizes the need for personalized medicine approaches that consider the specific genetic and sociodemographic factors affecting diverse populations.

8.2 Rheumatoid Arthritis

Rheumatoid arthritis (RA) is a chronic systemic disease associated with progressive joint damage and inflammation, diminished quality of life, significant disability, and premature mortality. In contrast to a number of chronic diseases where there is no doubt about the worse outcomes in African Americans, there is more controversy regarding the existence of disparities in RA. When objective clinical signs like rheumatoid nodules, joint deformities on radiographs, and tender joints are considered, there seem to be fewer differences between racial and ethnic groups [32]. In contrast, functional status in African Americans with RA generally shows decreased abilities and lower ranking of self-reported health when compared with the majority populations [3].

In a review of laboratory trends, African American RA patients tended to have rheumatoid factor-positive results in slightly more cases (80% of patients) compared with European Americans (74% of patients) [3].

In all patients with RA, early joint damage (within the first few years) is highly predictive of more damaging disease later and a clear indicator of the need for more aggressive treatment in all patients [33]. Advancing these patients to "disease-modifying antirheumatic drugs" (DMARDs) including hydroxychloroquine, sulfasalazine, methotrexate, and other newer options can slow progression and prevent deformities. Unfortunately, remission rates on DMARDs were comparatively lower in African Americans but still significantly beneficial [3].

8.3 Systemic Lupus Erythematosus

Systemic lupus erythematosus (SLE) is a chronic autoimmune disease that affects an array of organ systems including diffuse joint involvement, dermatitis, pleuritis, myocarditis, hepatitis, blood dyscrasias, and nephritis. African American women have a three- to fourfold increased presentation of SLE when compared with European American women, and like other chronic diseases have increased morbidity and mortality related to the disease [34–36]. SLE can present in a number of unusual fashions. So unusual that experts suggest that if you have an African American woman with a number of seemingly unrelated symptoms that wax and wane, a screen for SLE is a very reasonable diagnostic approach.

SLE Presentation
- Low-grade fever
- Malaise and fatigue
- Weight changes
- Sun-sensitive rash (malar rash)
- Arthritis affecting two or more joints
- Oral ulcers (painless)
- Pleuritis
- Proteinuria
- Seizures or psychosis
- Headaches
- Premature atherosclerosis
- Anemia
- Low WBC
- Low platelet count

Gender disparities also exist with SLE occurring far more often in women (8–10 times more prevalent than in men) [34, 36, 37].

A number of studies have confirmed a much more severe disease course in African Americans with an earlier onset, higher incidence of kidney failure, progression to dialysis, and kidney transplant complications [2, 35, 36]. Lymphadenopathy (LAD) is also a common feature with an increased risk of progression to lymphoma. LAD occurs in approximately 33.7% of patients and is associated with various clinical features, including fever, pericarditis, leukopenia, and membranous nephritis. Histologically, LAD in SLE can present as reactive/proliferative or necrotizing patterns, with necrotizing LAD being linked to more severe symptoms such as fever and malar rash. African Americans with SLE tend to have higher rates of autoantibodies, such as anti-Smith and anti-RNP, which are associated with more severe disease phenotypes, including LAD [38, 39]. Additionally, African Americans are more likely to develop lupus nephritis, a condition significantly associated with LAD.

The increased severity of SLE in African Americans, including the higher prevalence of lymphadenopathy, can be attributed to both genetic predispositions and socioeconomic factors. Genetic studies have shown that African Americans have a higher burden of genetic risk variants that predispose them to more severe SLE manifestations, and lower SES African Americans tend to have worse disease.

Arthritis is seen in 95% of SLE patients and frequently involves the wrists and hands [34, 40, 41]. Kidney involvement in the form of nephritis is the most common manifestation in SLE and is seen microscopically in over 90% of patients but results in significant disease in 50% of patients [42, 43]. The *APOL1* gene that results in increased kidney disease in African Americans (see Chap. 7) makes SLE-related kidney disease much more severe. This gene is so intertwined with renal decline that receiving a transplanted kidney from a donor with the *APOL1* gene makes recurrent kidney failure more common [44, 45].

A study by Franco and colleagues looked at predictors of kidney failure in African Americans and found that hypertension, elevated creatinine, proliferative nephritis, and decreased glomerular filtration rate (GFR) were all associated with an increased risk [45, 46]. The presence of APOL1 G1 and G2 nephropathy risk alleles significantly increases the risk of lupus nephritis progressing to end-stage renal disease (ESRD) [5, 44]. African Americans with these alleles have a higher likelihood of developing ESRD and a shorter time to progression compared to those without these alleles [5]. Consequently, early detection and targeted interventions are crucial for improving outcomes in African Americans with SLE. This includes regular monitoring for lupus nephritis and managing socioeconomic disparities to mitigate the impact of lower SES on disease severity. Proteinuria within the first year of SLE diagnosis strongly predicts ESRD. Additionally, low complement C3 levels are associated with an increased risk of renal failure [47].

There have also been significant investigations into environmental influences on SLE. Carroll et al. did an extensive evaluation of environmental exposures including water analysis, diet, lifestyle factors (smoking and pesticide use), industry proximity, soil chemical data, and more and statistically matched the presence, or development, of antinuclear antibodies (ANA) [48]. Increased exposure to pollutants positively correlated with increased occurrences of ANA status and SLE development. Unfortunately, African Americans are disproportionately exposed and impacted.

As far as treatment differences between races with SLE, African American patients are underrepresented in clinical trials, which limits the generalizability of trial results to this population and affects the availability of evidence-based treatments tailored to their needs [46]. Despite these deficiencies, African American patients have shown a favorable response to mycophenolate mofetil (MMF) for lupus nephritis compared with intravenous cyclophosphamide (IVC) [49, 50]. The American College of Rheumatology guidelines recommend MMF or IVC for induction therapy in lupus nephritis, noting that MMF may be more effective in African American patients [50]. African American patients are more likely to be on chronic glucocorticoid therapy compared with European American patients, which can lead to increased glucocorticoid-related morbidity [51, 52]. This persistent use is associated with higher disease activity and poorer outcomes. There are also indications that vitamin D supplementation may be useful in African American patients with SLE when decreased vitamin D levels were found compared with controls [53–55].

In terms of behaviors contributing to increased SLE risk, the Black Women's Health Study and others found that smoking increases the risk of developing the disease, whereas moderate alcohol consumption was associated with decreased risk [56–59].

Patients with systemic lupus erythematosus have a high prevalence of hypertension, accelerated atherosclerosis, and arterial stiffness that substantially increases their risk for cardiovascular-related death [60, 61]. SLE itself carries an independent risk for coronary artery disease even after adjustment for traditional Framingham risk factors [62, 63]. Garg and colleagues at the University of Wisconsin found that African American patients with SLE had a 19-fold higher risk of incident cardiovascular events in the first 12 years after diagnosis compared with non-African Americans [63]. Risk analyses for perioperative medical management of SLE patients show an increased risk for cardiac and venous thromboembolism in patients with total knee or hip replacement. These patients also had higher perioperative infections suggesting the need for withdrawing immunosuppressive medications earlier [64].

SLE-associated chronic immune-mediated inflammation and damage to the arterial walls causes aortic stiffness, which then leads to hypertension, which then promotes atherosclerosis. Studies have confirmed higher aortic stiffness in younger SLE patients that seems to be independent of age, blood pressure, renal function, and risk factors. In fact, SLE patients with normal blood pressure had consistently higher aortic stiffness [65].

As reviewed earlier, SLE can be tricky to diagnose as it can affect any organ, including musculoskeletal, skin, hematologic, renal, neuropsychiatric, cardiovascular, and respiratory systems. There is no typical order of presentation aside from fatigue and arthritis pain being pervasive complaints. Another clue is increased healthcare utilization in the form of higher-than-expected emergency department or urgent care visits. SLE should also be suspected in any patient who presents with unexplained manifestations involving two or more organ systems [66].

Glucocorticoids and antimalarial drugs form the foundation of SLE management, along with immunosuppressive medications and newer biologic therapies. As the pathogenesis of SLE becomes clearer, more targeted, and better tolerated, treatments will become available [49, 50, 52, 67].

8.4 Ankylosing Spondylitis

Ankylosing spondylitis (AS) is a debilitating spinal arthritic condition usually presenting before age 40, with male predominance, and a very low presentation in African Americans when compared with other racial groups [68]. African Americans with AS tend to exhibit higher disease activity, as evidenced by elevated erythrocyte sedimentation rate (ESR) and C-reactive protein (CRP) levels [68]. They also have a higher frequency of anterior uveitis, hypertension, diabetes, depression, and heart disease compared with European Americans. The prevalence of HLA-B27, a genetic marker strongly associated with AS, is lower in African Americans (approximately 48%) compared with European Americans (94%) [69]. This suggests that susceptibility to AS in African Americans is less closely linked to HLA-B27, and other genetic or environmental factors may play a significant role. African Americans with AS also experience more significant functional impairment and higher disease activity [68, 70].

Additionally, African Americans are at a higher risk of developing osteoporosis, with a significant association between elevated CRP levels and African American race. AS can present with acute uveitis, peripheral arthritis, enthesitis, psoriasis, aortic root inflammation, and gut irritation. Ankylosing spondylitis involves both inflammatory erosive osteopenia and unusual bony overgrowth [71]. To manage comorbidities in African Americans with AS, it is crucial to adopt a comprehensive treatment approach. This includes regular monitoring and control of inflammation through medication, such as NSAIDs and biologics, to reduce disease activity. Additionally, implementing lifestyle modifications like a balanced diet, regular exercise, and smoking cessation can help manage cardiovascular risk factors and improve overall health outcomes [72].

8.5 Primary Sjögren's Syndrome

Sjögren's syndrome is a chronic, slowly progressing autoimmune disease characterized by lymphocytic infiltration of the exocrine glands resulting in xerostomia and dry eyes. The majority of patients with Sjögren's syndrome have symptoms related to impaired tear formation and salivary gland function. The disease progression is slow and a majority of patients manage well. Like ankylosing spondylitis and polymyalgia rheumatica, this has a rare presentation in African Americans [73, 74].

Sjögren's syndrome in African Americans is characterized by a distinct clinical and serological profile compared with other ethnic groups. African American patients with Sjögren's syndrome tend to present with higher systemic disease activity at diagnosis, as measured by the EULAR Sjögren's Syndrome Disease Activity Index (ESSDAI) [75]. They exhibit higher frequencies of lymphadenopathy, joint pain, peripheral nervous system, central nervous system, and biological domain involvement [76]. Additionally, African Americans with primary Sjögren's syndrome are more likely to have hypergammaglobulinemia, elevated erythrocyte sedimentation rate (ESR), and parotid gland enlargement, which puts them at a higher risk of developing lymphomas [76]. The disease tends to be diagnosed earlier in African Americans compared with European American patients, and the female-to-male ratio is lower in African Americans. Several genetic factors may contribute to the distinct presentation of Sjögren's syndrome in African Americans. Studies have identified specific genetic polymorphisms that are more prevalent in African American populations, which may influence immune system regulation and disease susceptibility [77]. Understanding these genetic predispositions is crucial for developing targeted therapies and personalized treatment plans for African American patients with Sjögren's syndrome.

8.6 Scleroderma (Systemic Sclerosis)

Scleroderma, also known as systemic sclerosis (SSc) scleroderma, is a chronic disorder characterized by diffuse fibrosis of the skin and internal organs. Women are affected four times more frequently than men [78]. Scleroderma had a modestly higher prevalence among African Americans than European Americans. In most patients, the impact is limited to the face, neck, and extremities; however, some patients have more severe and wide-ranging involvement. Raynaud's phenomenon is frequently present, but GERD, pulmonary fibrosis, pulmonary hypertension, and renal problems occur as well. Raynaud's phenomenon generally precedes other disease manifestations and may be the presenting complaint. CREST syndrome is an acronym for scleroderma's commonly associated problems, including calcinosis cutis, Raynaud's phenomenon, esophageal dysmotility, sclerodactyly, and telangiectasia.

African Americans generally have more severe manifestations of scleroderma, and the aggressiveness of the disease seems to be linked to socioeconomic status. Higher SES African Americans have a milder disease, whereas poorer patients tend to have a more complicated course [79].

Duncan Moore, Virginia Steen, and colleagues at Georgetown University Hospital looked at scleroderma in a large retrospective evaluation of clinical outcomes by race. They found that African Americans with scleroderma tend to have worse disease outcomes with more severe pulmonary disease with increased fibrosis noted on imaging as well as decreased overall lung function [78]. Worse cardiac disease with increased pulmonary hypertension on right heart catheterization was also noted in African Americans [80]. African American patients are more likely to have the confirmatory markers, anti-Scl70 (antitopoisomerase) and anti-U1RNP antibodies, than European American patients. They were less likely to have anticentromere antibodies than majority populations. Overall, African Americans tended to be younger at disease onset and were hospitalized more frequently. Interestingly, their study found that after controlling for socioeconomic status, "African American race was not a statistically significant independent mortality risk factor and that a lower household income increased the risk of death during follow-up" [78].

The differences seen in scleroderma are not based on race but instead based on a social determinant of health. The opportunity to completely erase the significant disparities seen in scleroderma is completely within our reach [81].

8.7 Polymyalgia Rheumatica and Giant Cell Arteritis

Polymyalgia rheumatica (PMR) is an inflammatory condition that generally affects people over the age of 50 and can cause profound pain and stiffness in the proximal muscles of the shoulders, neck, and hip. Giant cell arteritis (GCA), or temporal arteritis, is an inflammatory disease affecting the large blood vessels of the scalp, neck, and arms which causes a narrowing of the blood vessels. Polymyalgia rheumatica and giant cell arteritis probably represent a spectrum of one disease: one localized and the other more systemic [82]. The vasculitic involvement of these arteries leads to the typical symptoms of GCA, such as temporal headache, jaw pain, scalp tenderness, or abnormal temporal arteries on biopsy. Both affect the same older population, and the incidence increases with advancing age. Women are affected two to three times more often than men. PMR and giant cell arteritis are distinctly less common in Asian, African American, and Latino/Hispanic populations, though all racial and ethnic groups can be affected [83]. Both PMR and GCA respond well to steroid administration.

8.8 Gout

Gout is the most common inflammatory arthritis in the United States and is more common in African Americans principally due to a higher prevalence of risk factors [84, 85]. The increased incidence of diabetes, obesity, hypertension, and chronic kidney disease in African Americans contributes to higher uric acid levels that directly increase the risk for gout attacks. African American diet trends that increase the risk for hyperuricemia include:

8.8 Gout

- Increased meat consumption that leads to excess purine that is degraded to uric acid.
- Increased sugary-sweetened beverages, whereby fructose metabolism leads to increased uric acid levels.
- Decreased vitamin C-containing fruits and vegetables leads to decreased uric acid clearing.
- Less overall alcohol consumed but when used, leads to increased uric acid production [84].
- Hypertension and the use of diuretics can increase serum urate levels.

Genome-wide association studies (GWAS) have identified several genetic loci associated with serum urate levels and gout in African Americans. Notably, variants in the *SLC2A9* and *SLC22A12* genes have been implicated. The *SLC2A9* gene, which encodes a urate transporter, has significant associations with serum urate levels in African Americans [86]. Additionally, a novel rare nonsynonymous variant in the *SLC22A12* gene (rs12800450) has been identified and replicated, demonstrating a large effect size on serum urate levels [86–88]. Furthermore, the *ABCG2* gene, which encodes another urate transporter, has been associated with gout risk. The Q141K polymorphism (rs2231142) in the *ABCG2* gene has been shown to significantly increase serum urate levels and gout risk in African Americans [89].

The disorders usually associated with gouty attacks are clinically time-consuming chronic diseases, including coronary artery disease, diabetes, kidney disease, and hypertension. In comparison, these more life-threatening diseases supplant gout complaints and any discussion of strategies for improvement in uric acid. Studies have shown that reducing uric acid levels has been associated with better overall outcomes, including lower cardiovascular mortality and slowed kidney failure [85, 90].

A number of studies have documented lower uric acid levels in younger African Americans (average age 24 in one case) when compared with European Americans, but after maturity, their low risk disappears [91]. Aside from diet, the environmental, genetic, and physiologic factors explaining the uric acid differences between African Americans and European Americans remain obscure. Uric acid excretion abnormalities are the most common causes of hyperuricemia and make sense, considering comorbidities seem to drive some of the increased risk [92].

Given the increased comorbidities, choosing the right medications can be a challenge. Hydrochlorothiazide is suggested as the first line for the treatment of hypertensive African Americans, yet also well known to increase uric acid levels [93, 94]. Furthermore, a study at Johns Hopkins found that metoprolol increased the serum uric acid in African Americans with kidney disease that were treated for hypertension [95]. The researchers found no increase with ACE inhibitors or amlodipine [95]. This basically leaves amlodipine as the lone best choice for treating African Americans with hypertension, renal insufficiency, and a risk for gout. It is well accepted that hyperuricemia is a risk factor for kidney disease progression, given its increased occurrence in African Americans; the uric acid level should be used as a risk screen even in the absence of gout attacks [96]. In addition, the use of allopurinol has been suggested to slow the progression of renal disease.

> **Lifestyle Modifications for African Americans with High Uric Acid and/or Gout**
> - Lose weight
> - Avoid fructose-containing sugary-sweetened beverages
> - Limit red meat (beef, pork, and lamb) and seafood
> - Limit certain vegetables, including potatoes, spinach, asparagus, peas, cauliflower, and mushrooms
> - Avoid alcohol (particularly beer and liquor)
> - Increase dairy intake (eggs, low-fat milk, yogurt, cheese) if not lactose intolerant
> - Get regular exercise and stay hydrated

Overall, the treatment of gout in African Americans is no different than any other racial group or ethnicity. Patients should be counseled regarding dietary and behavioral modifications first. Suggestions should be specific. African Americans should avoid fructose-containing sugary-sweetened beverages ("high fructose corn syrup") [84]. Red meat (beef, pork, and lamb) and seafood should be significantly limited. Certain vegetables also lead to higher uric acid levels, including potatoes, mushrooms, spinach, asparagus, cauliflower, and peas [84, 97]. Remember to assess the patient's alcohol intake, recommend a decrease, and particularly discourage beer [97]. Daily intake of coffee has been shown to be protective of gout [98], as has vitamin C and cherry juice [99]. Although there is increased lactose intolerance in African Americans, those not intolerant should increase their dairy intake in the form of skim milk, cheese, and eggs [97, 100]. A study by Dalbeth and colleagues found a decrease in uric acid levels of 10% in those that consumed milk [101]. Like in many disorders related to lifestyle habits, exercise and weight loss are always beneficial [100].

> **A Precision Medicine Approach to Rheumatic Diseases in African Americans**
> - Racial differences exist in clinical pain severity, functional limitations, and poor performance between African Americans and European Americans with osteoarthritis, but the differences are small.
> - Data in rheumatologic studies across the spectrum of diseases suggest that childhood low socioeconomic status increases the risk of later-life disease.
> - Flat feet (pes planus) are three times more common in African Americans, while high arches (pes cavus) are five times less common. African Americans were also more likely to have bunions (hallux valgus), hammer toes, and overlapping toes.
> - African American RA patients tended to have rheumatoid factor-positive results in slightly more cases (80% of patients) compared with European Americans (74% of patients).

(continued)

- The *APOL1* gene that results in increased kidney disease in African Americans makes SLE-related kidney disease much more severe.
- In all patients with RA, early joint damage (within the first few years) is very predictive of more damaging disease later and a clear indicator of the need for more aggressive treatment.
- Patients with SLE and hypertension, higher creatinine, and decreased GFR are at higher risk for dialysis.
- There is an environmental exposure and SLE outcome relationship such that the occurrence and severity of SLE are more prominent in urban industrial regions.
- The *APOL1* gene results in increased and earlier kidney disease progression in African Americans with SLE.
- Patients with SLE and hypertension, higher creatinine, proliferative nephritis, and decreased GFR as well as genetic, environmental, and socioeconomic factors were associated with increased ESRD requiring dialysis.
- Ankylosing spondylitis (AS) is a debilitating spinal arthritic condition related to HLA-B27 that is found in 2%–4% of African Americans.
- Sjögren's syndrome is a chronic, slowly progressing autoimmune disease that rarely occurs in African Americans.
- Scleroderma had a modestly higher prevalence among African Americans than European Americans.
- African Americans generally have more severe manifestations of scleroderma, and the aggressiveness of the disease seems to be linked to socioeconomic status. Higher SES African Americans have a milder disease, whereas poorer patients tend to have a more complicated course.
- Both PMR and GCA rarely occur in African Americans.
- African Americans start with a lower risk for gout but, as they age, develop a higher risk due to dietary, environmental, genetic, and physiologic factors.
- Hydrochlorothiazide increases the risk for hyperuricemia.
- Metoprolol increases the risk for hyperuricemia in African Americans with chronic kidney disease.

References

1. Benjamin NW, Barnes EL, Shilpa V, Kappelman MD, Curtis JR, Merkel PA, Shaw DG, Kalen L, Justin G, George MD. Racial and ethnic distribution of rheumatic diseases in health Systems of the National Patient-Centered Clinical Research Network. J Rheumatol. 2023;50(11):1503–8. https://doi.org/10.3899/jrheum.2022-1300.
2. Liang MH, Lew ER, Fraser PA, Cindy F, Hennis Edward H, Sang-Cheol B, Anselm H, Mohammed T, Neal RW. Choosing to end African American health disparities in patients with systemic Lupus Erythematosus. Arthritis Rheumatol. 76(6):823–35. https://doi.org/10.1002/art.42797.

3. Greenberg JD, Spruill T, Shan Y, et al. Racial and ethnic disparities in disease activity in rheumatoid arthritis patients. Am J Med. 2013;126(12):1089–98.
4. Baldassari AR, Cleveland RJ, Jonas BL, Conn DL, Moreland LW, Bridges SL, Callahan Leigh F. Socioeconomic disparities in the health of African Americans with Rheumatoid Arthritis from thie Southeastern United States. Arthritis Care Res. 66(12):1808–17. https://doi.org/10.1002/acr.22351.
5. Barry F I, Langefeld Carl D, Andringa Kelly K, Croker Jennifer A, Williams Adrienne H, Garner Neva E, Birmingham Daniel J, Hebert Lee A, Hicks Pamela J, Segal Mark S, Edberg Jeffrey C, Brown Elizabeth E, Alarcón Graciela S, Costenbader Karen H, Comeau Mary E, Criswell Lindsey A, Harley John B, James Judith A, Kamen Diane L, Sam LS, Merrill Joan T, Sivils Kathy L, Niewold Timothy B, Patel Neha M, Michelle P, Rosalind R-G, Reveille John D, Salmon Jane E, Tsao Betty P, Gibson Keisha L, Byers Joyce R, Vinnikova Anna K, Lea Janice P, Julian Bruce A, Kimberly Robert P. End-stage renal disease in African Americans with lupus nephritis is associated with APOL1. Arthritis Rheumatol. 66(2):390–6. https://doi.org/10.1002/art.38220.
6. Hanscombe Ken B, Morris David L, Noble Janelle A, Dilthey Alexander T, Philip T, Kaufman Kenneth M, Mary C, Langefeld Carl D, Alarcon-Riquelme Marta E, Gaffney Patrick M, Jacob Chaim O, Sivils Kathy L, Tsao Betty P, Alarcon Graciela S, Brown Elizabeth E, Jennifer C, Jeff E, Gary G, James Judith A, Kamen Diane L, Kelly Jennifer A, Joseph MC, Merrill Joan T, Michelle P, Rosalind R-G, Reveille John D, Salmon Jane E, Hal S, Tammy U, Wallace Daniel J, Weisman Michael H, Kimberly Robert P, Harley John B, Lewis Cathryn M, Criswell Lindsey A, Vyse Timothy J. Genetic fine mapping of systemic lupus erythematosus MHC associations in Europeans and African Americans. Hum Mol Genet. 2018;27(21):3813–24. https://doi.org/10.1093/hmg/ddy280.
7. Owen Katherine A, Andrew P, Hannah A, Aidukaitis Bryce N, Prathyusha B, Catalina Michelle D, Dittman James M, Howard Timothy D, Kingsmore Kathryn M, Labonte Adam C, Marion Miranda C, Robl Robert D, Zimmerman Kip D, Langefeld Carl D, Grammer Amrie C, Lipsky Peter E. Analysis of trans-ancestral SLE risk Loci identifies unique biologic networks and drug targets in African and European ancestries. Am J Human Genetics. 107(5):864–81. https://doi.org/10.1016/j.ajhg.2020.09.007.
8. Langefeld CD, Ainsworth HC, Cunninghame GDS, Kelly Jennifer A, Comeau Mary E, Marion Miranda C, Howard Timothy D, Ramos Paula S, Croker Jennifer A, Morris David L, Sandling Johanna K, Carlsson AJ, Acevedo-Vásquez Eduardo M, Alarcón Graciela S, Babini Alejandra M, Vicente B, Bengtsson Anders A, Berbotto Guillermo A, Marc B, Brown Elizabeth E, Hermine B I, Cardiel Mario H, Luis C, Ricard C, Cucho-Venegas Jorge M, Rantapää Sandra D'A, Martins DSB, de la Rúa Figueroa Iñigo, Andrea D, Edberg Jeffrey C, Emőke E, Esquivel-Valerio Jorge A, Fortin Paul R, Barry F I, Johan F, García Mercedes A, de la García TI, Gilkeson Gary S, Gladman Dafna D, Iva G, Guthridge Joel M, Huggins Jennifer L, James Judith A, Kallenberg Cees GM, Kamen Diane L, Karp David R, Kaufman Kenneth M, Kottyan Leah C, László K, Helle L, Lauwerys Bernard R, Quan-Zhen L, Maradiaga-Ceceña Marco A, Javier M, M MCJ, R. MWD, Merrill Joan T, Pedro M, Moctezuma José F, Nath Swapan K, Niewold Timothy B, Lorena O, Norberto O-C, Michelle P, Pineau Christian A, Pons-Estel Bernardo A, Janet P, Prithvi R, Rosalind R-G, Reveille John D, Russell Laurie P, Sabio José M, Aguilar-Salinas Carlos A, Scherbarth Hugo R, Raffaella S, Seldin Michael F, Christopher S, Elisabet S, Thompson Susan D, Toloza Sergio MA, Lennart T, Teresa T-L, Carlos V, Vilá Luis M, Wallace Daniel J, Weisman Michael H, Wither Joan E, Tushar B, Oksenberg Jorge R, Rioux John D, Gregersen Peter K, Ann-Christine S, Lars R, Criswell Lindsey A, Jacob Chaim O, Sivils Kathy L, Tsao Betty P, Schanberg Laura E, Behrens Timothy W, Silverman Earl D, Alarcón-Riquelme Marta E, Kimberly Robert P, Harley John B, Wakeland Edward K, Graham Robert R, Gaffney Patrick M, Vyse Timothy J. Transancestral mapping and genetic load in systemic lupus erythematosus. Nat Commun. 2017;8(1) https://doi.org/10.1038/ncomms16021.

9. Laufer Vincent A, Tiwari Hemant K, Reynolds Richard J, Danila Maria I, Jelai W, Edberg Jeffrey C, Kimberly Robert P, Kottyan Leah C, Harley John B, Mikuls Ted R, Gregersen Peter K, Absher Devin M, Langefeld Carl D, Arnett Donna K, Bridges SL Jr. Genetic influences on susceptibility to rheumatoid arthritis in African-Americans. Hum Mol Genet. 2018;28(5):858–74. https://doi.org/10.1093/hmg/ddy395.
10. Danila MI, Laufer VA, Reynolds RJ, Qi Y, Nianjun L, Gregersen Peter K, Annette L, Marlena K, Langefeld Carl D, Arnett Donna K, Louis BS. Dense genotyping of immune-related regions identifies loci for rheumatoid arthritis risk and damage in African Americans. Molecul Med. 23(1):177–87. https://doi.org/10.2119/molmed.2017.00081.
11. Okoro CA, Hollis ND, Cyrus AC, Griffin-Blake S. Prevalence of disabilities and health care access by disability status and type among adults — United States, 2016. MMWR Morb Mortal Wkly Rep. 2018;67:882–7. https://doi.org/10.15585/mmwr.mm6732a3External.
12. Kamp Dush CM, Schmeer KK, Taylor M. Chaos as a social determinant of child health: reciprocal associations? Soc Sci Med. 2013;95:69–76.
13. Brennan SL, Turrell G. Neighborhood disadvantage, individual-level socioeconomic position, and self-reported chronic arthritis: a cross-sectional multilevel study. Arthritis Care Res (Hoboken). 2012;14(5):721–8.
14. Cleveland RJ, Schwartz TA, Prizer LP, Randolph R, Schoster B, Renner JB, Jordan JM, Callahan LF. Associations of educational attainment, occupation, and community poverty with hip osteoarthritis. Arthritis Care Res (Hoboken). 2013;14(6):954–61.
15. Bengtsson C, Nordmark B, Klareskog L, Lundberg I, Alfredsson L. Socioeconomic status and the risk of developing rheumatoid arthritis: results from the Swedish EIRA study. Ann Rheum Dis. 2005;14(11):1588–94.
16. Morgan Banks L, Kuper H, Polack S. Poverty and disability in low- and middle-income countries: a systematic review. PLoS One. 2017;12(12):e0189996.
17. Allen KD, Helmick CG, Schwartz TA, DeVellis RF, Renner JB, Jordan JM. Racial differences in self-reported pain and function among individuals with radiographic hip and knee osteoarthritis: the Johnston County osteoarthritis project. Osteoarthr Cartil. 2009;17(9):1132–6.
18. Burns R, Graney MJ, Lummus AC, Nichols LO, Martindale-Adams J. Differences of self-reported osteoarthritis disability and race. JAMA. 2007;99(9):1046–51.
19. Andresen EM, Brownson RC. Disability and health status: ethnic differences among women in the United States. J Epidemiol Community Health. 2000;54(3):200–6.
20. Sherwin N, Carolina A, Renner JB, Golightly YM, Nelson AE. Features of knee and multijoint osteoarthritis by sex and race and ethnicity: a preliminary analysis in the Johnston County health study. J Rheumatol. 2024;51(1):75–83. https://doi.org/10.3899/jrheum.2023-0479.
21. Vaughn IA, Terry EL, Bartley EJ, Nancy S, Fillingim Roger B. Racial-ethnic differences in osteoarthritis pain and disability: a meta-analysis. J Pain. 20(6):629–44. https://doi.org/10.1016/j.jpain.2018.11.012.
22. Colbert CJ, Almagor O, Chmiel JS, Song J, Dunlop D, Hayes KW, Sharma L. Excess body weight and four-year function outcomes: comparison of African Americans and whites in a prospective study of osteoarthritis. Arthritis Care Res (Hoboken). 2013;65(1):5–14. https://doi.org/10.1002/acr.21811.
23. Youssef A, Olubowale Olayemi O, Hackshaw Kevin V. Racial disparities in osteoarthritis: Prevalence presentation and management in the United States. J National Med Assoc. 117(1):55–60. https://doi.org/10.1016/j.jnma.2025.01.007.
24. Jordan JM, Helmick CG, Renner JB, et al. Prevalence of knee symptoms and radiographic and symptomatic knee osteoarthritis in African Americans and Caucasians: the Johnston County osteoarthritis project. J Rheumatol. 2007;34(1):172–80.
25. Allen KD, Helmick CG, Schwartz TA, et al. Racial differences in self-reported pain and function among individuals with radiographic hip and knee osteoarthritis: the Johnston County osteoarthritis project. Osteoarthr Cartil. 2009;17(9):1132–6.
26. Golightly Y, Hannan MT, Dufour AB, Jordan JM. Racial differences in foot disorders and foot type. Arthritis Care Res (Hoboken). 2012;64(11):1756–9.

27. Vaughn IA, Terry EL, Bartley EJ, et al. Racial-ethnic differences in osteoarthritis pain and disability: a meta-analysis. J Pain. 2019;20:629–44. Pii: S1526–5900(18)30964–7
28. Cruz-Almeida Y, Sibille KT, Goodin BR, et al. Racial and ethnic differences in older adults with knee osteoarthritis. Arthritis Rheumatol. 2014;66(7):1800–10.
29. Burns R, Graney M, Lummus AC, et al. Differences of self-reported osteoarthritis disability and race. J Natl Med Assoc. 2007;99(9):1046–51.
30. Wu M, Ayden C, Billy K I, Cochrane Niall H, Nagy Gabriela A, Bolognesi Michael P, Seyler Thorsten M. Racial and ethnic disparities in the imaging workup and treatment of knee and hip osteoarthritis. J Arthropl. 37(8):S753–S760.e2. https://doi.org/10.1016/j.arth.2022.02.019.
31. Youfang L, Yau MS, Yerges-Armstrong LM, Duggan DJ, Renner JB, Hochberg MC, Mitchell BD, Jackson RD, Jordan JM. Genetic determinants of radiographic knee osteoarthritis in African Americans. J Rheumatol. 2017;44(11):1652–8. https://doi.org/10.3899/jrheum.161488.
32. Mikuls TR, Kazi S, Cipher D, et al. The association of race and ethnicity with disease expression in male US veterans with rheumatoid arthritis. J Rheumatol. 2007;34(7):1480–4.
33. Bridges SL, Causey ZL, Burgos PI, et al. Radiographic severity of rheumatoid arthritis in African Americans: results from the CLEAR registry. Arthritis Care Res (Hoboken). 2010;62(5):624–31.
34. Williams EM, Bruner L, Adkins A, et al. I too, am America: a review of research on systemic lupus erythematosus in African Americans. Lupus Sci Med. 2016;3(1):e000144.
35. Bilal H, Alice F, Sarfaraz H. Health disparities in systemic lupus erythematosus—a narrative review. Clin Rheumatol. 41(11):3299–311. https://doi.org/10.1007/s10067-022-06268-y.
36. Chae David H, Martz Connor D, Fuller-Rowell Thomas E, Spears Erica C, Gao STT, Hunter Evelyn A, Cristina D, Sam LS. Racial discrimination disease activity and organ damage: the black women's experiences living with lupus (BeWELL) study. Am J Epidemiol. 2019;188:1434. https://doi.org/10.1093/aje/kwz105.
37. Harley JB, Kelly JA. Genetic basis of systemic lupus erythematosus: a review of the unique genetic contributions in African Americans. J Natl Med Assoc. 2002;94(8):670–7.
38. April B, Carroll Robert J, Carolyn C, Lee W, Denny Joshua C, Crofford Leslie J. Phenome-wide association study identifies marked increased in burden of comorbidities in African Americans with systemic lupus erythematosus. Arthritis Res Therapy. 20(1) https://doi.org/10.1186/s13075-018-1561-8.
39. Samantha S-W, Kevin T, Miles S, Wagner CA, Susan M, Aleksandra B, Michele D, Mai D, Chang SE, Alex K, Peggie C, Laurynas K, Ananthakrishnan G, Denis D, Guthridge CJ, Wade DJ, Christian W, Foecke MH, Merrill JT, Eliza C, Cristina A, Maecker HT, Purvesh K, Utz PJ, James JA, Guthridge JM. Ancestry-based differences in the immune phenotype are associated with lupus activity. JCI Insight. 2023;8(16) https://doi.org/10.1172/jci.insight.169584.
40. Barbhaiya M, Feldman CH, Guan H, et al. Race/ethnicity and cardiovascular events among patients with systemic lupus erythematosus. Arthritis Rheumatol. 2017;69(9):1823–31.
41. Burgos PI, McGwin G Jr, Pons-Estel GJ, et al. US patients of Hispanic and African ancestry develop lupus nephritis early in the disease course: data from LUMINA, a multiethnic US cohort (LUMINA LXXIV). Ann Rheum Dis. 2011;70:393–4.
42. Alarcón GS, Bastian HM, Beasley TM, et al. Systemic lupus erythematosus in a multi-ethnic cohort (LUMINA) XXXII: [corrected] contributions of admixture and socioeconomic status to renal involvement. Lupus. 2006;15:26–31.
43. Contreras G, Lenz O, Pardo V, et al. Outcomes in African Americans and Hispanics with lupus nephritis. Kidney Int. 2006;69:1846–51.
44. Freedman BI, Limou S, Ma L, Kopp JB. APOL1-associated nephropathy: a key contributor to racial disparities in CKD. Am J Kidney Dis. 2018 Nov;72(5S1):S8–S16:S8.
45. Franco C, Yoo W, Franco D, et al. Predictors of end stage renal disease in African Americans with lupus nephritis. Bull Hosp Jt Dis. 2010;68:251–6.

46. Portalatin GM, Gebreselassie SK, Bobart SA. Lupus nephritis—an update on disparities affecting african americans. J Nat Med Assoc. 114(3):S34–42. https://doi.org/10.1016/j.jnma.2022.05.005.
47. Michelle P, Erik B, Magder LS. Risk of renal failure within 10 or 20 years of systemic lupus erythematosus diagnosis. J Rheumatol. 2021;48(2):222–7. https://doi.org/10.3899/jrheum.191094.
48. Carroll R, Lawson AB, Voronca D, et al. Spatial environmental modeling of autoantibody outcomes among an African American population. Int J Environ Res Public Health. 2014;11:2764–79.
49. David I, Appel GB, Gabriel C, Dooley MA, Ginzler EM, David J, Jorge S-G, Wofsy David Y, Xueqing SN. Influence of race/ethnicity on response to lupus nephritis treatment: the ALMS study. Rheumatology. 2009;49(1):128–40. https://doi.org/10.1093/rheumatology/kep346.
50. Hahn Bevra H, McMahon Maureen A, Alan W, Dean WW, David D I, FitzGerald John D, Karpouzas George A, Merrill Joan T, Wallace Daniel J, Jinoos Y, Rosalind R-G, Karandeep S, Mazdak K, Soo-In C, Maneesh G, Suzanne K, Mohammad K, Christine L, Martin William J, Sefali P, Justin P, Anjay R, Weiling C, Grossman Jennifer M. American college of rheumatology guidelines for screening treatment and management of lupus nephritis. Arthritis Care Res. 64(6):797–808. https://doi.org/10.1002/acr.21664.
51. Sullivan James K, Littlejohn Emily A. Utilization of glucocorticoids among White and Black patients with systemic lupus erythematosus: observations from the enrollment visit of a prospective registry. Lupus. 30(14):2298–303. https://doi.org/10.1177/09612033211055817.
52. Chandler MT, Santacroce LM, Costenbader KH, Kim SC, Feldman CH. Racial differences in persistent glucocorticoid use patterns among medicaid beneficiaries with incident systemic lupus erythematosus. Sem Arthritis Rheum:58152122. https://doi.org/10.1016/j.semarthrit.2022.152122.
53. Ravenell R, Kamen D, Spence J, et al. Premature atherosclerosis is associated with hypovitaminosis D and angiotensin-converting enzyme inhibitor non-use in lupus patients. Am J Med Sci. 2012;344:268–73.
54. Hoffecker BM, Raffield LM, Kamen DL, Nowling TK. Systemic lupus erythematosus and vitamin D deficiency are associated with shorter telomere length among African Americans: a case-control study. PLoS One. 2013;8(5):e63725.
55. Word AP, Perese F, Tseng LC, et al. 25-Hydroxyvitamin D levels in African-American and Caucasian/Hispanic subjects with cutaneous lupus erythematosus. Br J Dermatol. 2012;166:372–9.
56. Formica MK, Palmer JR, Rosenberg L, et al. Smoking, alcohol consumption, and risk of systemic lupus erythematosus in the black women's health study. J Rheumatol. 2003;30:1222–6.
57. Cozier YC, Barbhaiya M, Castro-Webb N, et al. Relationship of cigarette smoking and alcohol consumption to incidence of systemic lupus erythematosus in the black women's health study. Arthritis Care Res (Hoboken). 2018;71:671. https://doi.org/10.1002/acr.23703.
58. Kiyohara C, Wasakazu M, Horiuchi T, et al. Cigarette smoking, alcohol consumption, and risk of systemic lupus erythematosus: a case-control study in a Japanese population. J Rheumatol. 2012;39(7):1363–70.
59. Takvorian SU, Merola JF, Costenbader KH. Cigarette smoking, alcohol consumption and risk of systemic lupus erythematosus. Lupus. 2014;23(6):537–44.
60. Becker-Merok A, Nossent J. Prevalence, predictors and outcome of vascular damage in systemic lupus erythematosus. Lupus. 2009;18:508–15.
61. Liang MH, Mandl LA, Costenbader K, et al. Atherosclerotic vascular disease in systemic lupus erythematosus. J Natl Med Assoc. 2002;94:813–9.
62. Esdaile JM, Abrahamowicz M, Grodzicky T, et al. Traditional Framingham risk factors fail to fully account for accelerated atherosclerosis in systemic lupus erythematosus. Arthritis Rheum. 2001;44(10):2331–7.

63. Shivani G, Bartels CM, Gaobin B, Helmick CG, Cristina D, Sam LS. Timing and predictors of incident cardiovascular disease in systemic lupus erythematosus: risk occurs early and highlights racial disparities. J Rheumatol. 2023;50(1):84–92. https://doi.org/10.3899/jrheum.220279.
64. Goodman SM, Bass AR. Perioperative medical management for patients with RA, SPA, and SLE undergoing total hip and total knee replacement: a narrative review. BMC Rheumatol. 2018;2:2. https://doi.org/10.1186/s41927-018-0008-9.
65. Roldan CA, Joson J, Qualls CR, et al. Premature aortic stiffness in systemic lupus erythematosus by transesophageal echocardiography. Lupus. 2010;19(14):1599–605.
66. Pramanik B. Diagnosis of systemic lupus erythematosus in an unusal presentation: what a primary care physician should know. Curr Rheumatol Rev. 2014;10(2):81–6.
67. Sciascia S, Rdin M, Roccatello D, et al. Recent advances in the management of systemic lupus erythematosus. F1000Res. 2018;7:7.
68. Kaur SD, Magrey MN. Racial differences in clinical features and comorbidities in ankylosing spondylitis in the United States. J Rheumatol. 2020;47(6):835–8. https://doi.org/10.3899/jrheum.181019.
69. Khan MA, Braun WE, Kushner I, Grecek DE, Muir WA, Steinberg AG. HLA B27 in ankylosing spondylitis: differences in frequency and relative risk in American blacks and Caucasians. J Rheumatol. 2023 Jan;50(1):39–43.
70. Farokh J, Ward Michael M, Shervin A, Learch Thomas J, MinJae L, Gensler Lianne S, Brown Matthew A, Laura D, Amirali T, Rahbar Mohammad H, Weisman Michael H, Reveille John D. Ethnicity and disease severity in ankylosing spondylitis a cross-sectional analysis of three ethnic groups. Clin Rheumatol. 36(10):2359–64. https://doi.org/10.1007/s10067-017-3767-6.
71. Smith JA. Update on ankylosing spondylitis: current concepts in pathogenesis. Current concepts in pathogenesis. Curr Allergy Asthma Rep. 2015;15:489.
72. Ward MM, Atul D, Gensler LS, Dubreuil Maureen Y, David KM, Asim HN, David B, Runsheng W, Ann B, Fang MA, Grant L, Vikas M, Bernard N, Rosemary B, Michael P, Aakash SA, Nancy S, Marat T, Jeff O, Amy T, Maksymowych WP, Liron C. Update of the American college of rheumatology/spondylitis association of America/Spondyloarthritis research and treatment network recommendations for the treatment of ankylosing spondylitis and nonradiographic axial Spondyloarthritis. Arthritis Rheumatol. 2019;71(10):1599–613. https://doi.org/10.1002/art.41042.
73. Helmick CG, Felson DT, Lawrence RC, et al. Estimates of the prevalence of arthritis and other rheumatic conditions in the United States: part 1. Arthritis Rheum. 2008;58(1):15–25.
74. Brito-Zerón P, Acar-Denizli N, Zeher M. On behalf of the EULAR-SS task force big data consortium, et al. influence of geolocation and ethnicity on the phenotypic expression of primary Sjögren's syndrome at diagnosis in 8310 patients: a cross-sectional study from the big data Sjögren project consortium. Ann Rheum Dis. 2017;76:1042–50.
75. Pilar B-Z, Nihan A-D, Wan-Fai N, Fanny HI, Astrid R, Raphaele S, Xiaomei L, Chiara B, Jacques-Eric G, Debashish D, Luca Q, Roberta P, Gabriela H-M, Berkan A, Kruize Aike A, Seung-Ki K, Marika K, Sonja P, Damien S, Roberto G, Roser S, Maureen R, Thomas M, Yasunori S, David I, Valeria V, Piotr W, Gunnel N, Guadalupe F, Hendrika B, Hideki N, Roberto G, Valerie D-P, Benedikt H, Michele B, Moça TVF, Daniel H, Pasoto Sandra G, Soledad R, Gheita Tamer A, Fabiola A, Jacques M, Cristina V, Margit Z, Sivils Kathy X, Bei BS, Pulukool S, Salvatore DV, Antonina M, Jorge S-G, Levent K, van der Eefje H, Sung-Hwan P, Marie W-H, Xavier M, Manuel R-C. Epidemiological profile and north–south gradient driving baseline systemic involvement of primary Sjögren's syndrome. Rheumatology. 2019;59(9):2350–9. https://doi.org/10.1093/rheumatology/kez578.
76. Hal SR, Rohan S, Nathan P, Kelly Jennifer A, Lida R, Lewis David M, Erick KC, Sarah C, Judy H, Kiely G, Rhodus Nelson L, Wallace Daniel J, Weisman Michael H, Swamy V, Brennan Michael T, Koelsch Kristi A, Lessard Christopher J, Montgomery Courtney G, Sivils Kathy L, Astrid R. American Indians have a higher risk of Sjögren's syndrome and

more disease activity Than European Americans and African Americans. Arthritis Care Res. 72(8):1049–56. https://doi.org/10.1002/acr.24003.
77. Pilar B-Z, Nihan A-D, Margit Z, Astrid R, Raphaele S, Elke T, Xiaomei L, Chiara B, Jacques-Eric G, Debashish D, Luca Q, Roberta P, Gabriela H-M, Kruize Aike A, Valeria V, Marika K, Damien S, Roberto G, Sonja P, David I, Roser S, Maureen R, Seung-Ki K, Gunnel N, Yasunori S, Roberto G, Valerie D-P, Michele B, Benedikt H, Hendrika B, Brun Johan G, Guadalupe F, Carsons Steven E, Gheita Tamer A, Jacques M, Cristina V, Fabiola A, Soledad R, Fanny HI, Kathy S, Thomas M, Pulukool S, Salvatore DV, Jorge S-G, Eefje v d H, Moça TVF, Marie W-H, Xavier M, Manuel R-C. Influence of geolocation and ethnicity on the phenotypic expression of primary Sjögren's syndrome at diagnosis in 8310 patients: a cross-sectional study from the Big Data Sjögren Project Consortium. Annals Rheumatic Dis. 76(6):1042–50. https://doi.org/10.1136/annrheumdis-2016-209952.
78. Moore DF, Kramer E, Eltaraboulsi R, Steen VD. Increased morbidity and mortality of scleroderma in African Americans compared to non-African Americans. Arthritis Care Res. 2019;71(9):1154–63.
79. Gelber AC, Manno RL, Shah AA, et al. Race and association with disease manifestations and mortality in scleroderma: a 20-year experience at the Johns Hopkins scleroderma center and review of the literature. Medicine (Baltimore). 2013;92(4):191–205.
80. McNearney TA, Reveille JD, Fischbach M, Friedman AW, Lisse JR, Goel N, et al. Pulmonary involvement in systemic sclerosis: associations with genetic, serologic, sociodemo-graphic, and behavioral factors. Arthritis Rheum. 2007;57:318–26.
81. Morgan ND, Gelber AC. African Americans and scleroderma: examining the root cause of the association. Arthritis Care Res (Hoboken). 2019;71:1151. https://doi.org/10.1002/acr.23860.
82. Gonzalez-Gay MA, Matteson EL, Castaneda S. Polymyalgia rheumatica. Lancet. 2017;390(10103):1700–12.
83. Smith CA, Fidler WJ, Pinals RS. The epidemiology of giant cell arteritis. Report of a ten-year study in Shelby County, Tennessee. Arthritis Rheum. 1983;26(10):1214–9.
84. Kumar B, Lenert P. Gout and African Americans: reducing disparities. Cleve Clin J Med. 2016;83(9);665–74.
85. Natalie MC, Lu N, Chio Y, Joshi Amit D, Shanshan S, Lynn R, Warner Erica T, Nicola D, Merriman Tony R, Saag Kenneth G, Yuqing Z, Choi Hyon K. Racial and sex disparities in gout prevalence among US adults. JAMA Network Open. 5(8):e2226804. https://doi.org/10.1001/jamanetworkopen.2022.26804.
86. Adrienne T, Woodward OM, Linda KWH, Ching-Ti L, Xiaoning L, Nalls Michael A, Daniel S, Mariam S, Akylbekova Ermeg L, Wyatt Sharon B, Shih-Jen H, Qiong Y, Zonderman Alan B, Adeyemo Adebowale A, Cameron P, Yan M, Muredach R, Shlipak Michael G, David S, Evans Michele K, Rotimi Charles N, Flessner Michael F, Michael K, Adrienne CL, Fox Caroline S, Anna K. Genome-wide association study for serum urate concentrations and gout among African Americans identifies genomic risk loci and a novel URAT1 loss-of-function allele. Hum Mol Genet. 2011;20(20):4056–68. https://doi.org/10.1093/hmg/ddr307.
87. Guanjie C, Daniel S, Doumatey Ayo P, Jie Z, Bentley Amy R, Lin L, Adebowale A, Rotimi Charles N. Refining genome-wide associated loci for serum uric acid in individuals with African ancestry. Hum Mol Genet. 2019;29(3):506–14. https://doi.org/10.1093/hmg/ddz272.
88. Rule AD, de Andrade M, Matsumoto M, Mosley TH, Kardia S, Turner ST. Association between SLC2A9 transporter gene variants and uric acid phenotypes in African American and white families. Rheumatology. 2011;50(5):871–8. https://doi.org/10.1093/rheumatology/keq425.
89. Woodward OM, Anna K, Josef C, Eric B, Guggino William B, Michael K. Identification of a urate transporter ABCG2 with a common functional polymorphism causing gout. Proc Nat Acad Sci. 106(25):10338–42. https://doi.org/10.1073/pnas.0901249106.
90. Karis E, Crittenden DB, Pillinger MH. Hyperuricemia, gout, and related comorbities: cause and effect on a two-way street. South Med J. 2014;107:235–41.

91. Gaffo AL, Jacobs DR Jr, Lewis CE, Mikuls TR, Saag KG. Association between being African-American, serum urate levels and the risk of developing hyperuricemia: findings from the coronary artery risk development in young adults cohort. Arthritis Res Ther. 2012;14:R4.
92. Juraschek SP, Kovell LC, Miller ER, Gelber AC. Gout, urate-lowering therapy, and uric acid levels among adults in the United States. Arthritis Care Res. 2015;67(4):588–92.
93. Wright J, Probstfield JL, Cushman W, et al. ALLHAT findings revisited in the context of subsequent analyses, other trials, and meta-analyses. Arch Intern Med. 2009;169(9):832–42.
94. Musini VM, Nazer M, Bassett K, Wright JM. Blood pressure-lowering efficacy of monotherapy with thiazide for primary hypertension. Cochrane Database Syst Rev. 2014;5:CD003824.
95. Juraschek SP, Appel LJ, Miller ER. Metoprolol increases uric acid and risk of gout in African Americans with chronic kidney disease attributed to hypertension. Am J Hypertens. 2017;30(9):871–5.
96. Kumagai T, Ota T, Tamura Y, et al. Time to target uric acid to retard CKD progression. Clin Exp Nephrol. 2017;21(2):182–92.
97. Major TJ, Topless RK, Albeth N, Merriman TR. Evaluation of the diet wide contribution to serum urate levels: meta-analysis of population based cohorts. BMJ. 2018;363:k3951.
98. Park KY, Kim HJ, Ahn HS, et al. Effects of coffee consumption on serum uric acid: systematic review and meta-analysis. Semin Arthritis Rheum. 2016;45(5):580–6.
99. Martin KR, Coles KM. Consumption of 100% tart cherry juice reduces serum urate in overweight and obese adults. Curr Dev Nutr. 2019;3(5):nzz011:nzz011.
100. Richette P, Doherty M, Pascual E, et al. 2016 updated EULAR evidence-based recommendations for the management of gout. Ann Rheum Dis. 2017;76(1):29–42.
101. Dalbeth N, Wong S, Gamble GD, et al. Acute effect of milk on serum urate concentrations: a randomized controlled crossover trial. Ann Rheum Dis. 2010 Sep;69(9):1677–82.

Chapter 9
A Precision Medicine Approach to Pulmonary Diseases in African Americans

Contents

9.1 COPD (Emphysema and Chronic Bronchitis)... 166
9.2 Asthma... 169
9.3 Sarcoidosis... 171
9.4 Obstructive Sleep Apnea (OSA)... 173
References.. 175

Pulmonary disease in African Americans encompasses a range of respiratory conditions, with asthma and COPD being particularly prevalent. African Americans experience a higher incidence and severity of asthma compared to other ethnic groups, often attributed to factors such as socioeconomic status, environmental exposures, and genetic predisposition [1, 2]. For instance, urban living conditions may expose individuals to higher levels of air pollution and allergens, exacerbating asthma symptoms [2]. Additionally, disparities in healthcare access can lead to delayed diagnosis and inadequate management of these conditions, resulting in increased morbidity. COPD is another significant concern, with African American individuals often diagnosed at a younger age and exhibiting more severe symptoms than their white counterparts. Factors such as smoking rates, occupational exposures, and limited access to smoking cessation programs contribute to these disparities. Lung cancer, another critical pulmonary disease, also shows disparities [3]. African Americans also have a higher incidence of lung cancer and poorer survival outcomes due to lower rates of low-dose computed tomography screening and less access to high-quality treatment. Furthermore, pulmonary diseases are often compounded by comorbidities such as hypertension and diabetes, which are more prevalent in the African American community. Genetic factors play a significant role in the higher prevalence, morbidity, and mortality rates of pulmonary diseases such as asthma and

© The Author(s), under exclusive license to Springer Nature Switzerland AG 2025
G. L. Hall, *Precision Medicine for African Americans*,
https://doi.org/10.1007/978-3-031-95774-1_9

COPD in African Americans. For asthma, several genetic loci have been identified that are associated with increased risk in African American populations. The 17q12–21 locus, particularly variants in the GSDMB and ORMDL3 genes, is implicated in childhood-onset asthma [4–7]. Additionally, the 9p24.1 locus (rs10975467) and loci such as 11q13.4 (rs7480008) and 13q14.3 (rs1543525) have been identified as significant in African American populations [4–6]. These loci involve regulatory activities and gene expression relevant to asthma pathogenesis. For COPD, differential DNA methylation marks have been identified in African Americans, with genes such as MAML1 showing significant associations. MAML1 affects NOTCH-dependent angiogenesis, which is relevant to lung function and COPD pathophysiology [8]. Network modeling has also identified gene modules related to inflammatory pathways and lung development processes, which may contribute to COPD susceptibility and severity in African Americans [8]. These genetic factors, combined with environmental and socioeconomic influences, contribute to the observed disparities in pulmonary disease outcomes in African American populations.

9.1 COPD (Emphysema and Chronic Bronchitis)

Chronic Obstructive Pulmonary Disease (COPD) is a progressive lung condition that makes it difficult to breathe. It is characterized by long-term respiratory symptoms and airflow limitations, primarily caused by smoking and other inhaled irritants (fumes, allergens, or chemicals). Emphysema and chronic bronchitis are two of the common forms of COPD. Common symptoms include chronic cough, shortness of breath, wheezing, and frequent respiratory infections. In addition to smoking, other risk factors for COPD include long-term exposure to air pollutants, such as chemical fumes or dust in the workplace. A history of frequent respiratory infections during childhood can also predispose individuals to the disease [9]. Emphysema, a form of COPD, is a significant health concern among African Americans, characterized by the destruction of alveoli (air sacs) in the lungs, leading to breathing difficulties. While emphysema occurs more often in European Americans, who also have a higher mortality rate (see Fig. 9.1 [10]), studies indicate that African Americans often develop emphysema at a younger age and, when it occurs, experience more severe symptoms compared to European American populations [2, 11]. Contributing factors include higher rates of smoking, occupational exposures to pollutants, and socioeconomic disparities that limit access to healthcare and smoking cessation programs. For example, African American smokers are less likely to receive smoking cessation support, which exacerbates the progression of the disease [2]. The lack of awareness and education about emphysema further impedes early diagnosis and effective treatment. African Americans, particularly men, have a higher prevalence of lower-grade emphysema compared to European Americans, even among those with normal spirometry results. A study found that African American men had a 3.9-fold higher prevalence of emphysema than European American men when their FEV1 was between 80% and 99% of predicted

9.1 COPD (Emphysema and Chronic Bronchitis)

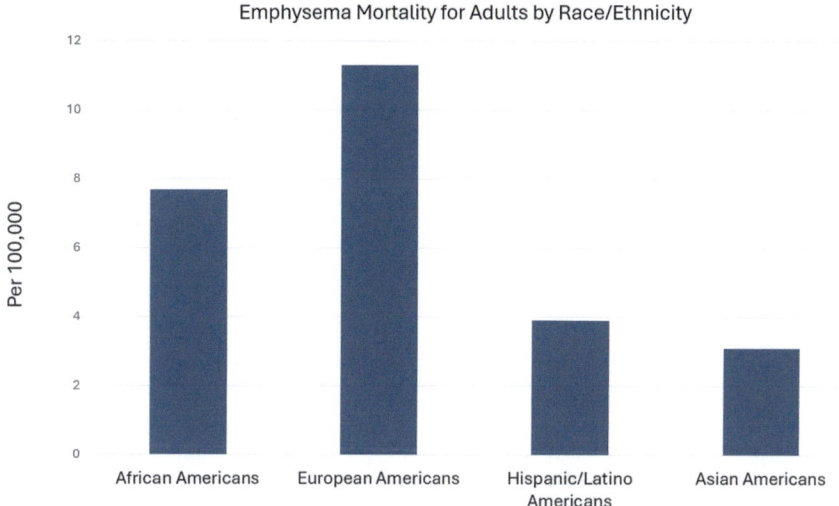

Fig. 9.1 Emphysema mortality by race/ethnicity *Saeed* et al.

[2, 12]. Additionally, another study highlighted that African Americans had a higher percentage of emphysema and air trapping on CT metrics compared to European Americans, even after adjusting for individual and neighborhood socioeconomic status [12]. These patients with a smoking history and low-grade emphysema frequently also have poorly controlled hypertension, diabetes, heart disease, and PVD with related complaints that more significantly impair their daily activities. The management of their comorbidities slows the attention we pay to their breathing status and our interventions to improve it.

Chronic bronchitis, another form of COPD, is characterized by inflammation of the bronchial tubes, leading to persistent coughing and mucus production. When combined with emphysema, which involves damage to the lung alveoli, the overall impact on lung function is significantly compounded. This makes it difficult to breathe appropriately. Chronic bronchitis is also less prevalent among African Americans compared to European Americans. According to a study, African Americans had a lower prevalence of chronic bronchitis than European Americans, with adjusted odds ratios indicating a significant difference [13, 14]. Genetic factors contribute to the lower prevalence of chronic bronchitis in African Americans. One significant factor is the differential DNA methylation patterns observed in African Americans with COPD. A study identified specific differentially methylated CpG sites associated with COPD in African Americans, including genes involved in inflammatory pathways and lung development processes, such as MAML1 and FXYD1/LGI4 [8]. These genetic variations may influence the susceptibility to chronic bronchitis and other COPD-related conditions [8, 15]. Additionally, genetic variations in antioxidant enzymes play a role. Variants in genes encoding antioxidant enzymes, such as SOD3 and GLRX2, have been associated with lung function and COPD risk in African Americans [15]. These genetic differences may provide some protective effects against the development of chronic bronchitis. Furthermore, genomic regions such as 10q22.2, 17q21.31, and 2p23.1 have been linked to lower lung function in African descent populations, which may contribute to the observed differences in chronic bronchitis prevalence. These regions are associated with airway function and may modulate the risk of developing chronic bronchitis [16].

While COPD has historically been considered a "white male smoker's disease," newer data and migrating smoking demographics have shown an increased prevalence in woman and a rapidly growing incidence in African Americans. Chronic obstructive pulmonary disease disproportionately affects ethnic minorities and low socioeconomic groups not just in the United States but across the world. Because of disproportional poverty and urban living, African Americans have an increased exposure to indoor and outdoor pollution, occupational and environmental hazards, and tobacco smoke, which contribute to disparities in the prevalence and outcomes of COPD. In short, the social determinants of health (healthcare access, educational opportunities, economic stability, and social and community environment) complicate the course of COPD for too many African Americans [17].

A study by Hardin et al. at Harvard Medical School showed that African Americans had a significantly higher history of asthma and therefore were more likely to have more frequent COPD exacerbations [18].

COPD is an independent risk factor for lung cancer, with chronic bronchitis and/or emphysema increasing lung cancer risk by two- to fivefold as compared to smokers with normal spirometry. African Americans are at higher risk for developing COPD and lung cancer [19]. Research done by Mark Dransfield showed that African Americans (women in particular) are more susceptible to the damaging effects of tobacco smoke when compared to European American men [20]. Therefore, while all tobacco smokers may be at comparable risk for the development of COPD, African Americans and women who develop COPD may be particularly susceptible to progressive disease [21, 22]. These added adverse events make smoking cessation counseling critical.

Another study by Han et al. looked at quality of life and related it to COPD exacerbations and found that African Americans had more frequent hospitalizations despite similar quality of life indexes [23]. The same study noted disparities in home oxygen prescriptions, influenza vaccination administrations, and referral for smoking cessation counseling, which were surmised to be contributing to the increased hospitalizations [23].

Hyun Lee and colleagues looked at NHANES data for COPD-related comorbidities to see if racial differences existed and found some interesting trends [24]. African Americans had a number of comorbidities including a high prevalence of current smokers, a history of asthma, hypertension, stroke, diabetes, anemia, and rheumatoid arthritis [24].

Finally, Tadahiro Goto at Massachusetts General looked at the readmission rates for patients with COPD. Overall there was a 20% 30-day readmission rate for patients with COPD. When examined by race, he found that African American patients had a higher rate of asthma-COPD overlap with asthma as a predominant cause for readmission. Using COPD as a sole metric, Nastars and colleagues at the

University of Texas looked at 30-day readmission rates in Medicare beneficiaries and, despite worse clinical profiles, found comparable readmission rates across populations [25]. COPD patients with asthma had significantly more exacerbations and readmissions. Because of the asthma component, the authors presumed that long-acting beta2-agonist and inhaled corticosteroid use would benefit these patients more [26]. When African American patients present with COPD, it is critical to determine if they have a history of asthma.

9.2 Asthma

Asthma is a chronic respiratory condition that disproportionately affects African Americans, who experience higher prevalence rates, more severe symptoms, and greater mortality compared to other racial and ethnic groups. African Americans have a 1.5- to twofold greater prevalence of asthma and a two- to threefold greater risk of emergency department visits, hospitalizations, and mortality due to asthma compared to European Americans [1, 3]. Several factors contribute to these disparities, including environmental influences such as urban air pollution, inadequate housing conditions, and socioeconomic challenges that limit access to healthcare.

Asthma occurs in almost 14% of African American children with a higher prevalence in girls (15.7% compared to 11.4%) [27]. African American adults are three times more likely to die from asthma. In fact, mortality rates are highest in African American women, whose rate is more than two times higher than that of European American women. African American children have a death rate ten times that of European American children [27]. Despite the high mortality, increased ED visits and hospitalizations, and poor outcomes, African Americans have lower physician office visits, lower specialty office visits, and lower levels of asthma care as recommended by guidelines [28–30]. Because of the fewer referrals to pulmonologists, there is less pulmonary function testing and diagnosis confirmation. Given the worse outcomes yet less intensive interventions, frontline providers have a unique opportunity to make a big difference in the quality of care of asthma in this population.

Risk factors for increased mortality in patients with asthma include multiple emergency department visits or hospitalizations, history of intubation or ICU admission in the past 5 years, nonuse of inhaled corticosteroids, current smoking, psychosocial stress and depression, socioeconomic factors, and negative attitudes and beliefs regarding the benefit of medications [31]. Unfortunately, African Americans disproportionately have these comorbidities, factors, and beliefs.

As in COPD, environmental factors also play a prominent role in the frequency and severity of asthma. Because African Americans live disproportionately in urban areas where industrial pollutants and occupational exposures occur, asthma occurrence and severity are worse. Differences in housing, with a higher rate of living in poverty, also increase the exposure to asthma-inducing antigens (dust, dust mites, mold, cockroaches, mice, rats, and more). Rates of asthma were also significantly higher among children whose home exteriors and interiors were described as being in "poor condition" [32]. Essentially, social and economic variables working at the individual, household, and neighborhood level can greatly impact the occurrence and severity of asthma [33].

Obesity is another important modifiable risk factor. Higher BMI is associated with more uncontrolled asthma, increased severity of asthma, and increased number of medications [34–36]. Weight loss is associated with improved outcomes [34]. Addressing obesity and its impact on asthma with our patients is important.

A study by Brehm et al. at Brigham and Woman's Hospital found that vitamin D deficiency was associated with increased asthma severity [37]. The vitamin D insufficiency occurred more often with older age, higher BMI, and African American race. When the vitamin D level exceeded 30 ng/mL, the likelihood of an asthma exacerbation decreased. The odds of any hospitalization or emergency department visit were higher in patients with low vitamin D even after adjusting for age, sex, BMI, and baseline asthma severity [37]. A majority of African Americans have low vitamin D levels [38]. Note that a number of other researchers have also looked at the connection between vitamin D and asthma and not found either a true connection, or benefit from vitamin D supplementation [39].

Another curious finding was the positive association with breast feeding and a lower prevalence of asthma exacerbations, even after controlling for socioeconomic status, maternal smoking, BMI, and a number of other factors [40]. One-third of African American children are never breast fed and are also at increased risk for worse asthma outcomes [40].

The pharmacological treatment of asthma is essentially the same across racial groups with a long-acting beta2-agonist and inhaled corticosteroid combination resulting in greater improvements in pulmonary function and asthma control [27]. Improving asthma outcomes in African Americans requires a multifaceted approach that addresses both medical and social determinants of health. Effective interventions include culturally tailored education programs that empower individuals to understand their condition, recognize triggers, and adhere to treatment plans. For example, community health worker-led initiatives have been shown to enhance asthma management by providing personalized support and education in a culturally relevant context [3, 41]. Environmental control interventions that involve reducing exposure to asthma triggers such as dust mites, cockroaches, mold, and mouse allergens are crucial. Programs that focus on improving the structural soundness of homes and reducing allergen and pollutant exposures have also been effective [3]. Additionally, increasing access to preventive medications, such as inhaled corticosteroids, is crucial; studies have indicated that African Americans are less likely to receive these medications, contributing to poorer asthma control [42]. Implementing school-based asthma management programs can also be beneficial, as they provide children with education on self-management and facilitate communication between families and healthcare providers. Moreover, addressing environmental factors through policies that reduce exposure to pollutants and allergens—such as improving housing conditions and reducing tobacco smoke exposure—can significantly impact asthma outcomes [43]. Overall, a combination of education, medication access, environmental interventions, and community support systems is essential for effectively improving asthma outcomes in African Americans and reducing health disparities associated with this chronic condition.

9.3 Sarcoidosis

Sarcoidosis is a multisystem chronic inflammatory disease of unknown origin characterized by non-caseating granulomatous inflammation at the affected site (particularly the lungs, lymph nodes, skin, and eyes). Studies have shown that African Americans are three to four times more likely to develop sarcoidosis than European Americans [44]. This increased prevalence may be due to genetic factors, environmental influences, or a combination of both, but the exact cause remains unclear. Research suggests that certain genetic markers, such as variations in the BTNL2 and HLA genes, may contribute to the higher incidence of sarcoidosis among African Americans [44, 45]. These genetic factors might influence immune system responses, making individuals more susceptible to the disease. These affected genes regulate the immune system's response to inflammation. Variations in these genes can lead to an overactive immune response, which causes the body to form granulomas—clusters of immune cells—in various organs, characteristic of sarcoidosis [46]. This dysregulated immune activity can result in the chronic inflammation seen in the disease. Although any organ can be involved, the disease most commonly (>90%) affects the lungs and intrathoracic lymph nodes. Mortality rates are highest in African Americans, and they tend to have more severe lung involvement [47–49]. Environmental exposures are also linked to sarcoidosis due to a clustering of outbreaks during flu seasons. Geographic variations with increased occurrences in the southeast and coastal areas also support the role of environmental factors in sarcoidosis. Some scientists suggest that exposure to molds, mildew, and musty odors at home or work conveys a small increased risk [50].

It remains unclear how much racial differences are due to genetics, socioeconomic factors, or a combination of the two. Researchers have found specific genes in African Americans that are associated with more severe disease and worse outcomes and another set of genes in European Americans that are associated with milder disease [51]. Data show that lower socioeconomic status patients have more advanced and persisting disease with African Americans comprising a greater proportion of these patients [52].

Löfgren's syndrome is a specific acute presentation of sarcoidosis characterized by the triad of erythema nodosum, bilateral hilar adenopathy, and polyarthralgia or polyarthritis, often accompanied by fever. It is generally associated with a favorable prognosis and often resolves spontaneously within 2 years, particularly in patients who are HLA-DRB1*03–positive [44, 51]. Löfgren's syndrome, however, is less common in African Americans compared to other ethnic groups [44, 53]. When it does occur, it still tends to follow a more favorable course compared to other forms of sarcoidosis. The acute inflammatory nature of Löfgren's syndrome, characterized by its rapid onset and resolution, contrasts with the typically more chronic and severe course of sarcoidosis seen in African Americans [54].

Sarcoidosis lung involvement is more obvious with African American patients having decreased forced vital capacity and increased shortness of breath. African Americans have higher granuloma density compared with other races despite similar stages of disease and are diagnosed approximately 10 years earlier than European American patients, due to earlier onset of symptoms [52].

A study by Mirsaeidi and colleagues of mortality in patients with sarcoidosis found dramatically more deaths due to respiratory failure, cardiac arrest, pulmonary hypertension, heart failure, pulmonary fibrosis, hypertension, diabetes, and renal failure [52]. Overall African Americans had an eightfold higher mortality rate compared to European Americans. This study also found a different geographical distribution for African Americans with increased cases in the District of Columbia, North and South Carolina, Pennsylvania, and New Jersey [52].

There are also differences in outcomes based on ethnicity and gender among families with sarcoidosis with African American women dying at a higher rate and younger age than European Americans. Yvette Cozier and colleagues at the Slone Epidemiology Center at Boston University looked closely at sarcoidosis in African American women as part of the Black Women's Health Study [48]:

> the lung was the organ most commonly involved in the disease process, with 61% of women having lung involvement, followed by intrathoracic lymph nodes (35%); 96% had intrathoracic involvement. There was also substantial extrapulmonary disease; sites affected most often were the skin (including erythema nodosum) (20%), and eyes (16%). Cardiac sarcoidosis was reported for only one woman. Chest radiograph was reported as the method of diagnosis for 73% of women, followed by biopsy (54%), and chest CT scan (31%). Sixty percent of women with a diagnostic chest radiograph were classified by their physicians as stage II or higher. Comorbid illness was noted for 56% of cases: conditions reported by physicians included asthma, hypertension, type 2 diabetes, cancer, scleroderma, lupus, obesity, hypercholesterolemia, and depression [48].

In terms of clinical presentation, patients in this study presented with shortness of breath (45%), fatigue (41%), and cough (40%) most frequently [48]. Twenty-five percent presented with sinus congestion and 20% had chest pain. Palpitations as a presenting complaint are highly suggestive of sarcoid cardiac involvement [55]. Pulmonary hypertension, which occurs more often in African Americans, heralds a poor prognosis when developed [56, 57].

There is general consensus that patients with sarcoidosis and no evidence of end-organ impairment and minimal respiratory symptoms should not be treated [44, 58–60]. Because African Americans tend to have more severe disease with more varied organ involvement, it is going to be critical that these patients be followed closely. If more advanced disease is determined, the treatment generally involves steroids for an extended period of time. Steroid-sparing medications (methotrexate, azathioprine, mycophenolate mofetil, etc.) are gaining popularity and are used more frequently in African Americans [61].

9.4 Obstructive Sleep Apnea (OSA)

Obstructive Sleep Apnea (OSA) is a common sleep disorder marked by repeated interruptions in breathing during sleep due to the relaxation of throat muscles. African Americans have a higher prevalence and severity of OSA than other racial and ethnic groups, influenced by a mix of genetic, environmental, and socioeconomic factors. Studies show that African American adults are more likely to have higher body mass indices (BMIs), which is a significant risk factor for OSA. Moreover, anatomical differences, such as a narrower airway or larger neck circumference, add to the increased risk [62–64].

A study by Chen et al. at the Harvard School of Public Health confirmed there are more sleep apnea, interrupted sleep, and daytime sleepiness in African Americans than in European Americans [58]. The lost sleep leads to daytime sleepiness, fatigue, poor concentration, poor energy, increased hypertension, heart disease, poor digestion and metabolism, and more [65, 66].

A number of studies have found increased sleep-disordered breathing in African Americans, and these disparities persist even after controlling for BMI [67–69]. While increased obesity does directly increase the occurrence of OSA in African Americans, it is likely not the entire cause. In terms of risk factors, African Americans tend to have craniofacial soft tissue features that contribute to obstructive sleep apnea including a larger tongue area. For those significantly obese patients, weight loss can reverse obstructive sleep apnea in some [70].

There is also a significant disparity with African American children having 20% more sleep apnea severity and oxygen desaturation [67].

> African American children are 4-6 times more likely to have OSA compared to white children. Even among young adults less than 26 years of age, African Americans are 88% more likely to have OSA as compared to whites. Among middle-aged populations, the evidence for a disparity in OSA prevalence is weaker as differences in OSA prevalence from community based studies are evident in some but not all studies. In contrast, data from older populations suggests a disparity may re-emerge in this age group. While African Americans had similar prevalence of OSA as whites (32% and 30% respectively) in a community-based survey of individuals 65 years of age and older, this group was 2.1 times more likely to have severe OSA [67].

Chen also found significantly increased sleep apnea patterns with more snoring, more obesity, and worse global functioning in African Americans. They also showed decreased formally diagnosed sleep apnea in African Americans despite the disproportional increased occurrence [65].

African Americans have a poorer sleep quality overall associated with shortest sleep duration and the highest levels for excessive daytime sleepiness [71]. With prolonged loss of sleep, the risk for hypertension and resultant strokes, heart disease, and kidney failure ensues [66, 72, 73].

Continuous positive airway pressure (CPAP) therapy is the treatment of choice for mild, moderate, and severe obstructive sleep apnea. CPAP reduces daytime sleepiness, depression, and hypertension and improves alertness and global quality of life [74].

Schwartz and colleagues at the University of South Florida looked at veteran data and found that only a fraction of patients with sleep apnea and a CPAP machine use it. In African Americans, the use of this technology is even worse. African Americans were over five times more likely to not use their CPAP machine than European Americans [75]. They also found that when African Americans had severe OSA, they were three times more likely to use CPAP than African Americans with mild or moderate symptoms [75].

Addressing poor compliance with CPAP usage has been a growing medical concern. Jessie Bakker and colleagues at Harvard Medical School looked at an array of published approaches to improved compliance with CPAP and concluded that remote monitoring associated with a personalized behavioral modification plan would likely be part of the solution to this difficult and pervasive problem [76].

> To be implemented clinically, it is critical that an adjunct therapy to promote CPAP adherence be cost-effective, feasible in a wide range of settings, and scalable to large and diverse patient populations. The most efficacious interventions tested to date have been behavioral in nature; when combined with the remote-monitoring capabilities available in modern CPAP machines, these theory-driven methods could hold the answer to increasing real-world CPAP adherence rates [76].

Patients with sleep apnea will need a compliance discussion on follow-up visits that includes an assessment of their CPAP comfort including mask style, sleeping position, and what approaches they have used to improve compliance. A study by Shaw and colleagues at the Brooklyn Health Disparities Center highlighted that African Americans often face barriers related to the confining nature of the CPAP device, discomfort while wearing the mask, and concerns about their partner's perceptions of the treatment [77]. These factors can significantly impact mask preference and adherence. Additionally, another study compared different CPAP interfaces and found that nasal masks were generally preferred over oronasal masks due to better comfort, fewer leak issues, and higher patient satisfaction [78]. This preference for nasal masks may be particularly relevant for African Americans, who may experience similar mask fit and comfort issues.

It is also worth reviewing the significant improvement in sleep apnea comorbidities (hypertension, cardiovascular, daytime alertness, etc.) when emphasizing CPAP use.

A Precision Medicine Approach to Pulmonary Diseases in African Americans
- Because of disproportional poverty and urban living, African Americans have an increased exposure to indoor and outdoor pollution, occupational and environmental hazards, and tobacco smoke, which contribute to disparities in prevalence and outcomes of COPD.
- African American patients had a higher rate of asthma-COPD overlap with asthma as a predominant cause for resistant treatment and hospital readmission.

(continued)

- African Americans have a higher rate of chronic bronchitis and a lower rate of emphysema when compared to European Americans.
- Vitamin D insufficiency is associated with higher odds of severe asthma exacerbation, and having a vitamin D level greater than 30 ng/mL is protective against severe asthma exacerbations.
- African Americans with COPD are significantly younger, smoke less, report concurrent asthma more frequently, and have less radiographic emphysema on volumetric computed tomography.
- There is more sleep apnea, interrupted sleep, and daytime sleepiness in African Americans than in European Americans.
- African Americans had a significantly higher history of asthma and were more likely to have more frequent COPD exacerbations.
- African Americans (women in particular) are more susceptible to the damaging effects of tobacco smoking when compared to European American men.
- Asthma occurs in almost 14% of African American children with a higher prevalence in girls.
- African American mortality rate, emergency department visit rate, and hospital admission rate for asthma are all multiple times higher than European Americans.
- Obesity is associated with more uncontrolled asthma, increased severity of asthma, and increased number of medications.
- Breast feeding is associated with a lower prevalence and severity of asthma.
- Sarcoidosis is more severe (eight times higher mortality) with more end-organ damage in African Americans with an increased occurrence in woman.
- African Americans have a poorer sleep quality overall, associated with worse insomnia levels and the highest levels of excessive daytime sleepiness.
- African Americans were over five times more likely to not use their CPAP machine than European Americans.
- African Americans often prefer nasal (CPAP) masks due to their better comfort and fewer leak issues.

References

1. Burbank AJ, Hernandez ML, Jefferson A, Perry TT, Phipatanakul W, Poole J, Matsui EC. Environmental justice and allergic disease: a work group report of the AAAAI environmental exposure and respiratory health committee and the diversity equity and inclusion committee. J Allergy Clin Immunol. 2023;151(3):656–70. https://doi.org/10.1016/j.jaci.2022.11.025.
2. Ejike CO, Woo H, Galiatsatos P, Paulin LM, Krishnan JA, Cooper CB, Couper DJ, Kanner RE, Bowler RP, Hoffman EA, Comellas AP, Criner GJ, Barr RG, Martinez FJ, Han MK, Martinez CH, Ortega VE, Parekh TM, Christenson SA, Thakur N, Baugh A, Belz DC, Raju S, Gassett

AJ, Kaufman JD, Putcha N, Hansel NN. Contribution of individual and neighborhood factors to racial disparities in respiratory outcomes. Am J Respir Crit Care Med. 2021;203(8):987–97. https://doi.org/10.1164/rccm.202002-0253OC.
3. Davis CM, Apter AJ, Casillas A, Foggs MB, Louisias M, Morris EC, Nanda A, Nelson MR, Ogbogu PU, Walker-McGill CL, Wang J, Perry TT. Health disparities in allergic and immunologic conditions in racial and ethnic underserved populations: a work group report of the AAAAI Committee on the underserved. J Allergy Clin Immunol. 2021;147(5):1579–93. https://doi.org/10.1016/j.jaci.2021.02.034.
4. Ober C, CG MK, Magnaye KM, Altman MC, Washington C 3rd, Stanhope C, Naughton KA, Rosasco MG, Bacharier LB, Billheimer D, Gold DR, Gress L, Hartert T, Havstad S, Khurana Hershey GK, Hallmark B, Hogarth DK, Jackson DJ, Johnson CC, Kattan M, Lemanske RF, Lynch SV, Mendonca EA, Miller RL, Naureckas ET, O'Connor GT, Seroogy CM, Wegienka G, White SR, Wood RA, Wright AL, Zoratti EM, Martinez FD, Ownby D, Nicolae DL, Levin AM, Gern JE, Environmental Influences on Child Health Outcomes-Children's Respiratory Research Workgroup. Expression quantitative trait locus fine mapping of the 17q12–21 asthma locus in African American children: a genetic association and gene expression study. Lancet Respir Med. 2020;8(5):482–92. https://doi.org/10.1016/S2213-2600(20)30011-4.
5. Gui H, Levin AM, Hu D, Sleiman P, Xiao S, ACY M, Yang M, Barczak AJ, Huntsman S, Eng C, Hochstadt S, Zhang E, Whitehouse K, Simons S, Cabral W, Takriti S, Abecasis G, Blackwell TW, Kang HM, Nickerson DA, Germer S, Lanfear DE, Gilliland F, Gauderman WJ, Kumar R, Erle DJ, Martinez FD, Hakonarson H, Burchard EG, Williams LK. Mapping the 17q12–21.1 locus for variants associated with early-onset asthma in African Americans. Am J Respir Crit Care Med. 2021;203(4):424–36. https://doi.org/10.1164/rccm.202006-2623OC.
6. Washington C 3rd, Dapas M, Biddanda A, Magnaye KM, Aneas I, Helling BA, Szczesny B, Boorgula MP, Taub MA, Kenny E, Mathias RA, Barnes KC, CAAPA, Khurana Hershey GK, Kercsmar CM, Gereige JD, Makhija M, Gruchalla RS, Gill MA, Liu AH, Rastogi D, Busse W, Gergen PJ, Visness CM, Gold DR, Hartert T, Johnson CC, Lemanske RF Jr, Martinez FD, Miller RL, Ownby D, Seroogy CM, Wright AL, Zoratti EM, Bacharier LB, Kattan M, O'Connor GT, Wood RA, Nobrega MA, Altman MC, Jackson DJ, Gern JE, CG MK, Ober C. African-specific alleles modify risk for asthma at the 17q12-q21 locus in African Americans. Genome Med. 2022;14(1):112. https://doi.org/10.1186/s13073-022-01114-x.
7. Chang X, March M, Mentch F, Qu H, Liu Y, Glessner J, Sleiman P, Hakonarson H. Genetic architecture of asthma in African American patients. J Allergy Clin Immunol. 2023;151(4):1132–6. https://doi.org/10.1016/j.jaci.2022.09.001.
8. Busch R, Qiu W, Lasky-Su J, Morrow J, Criner G, DeMeo D. Differential DNA methylation marks and gene comethylation of COPD in African-Americans with COPD exacerbations. Respir Res. 2016;17(1):143. https://doi.org/10.1186/s12931-016-0459-8.
9. Venkatesan P. GOLD COPD report: 2025 update. Lancet Respir Med. 2025;13(1):e7–8. https://doi.org/10.1016/S2213-2600(24)00413-2.
10. Saeed H, Arshad MK, Shahnoor S, Abdullah WA, Mahmood H, Zabeehullah SA, Daoud M. Temporal trends gender and ethnoracial disparities in mortality from pulmonary emphysema: a retrospective nationwide analysis. Medicine. 2024;103(52):e41032. https://doi.org/10.1097/MD.0000000000041032.
11. Regan EA, Lowe ME, Make BJ, Curtis JL, Chen QG, Crooks JL, Wilson C, Oates GR, Gregg RW, Baldomero AK, Bhatt SP, Diaz AA, Benos PV, O'Brien JK, Young KA, Kinney GL, Conrad DJ, Lowe KE, DL DM, Non A, Cho MH, Kallet J, Foreman MG, Westney GE, Hoth K, NR MI, Hanania NA, Wolfe A, Amaza H, Han M, Beaty TH, Hansel NN, McCormack MC, Balasubramanian A, Crapo JD, Silverman EK, Casaburi R, Wise RA. Early evidence of chronic obstructive pulmonary disease obscured by race-specific prediction equations. Am J Respir Crit Care Med. 2024;209(1):59–69. https://doi.org/10.1164/rccm.202303-0444OC.
12. Liu GY, Khan SS, Colangelo LA, Meza D, Washko GR, PHS S, Jacobs DR Jr, Dransfield MT, Carnethon MR, Kalhan R. Comparing racial differences in emphysema prevalence among adults with normal spirometry: a secondary data analysis of the CARDIA lung study. Ann. Intern. Med. 2022;175(8):1118–25. https://doi.org/10.7326/M22-0205.

13. Sood A, Petersen H, Liu C, Myers O, Shore XW, Gore BA, Vazquez-Guillamet R, Cook LS, Meek P, Tesfaigzi Y. Racial and ethnic minorities have a lower prevalence of airflow obstruction than non-hispanic whites. COPD J Chron Obstruct Pulmon Dis. 2022;19(1):61–8. https://doi.org/10.1080/15412555.2022.2029384.
14. Choi JY, Yoo KH, Jung KS, Kim V, Rhee CK. Clinical significance of chronic bronchitis in different racial groups. BMC Pulm Med. 2024;24(1):282. https://doi.org/10.1186/s12890-024-03100-y.
15. Tang W, Bentley AR, Kritchevsky SB, Harris TB, Newman AB, Bauer DC, Meibohm B, Cassano PA. Genetic variation in antioxidant enzymes cigarette smoking and longitudinal change in lung function. Free Radic Biol Med. 2013;63:304–12. https://doi.org/10.1016/j.freeradbiomed.2013.05.016.
16. Fonseca H, da Silva TM, Saraiva M, Santolalla ML, Sant'Anna HP, Araujo NM, Lima NP, Rios R, Tarazona-Santos E, Horta BL, Cruz A, Barreto ML, Figueiredo CA. Genomic regions 10q22.2 17q21.31 and 2p23.1 can contribute to a lower lung function in African descent populations. Genes. 2020;11(9):1047. https://doi.org/10.3390/genes11091047.
17. Pleasants RA, Riley IL, Mannino DM. Defining and targeting health disparities in chronic obstructive pulmonary disease. Int J Chron Obstruct Pulmon Dis. 2016;11:2475–96.
18. Hardin M, Silverman EK, Barr RG, et al. The clinical features of the overlap between COPD and asthma. Respir Res. 2011;12:127. https://doi.org/10.1186/1465-9921-12-127.
19. Mina N, Soubani AO, Cote ML, et al. The relationship between COPD and lung cancer in African American patients. Clin Lung Cancer. 2012;13(2):149–56.
20. Dransfield MT, Davis JJ, Gerald LB, Bailey WC. Racial and gender differences in susceptibility to tobacco smoke among patients with chronic obstructive pulmonary disease. Respir Med. 2006;100(6):1110–6.
21. Kirkpatrick DP, Dransfield MT. Racial and sex differences in chronic obstructive pulmonary disease susceptibility, diagnosis, and treatment. Curr Opin Pulm Med. 2009;15(2):100–4.
22. Kamil F, Pinzon I, Foreman MG. Sex and race factors in early-onset COPD. Curr Opin Pulm Med. 2013;19(2):140–4.
23. Han MK, Curran-Everett D, Dransfield MT, et al. Racial differences in quality of life in patients with COPD. Chest. 2011;140(5):1169–76.
24. Lee H, Shin SH, Gu S, et al. Racial differences in comorbidity profile among patients with chronic obstructive pulmonary disease. BMC Med. 2018;16:178.
25. Nastars DR, Rojas JD, Ottenbacher KJ, Graham JE. Race/ethnicity and 30-day readmission rates in medicare beneficiaries with COPD. Respiratory Care. 2019;64(8):931–6. https://doi.org/10.4187/respcare.06475.
26. Goto T, Faridi MK, Gibo K, et al. Sex and racial/ethnic differences in the reason for 30-day readmission after COPD hospitalization. Respir Med. 2017;131:6–10.
27. Asthma and African Americans. U.S. Department of Health and Human Services Office of Minority Health. 2018. https://minorityhealth.hhs.gov/omh/browse.aspx?lvl=4&lvlid=15. Accessed 12 June 2019.
28. Krishnan JA, Diette GB, Skinner EA, et al. Race and sex differences in consistency of care with national asthma guidelines in managed care organizations. Arch Intern Med. 2001;161(13):1660–8.
29. Trivedi M, Fung V, Kharbanda EO, Larkin EK, Butler MG, Horan K, Lieu TA, Wu AC. Racial disparities in family-provider interactions for pediatric asthma care. J Asthma. 2018;55(4):424–9. https://doi.org/10.1080/02770903.2017.1337790.
30. Fitzpatrick AM, Gillespie SE, Mauger DT, Phillips BR, Bleecker ER, Israel E, Meyers DA, Moore WC, Sorkness RL, Wenzel SE, Bacharier LB, Castro M, Denlinger LC, Erzurum SC, Fahy JV, Gaston BM, Jarjour NN, Larkin A, Levy BD, Ly NP, Ortega VE, Peters SP, Phipatanakul W, Ramratnam S, Teague WG. Racial disparities in asthma-related health care use in the National Heart Lung and Blood Institute's Severe Asthma Research Program. J Allergy Clin Immunol. 2019;143(6):2052–61. https://doi.org/10.1016/j.jaci.2018.11.022.

31. Brown RW, Cappelletti CS. Reaching beyond disparity: safely improving asthma control in the at-risk African American population. J Natl Med Assoc. 2013;105(2):138–49.
32. Holt EW, Theall KP, Rabito FA. Individual, housing, and neighborhood correlates of asthma among young urban children. J Urban Health. 2013;90(1):116–29.
33. Bruzzese JM, Kingston S, Falletta KA, et al. Individual and neighborhood factors associated with undiagnosed asthma in a large cohort of urban adolescents. J Urban Health. 2019;96(2):252–61.
34. Loman DG, Kwong CG, Henry LD, et al. Asthma control and obesity in urban African American children. J Asthma. 2017;54(6):578–83.
35. Camargo CA Jr, Sutherland ER, Bailey W, Castro M, Yancey SW, Emmett AH, Stempel DA. Effect of increased body mass index on asthma risk impairment and response to asthma controller therapy in African Americans. Curr Med Res Opin. 2010;26(7):1629–35. https://doi.org/10.1185/03007995.2010.483113.
36. ME MG, Castellanos E, Thakur N, Oh SS, Eng C, Davis A, Meade K, MA LN, Avila PC, Farber HJ, Serebrisky D, Brigino-Buenaventura E, Rodriguez-Cintron W, Kumar R, Bibbins-Domingo K, Thyne SM, Sen S, Rodriguez-Santana JR, Borrell LN, Burchard EG. Obesity and bronchodilator response in black and hispanic children and adolescents with asthma. Chest. 2015;147(6):1591–8. https://doi.org/10.1378/chest.14-2689.
37. Brehm JM, Schuemann B, Fuhlbrigge AL, et al. Serum vitamin D and severe asthma exacerbations in the childhood asthma management program study. J Allergy Clin Immunol. 2010;126(1):52–56.e5.
38. Harris SS. Vitamin D and African Americans. J Nutr. 2006;136(4):1126–9.
39. Hall SC, Agrawal DK. Vitamin D and bronchial asthma: an overview of the last five years. Clin Ther. 2017;39(5):917–29.
40. Oh S, Du R, Zeiger AM, et al. Breastfeeding associated with higher lung function in African American youths with asthma. J Asthma. 2017;54(8):856–65.
41. Nanda A, Siles R, Park H, Louisias M, Ariue B, Castillo M, Anand MP, Nguyen AP, Jean T, Lopez M, Altisheh R, Pappalardo AA. Ensuring equitable access to guideline-based asthma care across the lifespan: tips and future directions to the successful implementation of the new NAEPP 2020 guidelines a work group report of the AAAAI asthma cough diagnosis and treatment committee. J Allergy Clin Immunol. 2023;151(4):869–80. https://doi.org/10.1016/j.jaci.2023.01.017.
42. Ebell MH, Hall SP, Rustin RC, Powell-Threets K, Munoz L, Toodle K, Meng ML, O'Connor J. A multicomponent multi-trigger intervention to enhance asthma control in high-risk African American children. Prev Chronic Dis. 2019;16:E69. https://doi.org/10.5888/pcd16.180387.
43. Patel MR, Song PX, Sanders G, Nelson B, Kaltsas E, Thomas LJ, Janevic MR, Hafeez K, Wang W, Wilkin M, Johnson TR, Brown RW. A randomized clinical trial of a culturally responsive intervention for African American women with asthma. Ann Allergy Asthma Immunol. 2017;118(2):212–9. https://doi.org/10.1016/j.anai.2016.11.016.
44. Drent M, Crouser ED, Grunewald J. Challenges of sarcoidosis and its management. N Engl J Med. 2021;385(11):1018–32. https://doi.org/10.1056/NEJMra2101555.
45. Jain R, Yadav D, Puranik N, Guleria R, Jin JO. Sarcoidosis: causes diagnosis clinical features and treatments. J Clin Med. 2020;9(4):1081. https://doi.org/10.3390/jcm9041081.
46. Crouser ED, Maier LA, Wilson KC, Bonham CA, Morgenthau AS, Patterson KC, Abston E, Bernstein RC, Blankstein R, Chen ES, Culver DA, Drake W, Drent M, Gerke AK, Ghobrial M, Govender P, Hamzeh N, James WE, Judson MA, Kellermeyer L, Knight S, Koth LL, Poletti V, Raman SV, Tukey MH, Westney GE, Baughman RP. Diagnosis and detection of sarcoidosis. An Official American Thoracic Society Clinical Practice Guideline. Am J Respir Crit Care Med. 2020;201(8):e26–51. https://doi.org/10.1164/rccm.202002-0251ST.
47. Gerke AK, Judson MA, Cozier YC, et al. Disease burden and variability in sarcoidosis. Ann Am Thorac Soc. 2017;14(Suppl 6):S421–8.
48. Cozier YC, Berman JS, Palmer JR, Boggs DA, Serlin DM, Rosenberg L. Sarcoidosis in black women in the United States: data from the Black Women's Health Study. Chest. 2011;139:144–50.

References

49. Gideon NM, Mannino DM. Sarcoidosis mortality in the United States 1979–1991: an analysis of multiple-cause mortality data. Am J Med. 1996;100:423–7.
50. Newman LS, Rose CS, Bresnitz EA, ACCESS Research Group, et al. A case control etiologic study of sarcoidosis: environmental and occupational risk factors. Am J Respir Crit Care Med. 2004;170:1324–30.
51. Levin AM, Adrianto I, Datta I, et al. Association of HLA-DRB1 with sarcoidosis susceptibility and progression in African Americans. Am J Respir Cell Biol. 2015;53(2):206–16.
52. Mirsaeidi M, Machado RF, Schraufnagel D, et al. Racial difference in sarcoidosis mortality in the United States. Chest. 2015;147(2):438–49.
53. Brito-Zerón P, Kostov B, Superville D, Baughman RP, Ramos-Casals M. Autoimmune big data study group. Geoepidemiological big data approach to sarcoidosis: geographical and ethnic determinants. Clin Exp Rheumatol. 2019;37(6):1052–64. Epub 2019 Aug 26
54. Sève P, Pacheco Y, Durupt F, Jamilloux Y, Gerfaud-Valentin M, Isaac S, Boussel L, Calender A, Androdias G, Valeyre D, El Jammal T. Sarcoidosis: a clinical overview from symptoms to diagnosis. Cells. 2021;10(4):766. https://doi.org/10.3390/cells10040766.
55. Mehta D, Lubitz SA, Frankel Z, et al. Cardiac involvement in patients with sarcoidosis: diagnostic and prognostic value of outpatient testing. Chest. 2008;133(6):1426–35.
56. Judson MA, Boan AD, Lackland DT. The clinical course of sarcoidosis: presentation, diagnosis, and treatment in a large white and black cohort in the United States. Sarcoidosis Vasc Diffuse Lung Dis. 2012;29:119–27.
57. Rabin DL, Richardson MS, Stein SR, Yeager H. Sarcoidosis severity and socioeconomic status. Eur Respir J. 2001;18:499–506.
58. Beegle SH, Barba K, Gobunsuy R, Judson MA. Current and emerging pharmacological treatments for sarcoidosis: a review. Drug Des Devel Ther. 2013;7:325–38.
59. Baughman RP, Scholand MB, Rahaghi FF. Clinical phenotyping: role in treatment decisions in sarcoidosis. Eur Respir Rev. 2020;29(155):190145. https://doi.org/10.1183/16000617.0145-2019.
60. Belperio JA, Shaikh F, Abtin FG, Fishbein MC, Weigt SS, Saggar R, Lynch JP 3rd. Diagnosis and treatment of pulmonary sarcoidosis. JAMA. 2022;327(9):856. https://doi.org/10.1001/jama.2022.1570.
61. Duvall C, Pavlovic N, Rosen NS, Wand AL, Griffin JM, Okada DR, Tandri H, Kasper EK, Sharp M, Chen ES, Chrispin J, Gilotra NA. Sex and race differences in cardiac sarcoidosis presentation treatment and outcomes. J Card Fail. 2023;29(8):1135–45. https://doi.org/10.1016/j.cardfail.2023.03.022.
62. Johnson DA, Guo N, Rueschman M, Wang R, Wilson JG, Redline S. Prevalence and correlates of obstructive sleep apnea among African Americans: the Jackson Heart Sleep Study. Sleep. 2018;41(10):zsy154. https://doi.org/10.1093/sleep/zsy154.
63. Dong L, Dubowitz T, Haas A, Ghosh-Dastidar M, Holliday SB, Buysse DJ, Hale L, Gary-Webb TL, Troxel WM. Prevalence and correlates of obstructive sleep apnea in urban-dwelling low-income predominantly African-American women. Sleep Med. 2020;73:187–95. https://doi.org/10.1016/j.sleep.2020.06.022.
64. Thornton JD, Dudley KA, Saeed GJ, Schuster ST, Schell A, Spilsbury JC, Patel SR. Differences in symptoms and severity of obstructive sleep apnea between black and white patients. Ann Am Thorac Soc. 2022;19(2):272–8. https://doi.org/10.1513/AnnalsATS.202012-1483OC.
65. Chen X, Wang R, Zee P, et al. Racial/ethnic differences in sleep disturbances: the Multi-Ethnic Study of Atherosclerosis (MESA). Sleep. 2015;38(6):877–88.
66. Ullah MI, Tamanna S. Racial disparity in cardiovascular morbidity and mortality associated with obstructive sleep apnea: the sleep heart health study. Sleep Med. 2023;101:528–34. https://doi.org/10.1016/j.sleep.2022.12.007.
67. Dudley KA, Patel SR. Disparities and genetic risk factors in obstructive sleep apnea. Sleep Med. 2016;18:96–102.
68. Ruiter ME, DeCoster J, Jacobs L, Lichstein KL. Sleep disorders in African Americans and Caucasian Americans: a meta-analysis. Behav Sleep Med. 2010;8(4):246–59.

69. Scharf SM, Seiden L, DeMore J, Carter-Pokras O. Racial differences in clinical presentation of patients with sleep-disordered breathing. Sleep Breath. 2004;8:173–83.
70. Joosten SA, Khoo JK, Edwareds BA, et al. Improvement in obstructive sleep apnea with weight loss in dependent on body position during sleep. Sleep. 2017;40(5):zsx047. https://doi.org/10.1093/sleep/zsx047.
71. Hayes AL, Spilsbury JC, Patel SR. The Epworth score in African American populations. J Clin Sleep Med. 2009;5:344–8.
72. Jhamb M, Unruh M. Bidirectional relationship of hypertension with obstructive sleep apnea. Curr Opin Pulm Med. 2014;20(6):558–64.
73. Johnson DA, Thomas SJ, Abdalla M, Guo N, Yano Y, Rueschman M, Tanner RM, Mittleman MA, Calhoun DA, Wilson JG, Muntner P, Redline S. Association between sleep apnea and blood pressure control among blacks. Circulation. 2019;139(10):1275–84. https://doi.org/10.1161/CIRCULATIONAHA.118.036675.
74. Epstein LJ, Kristo D, Strollo PJ Jr, et al. Clinical guideline for the evaluation, management and long-term care of obstructive sleep apnea in adults. J Clin Sleep Med. 2009;5(3):263–76.
75. Schwartz SW, Sebastiao Y, Rosas J, et al. Racial disparity in adherence to positive airway pressure among US veterans. Sleep Breath. 2016;20(3):947–55.
76. Bakker JP, Weaver TE, Parthasarathy S, Aloia MS. Adherence to CPAP: what should we be aiming for, and how can we get there? Chest. 2019;155(6):1272–87.
77. Shaw R, McKenzie S, Taylor T, Olafiranye O, Boutin-Foster C, Ogedegbe G, Jean-Louis G. Beliefs and attitudes toward obstructive sleep apnea evaluation and treatment among blacks. J Natl Med Assoc. 2012;104(11–12):510–9. https://doi.org/10.1016/S0027-9684(15)30217-0.
78. Rowland S, Aiyappan V, Hennessy C, Catcheside P, Chai-Coezter CL, RD ME, Antic NA. Comparing the efficacy mask leak patient adherence and patient preference of three different CPAP interfaces to treat moderate-severe obstructive sleep apnea. J Clin Sleep Med. 2018;14(01):101–8. https://doi.org/10.5664/jcsm.6892.

Chapter 10
A Precision Medicine Approach to Laboratory Results and Hematological Disorders in African Americans

Gregory L. Hall and Keesha Powell-Roach

Contents

10.1	Creatinine and GFR Controversy...	182
10.2	Laboratory Results..	183
	10.2.1 CBC...	183
	10.2.2 Benign Ethnic Neutropenia (Typical Neutrophil Count with Fy(a-b-) Status)..	184
	10.2.3 Metabolic Panel..	185
	10.2.4 Thyroid-Stimulating Hormone (TSH)...	186
	10.2.5 Lipid Profile...	187
10.3	Cancer Markers..	187
	10.3.1 Prostate-Specific Antigen (PSA)..	187
	10.3.2 Cancer Antigen 125 (CA-125)..	188
	10.3.3 Alpha-Fetoprotein (AFP)..	189
	10.3.4 Carbohydrate Antigen 19-9 (CA 19-9)..	189
10.4	Vitamin Blood Levels..	190
	10.4.1 Vitamin B12...	190
	10.4.2 Folate..	190
	10.4.3 Vitamin A...	191
	10.4.4 Vitamin C...	191
	10.4.5 Vitamin E...	192
10.5	Sickle Cell Disease..	193
	10.5.1 Renal Complications..	194
	10.5.2 Pulmonary Hypertension..	195
	10.5.3 Eye Complications..	196
	10.5.4 Priapism...	196
	10.5.5 Stroke..	197
	10.5.6 Aplastic Crisis...	197
	10.5.7 Acute Chest Syndrome..	198
	10.5.8 Splenic Sequestration...	199
	10.5.9 Vaso-Occlusive Pain Management..	200

© The Author(s), under exclusive license to Springer Nature Switzerland AG 2025
G. L. Hall, *Precision Medicine for African Americans*,
https://doi.org/10.1007/978-3-031-95774-1_10

10.6 Thalassemia (Alpha and Beta)... 202
10.7 Glucose-6-Phosphate Dehydrogenase Deficiency (G6PD)............................. 204
References... 206

Before addressing the few hematological diseases specific to African Americans, it is sensible to review the differences in hematology laboratory results between African Americans and majority patients. Many providers face challenges when making decisions regarding laboratory test results that fall outside the normal range. Slight deviations from the reference range can occasionally result in additional lab tests, unnecessary referrals, and unjustified investigations. Although differences in laboratory reference intervals based on race (and gender) have been acknowledged for many years, clinical laboratories have been slow to implement race- or gender-specific reference ranges [1].

10.1 Creatinine and GFR Controversy

When race was included in the Glomerular Filtration Rate (GFR) and creatinine reference range, experts criticized its use and changed their position. The race-based GFR controversy focused on using race as a factor in estimating kidney function, mainly through formulas like the Modification of Diet in Renal Disease (MDRD) and the Chronic Kidney Disease Epidemiology Collaboration (CKD-EPI) equations [2, 3]. These formulas traditionally included a race coefficient that adjusted GFR estimates for African American patients, reflecting historical assumptions that Black individuals have higher muscle mass and, consequently, higher creatinine levels. The inclusion of race in these equations has faced increasing scrutiny. Critics argue that this practice perpetuates racial stereotypes and can lead to misdiagnoses or delayed treatment for kidney disease in this population. For instance, an African American patient might be deemed to have a normal GFR when they actually have kidney disease, potentially affecting their access to care and treatment options. The National Kidney Foundation (NKF) and the American Society of Nephrology (ASN) have recommended the removal of the race coefficient from GFR estimating equations, advocating for the use of race-neutral equations [3, 4]. The KDIGO 2024 Clinical Practice Guideline for the Evaluation and Management of Chronic Kidney Disease also advises against using race in eGFR calculations [3].

This shift aims to improve health equity and ensure that all patients receive appropriate care regardless of their racial or ethnic background, but if a difference exists, should not we consider it?

The genetic basis for differences in creatinine levels among various racial groups is multifactorial, involving both genetic and nongenetic factors. Elevated serum creatinine levels in individuals of African ancestry have been linked to several determinants. Genetic ancestry plays a significant role. Studies have shown that African ancestry correlates with higher serum creatinine levels. For example, every 10% increase in African ancestry is linked to a 1.3% rise in serum creatinine levels [2]. This association persists even after adjusting for measured GFR, suggesting that genetic factors contribute to these differences. Secondly, non-GFR determinants such as increased muscle mass, body mass index (BMI) [5], body surface area [5], and 24-h urinary excretion of creatinine are more common among individuals of African ancestry and contribute to elevated serum creatinine levels. These factors indicate higher muscle mass and creatinine production [2]. Additionally, APOL1 gene variants (G1 and G2) are recognized as significant genetic factors linked to an increased risk of chronic kidney disease (CKD) and elevated serum creatinine levels in individuals of African descent. These variants are believed to have evolved to offer protection against certain infectious diseases, yet they also heighten susceptibility to kidney disease [6].

On one hand, correcting for influences that lead to higher creatinine levels makes sense, as overall creatinine is elevated in the typical African American population [2]. On the other hand, the APOL1 gene, present in 13% of the African American population, is linked to a greater risk of developing chronic kidney disease, which results in elevated creatinine levels and indicates damage that should not be overlooked [7, 8]. A more nuanced approach is warranted.

10.2 Laboratory Results

In a report by the Mayo Clinic, 60–70% of clinical decisions regarding a patient's diagnosis, treatment, hospital admission, and discharge were based on laboratory results [9]. Clinicians also "routinely experience uncertainty and challenges in ordering and interpreting diagnostic laboratory tests" [10]. Traditionally, reference intervals used in clinical laboratories have been determined using predominantly European American reference individuals. However, variances in reference range values have routinely been noted between racial/ethnic groups. Despite many calls for more nuanced reference range options tailored for specific populations, having race-based reference ranges have been controversial. Below is a consolidation of the adjustments and trends that should be considered when interpreting an African American patient's laboratory report.

10.2.1 CBC

Eunjung Lim and colleagues at the Office of Biostatistics and Quantitative Health Sciences at the University of Hawaii looked at the reference intervals for common clinical laboratory results and found significant differences in gender and racial/

ethnic subpopulations that could impact decision-making. Compared to European Americans, the normal range for African Americans significantly shifted to lower values in hemoglobin (HGB), hematocrit (HCT), mean corpuscular hemoglobin (MCH),, and mean corpuscular hemoglobin concentration (MCHC) [11, 12]. A number of studies have also shown lower total white blood cell (CBC) counts, neutrophil count, monocyte count, and platelet counts in African Americans when compared to European Americans [13–21].

CBC Trends in African Americans	
WBC	*Lower*
HGB	*Lower*
HCT	*Lower*
MCH	*Lower*
MCHC	*Lower*
Neutrophils	*Lower*
Monocytes	*Lower*
Lymphocytes	*Higher*
Eosinophils	*Same*
Platelet count	*Lower*

10.2.2 Benign Ethnic Neutropenia (Typical Neutrophil Count with Fy(a-b-) Status)

Benign ethnic neutropenia (typical neutrophil count with Fy(a-b-) status.) is a condition characterized by a lower-than-average absolute neutrophil count (defined as between 1.0×10^9 cell/Liter and 1.5×10^9 cell/liter) in individuals of specific ethnic backgrounds, particularly those of African, Middle Eastern, and West Indian descent [22, 23]. Despite the reduced neutrophil count, individuals with benign ethnic neutropenia do not have an increased risk of infections, distinguishing it from other forms of neutropenia that are clinically significant. The condition is primarily associated with the Duffy antigen receptor for chemokines (DARC) gene, specifically the DARC-null phenotype, which is prevalent in these populations. This genetic variation is thought to cause neutrophils to redistribute from the peripheral blood to tissues such as the spleen, rather than indicating a true deficiency in neutrophil production [24, 25]. Clinically, benign ethnic neutropenia is often identified incidentally during routine blood tests, and it is important for healthcare providers to recognize this condition to avoid unnecessary diagnostic evaluations and interventions. Many healthy African Americans with low neutrophil counts undergo costly investigations, as well as delayed treatment, for a condition that has been demonstrated to be completely benign. Matthew Hsieh and colleagues looked at NHANES data and noted statistically significant differences in neutropenia by race. One in 22 African American men and 1 in 40 African American women have benign ethnic neutropenia [14]. In sharp contrast, European Americans have a neutropenia prevalence of 1 in 126.

The low neutrophil counts were tracked to a specific chromosome containing a receptor that influenced white blood cell production, and particularly neutrophils, in African Americans [23]. Rahul Lakhotia from the National Institute of Health looked at this phenomenon and "confirmed that the clinical nature for this condition was benign" [23]. The patients in his review with low neutrophil counts actually had low rates of infections as well as lower chronic disorders including hypertension and diabetes [23].

Benign ethnic neutropenia usually follows a hereditary pattern, and so a more detailed family history in neutropenic patients may reveal this cause [26, 27].

Patients with benign ethnic neutropenia do not require extensive monitoring or evaluation once this is discovered and incorporated into their past medical history. Otherwise if incidentally discovered, repeat the absolute neutrophil count three times within an interval of 2 weeks looking for count variations or signs/symptoms of infection. When determining the need for a diagnostic evaluation for neutropenia, clinicians should consider the patient's age, sex, and ethnicity [27, 28].

Lauren Merz and Maureen Achebe at Brigham and Women's Hospital in Boston criticized the term "benign ethnic neutropenia" as suggesting that somehow there is something wrong and strongly advocated for a more appropriate term: *typical neutrophil count with Fy(a-b-) status:*

> It is no surprise that systemic racism, structures of discriminatory policies and practices that assign privilege on the basis of skin color, is insidiously embedded in systems that we blithely invoke in our daily practice. We need to examine why we ascribe labels to clinically insignificant variants, labeling as conditions differences that predominantly affect non-White communities. Systemic racism was purposely construed; therefore, deliberate actions are crucial to its abolishment. Thus, we advocate for "benign ethnic neutropenia" to be referred to as "typical neutrophil count with Fy(a-b-) status." This is a more accurate description of the genetic driver of the lower ANCs and avoids the suggestion that ethnicity alone is causal or that this common variant is abnormal [29].

10.2.3 Metabolic Panel

Houman Tahmasebi and Khosrow Adeli of the CALIPER Program in Toronto, Canada, looked at the influence of race/ethnicity on population laboratory reference values and its impact on care [30]:

> Using RIs (reference intervals) established from a predominantly Caucasian population to interpret laboratory test results from a non-Caucasian or multi-ethnic patient population may lead to inaccurate interpretation of test results and, ultimately, missed diagnosis. For example, creatine kinase (CK) is commonly used as a biomarker for monitoring statin-induced myopathy to determine whether an individual can safely undergo or continue statin therapy. The median CK activity for healthy Black adult males and females is approximately double that of Caucasian adult males and females, respectively. The lack of an appropriate ethnic-specific RI for Black patients could result in termination of statin treatment in the absence of muscle toxicity, simply because their CK levels are above a RI established using a predominantly Caucasian reference population. In the absence of robust RIs that are ethnic-specific, clinicians are not able to provide the best possible healthcare for all patients [30].

Laboratory Trends in African Americans	
TSH	*Lower*
CRP	*Higher*
Creatine kinase (CK)	*Higher*
Creatinine	*Higher*
GGT	*Higher*
Total protein	*Higher*
Transferrin	*Lower*
PTH	*Higher*

When considering the general electrolytes, a number of studies have shown no significant difference in results in sodium, potassium, chloride, calcium, phosphorus, or magnesium between African Americans and European Americans [31].

10.2.4 Thyroid-Stimulating Hormone (TSH)

Thyroid-stimulating hormone (TSH) results in African Americans tend to be lower compared to other racial/ethnic groups. Several studies have demonstrated this difference [32–35]. For instance, the National Health and Nutrition Examination Survey (NHANES III) found that the mean serum TSH was significantly lower in African Americans (1.18 mIU/L) compared to European Americans (1.57 mIU/L) [33]. Additionally, genetic studies have shown that the distribution of TSH values is shifted toward lower values in African Americans. Genome-wide association studies (GWAS) have identified several genetic variants associated with TSH levels that differ between populations of African and European ancestry. For example, the study by Wade et al. found that the genetic associations with TSH levels differ significantly between individuals with genetic similarities to African reference populations (GSA) and those with similarities to European reference populations (GSE) [34]. Specifically, the PDE8B locus, which is strongly associated with TSH levels in European populations, does not show the same association in African American populations. This suggests that the genetic architecture influencing TSH levels varies between these groups. Additionally, Malinowski and colleagues reported that while some known TSH-associated variants, such as those in PDE8B, were nominally significant in African Americans, they did not reach genome-wide significance, indicating potential differences in the genetic determinants of TSH levels between racial/ethnic groups [35]. The American Association of Clinical Endocrinologists and the American Thyroid Association guidelines also acknowledge these racial differences in TSH levels, suggesting that race-specific reference ranges may be necessary to avoid misclassification of thyroid dysfunction [35].

Laura Boucai at Albert Einstein College of Medicine examined thyroid-stimulating hormone (TSH) levels in European Americans and African Americans using NHANES data and found statistically significant differences in the "normal" reference ranges for these racial/ethnic groups. Generally, African Americans exhibit lower TSH levels, with a range of 0.37–3.46 mIU/L, compared to the overall reference interval of 0.512–5.22 mIU/L [36]. When a lower TSH level is detected, it may prompt follow-up laboratory tests (e.g., T3 and T4) and the associated costs. A clear understanding that African Americans have a lower reference interval for TSH can be reassuring and save time and money.

Lipid Profile Trends in African Americans	
Total cholesterol	*Lower*
HDL	*Higher*
LDL	*Lower*
Triglyceride	*Lower*

10.2.5 Lipid Profile

As is mentioned in the cardiovascular section, the lipid profile in African Americans is generally more favorable with a higher HDL and lower total cholesterol, LDL, and triglycerides (TG) [37–39]. Several studies have identified genetic variants that influence lipid levels in African Americans. For instance, variants in the lipoprotein lipase (LPL) gene, such as rs328, have been associated with higher HDL-C and lower TG levels in African Americans [40–42]. Additionally, admixture mapping studies have shown that European ancestry is negatively correlated with HDL-C and positively correlated with TG levels, suggesting that genetic factors specific to African ancestry contribute to the favorable lipid profiles [42]. Moreover, the National Lipid Association highlights distinctive features of lipoprotein metabolism in African Americans, including increased post-heparin lipoprotein lipase activity and less inhibition of lipoprotein lipase by apo C3 and insulin resistance, which contribute to lower TG levels [40].

This seemingly better profile is in stark contrast to worse cardiovascular outcomes for African Americans and should be considered when deciding who needs cholesterol-lowering medications and what criteria is used [40].

10.3 Cancer Markers

10.3.1 Prostate-Specific Antigen (PSA)

As reviewed in the cancer chapter, the prostate-specific antigen (PSA) is a better and more sensitive detector of prostate cancer in African Americans [43]. PSA also tends to range higher in cancer-free African Americans [44]. Veda Giri at Fox Chase Cancer Center in Philadelphia PA found that at any given PSA, African Americans are at a higher risk for prostate cancer than European Americans. For example, a PSA of 3 gives a higher risk for prostate cancer to an African American than a matched European American with the same PSA [45]. The increased prostate cancer risk supports the need to follow "accelerating" PSAs, one that is rising over time yet still within normal limits, more closely in African Americans as this pattern is more associated with prostate cancer diagnosis [46]. PSA velocity, as it is also called, predicted more aggressive prostate cancer and a higher risk for death in African Americans [46]. In contrast, the study also found that PSA velocity did not add any significant utility over static PSA testing in European Americans or Asian Americans [46, 47].

Genome-wide association studies (GWAS) have identified several genetic loci that influence PSA levels, with genetic variants accounting for 5.5–9.5% of the variance in PSA levels among African American men [48]. This genetic component indicates that PSA levels in African Americans may inherently vary due to these genetic factors, independent of the presence of prostate cancer. The American Urological Association recommends that individuals with increased risk factors, such as African American ancestry, could benefit from earlier and more frequent PSA screening [49]. Evidence supports that African American men face a higher risk of developing aggressive prostate cancer and possess a higher mortality rate compared to other racial groups [50, 51].

10.3.2 Cancer Antigen 125 (CA-125)

CA-125 levels are a marker used to detect and monitor certain types of cancer, particularly ovarian cancer. Elevated levels of CA-125 may indicate the presence of cancer, but they can also be caused by other conditions such as endometriosis or pelvic inflammatory disease. CA-125 levels in African Americans are generally lower than in other racial and ethnic groups. Specifically, studies have shown that African American women tend to have significantly lower CA-125 levels than European American women [52, 53]. For instance, one study found that African American women had an average CA-125 level that was 29.0% lower than that of European American women [52]. This difference is crucial to consider in clinical settings, as current CA-125 thresholds for ovarian cancer screening and diagnosis were primarily developed based on data from majority populations, potentially leading to underdiagnosis or delayed diagnosis in African American women. Additionally, the lower CA-125 levels in African American women have been observed both in healthy individuals and in those diagnosed with ovarian cancer [54]. This suggests that race/ethnicity should be taken into account when interpreting CA-125 levels to avoid disparities in cancer detection and treatment.

10.3.3 Alpha-Fetoprotein (AFP)

Alpha-fetoprotein (AFP) levels are utilized to screen for liver cancer and can assist in detecting it at an early stage. Elevated AFP levels in the blood may suggest the presence of liver cancer (hepatocellular carcinoma), although other conditions, such as hepatitis or cirrhosis, may also lead to increased AFP levels.

Regarding hepatocellular carcinoma (HCC), African American patients often exhibit higher rates of elevated AFP levels compared to other racial groups [55, 56]. A study in Cancer Medicine reported that African American HCC patients had a significant prevalence of elevated AFP levels, which serves as an important prognostic factor for overall survival [55]. Furthermore, another study in Hepatology found that AFP is less sensitive for diagnosing HCC in African Americans with hepatitis C virus infection compared to other ethnic groups [56].

10.3.4 Carbohydrate Antigen 19-9 (CA 19-9)

Carbohydrate Antigen 19-9 (CA 19-9) levels serve as a tumor marker for detecting pancreatic cancer. Elevated CA 19-9 levels in the blood can indicate the presence of pancreatic cancer; however, other conditions, such as biliary tract diseases, may also lead to increased CA 19-9 levels.CA 19-9 levels in African Americans can show significant differences compared to those in other racial groups [57, 58]. Specifically, African Americans are more likely to be CA 19-9 nonproducers due to a higher prevalence of the Lewis (a-b-) genotype in this population, which results in an inability to synthesize CA 19-9 [59] As a consequence, these patients have an undetectable CA 19-9 level regardless of their actual cancer status. In a study presented at the 2024 ASCO Annual Meeting, researchers found that African American patients with advanced pancreatic ductal adenocarcinoma were significantly more likely to be CA 19-9 nonproducers compared to European American patients [57]. Another study indicated that African American patients with localized pancreatic cancer were also more likely to be CA 19-9 nonproducers and experienced significantly worse rates of major pathologic response following neoadjuvant chemotherapy [58]. Patients sometimes request specific lab tests by name to screen for cancer, and African American patients should be aware of the higher prevalence of CA 19-9 nonproducers in their population.

Cancer Marker Differences in African Americans	
PSA	*Higher*
CA-125	*Lower*
Alpha-fetoprotein (AFP)	*Higher*
CA 19-9	*May be unable to synthesize*

10.4 Vitamin Blood Levels

The vitamin level differences in African Americans, with the exception of vitamin D, which is related to sun exposure and skin pigmentation and covered extensively in Chap. 14, have primarily been attributed to dietary differences [60–63]. Curiously, the genetic drivers of these vitamin level differences get much less attention but do, nonetheless, exist. For example, vitamin B6 has consistently been found to be lower in populations of African descent [64].

10.4.1 Vitamin B12

In contrast, vitamin B12 levels are generally, and curiously, higher [65–67]. This phenomenon is likely influenced by genetic variations, such as polymorphisms in genes related to vitamin B12 metabolism, including transcobalamin II (TC-II) [65, 68]. Additionally, a study by O'Logbon et al. found that African patients, particularly those of Nigerian descent, had significantly higher serum vitamin B12 concentrations compared to patients of Asian and European descent [65]. This indicates that genetic factors significantly contribute to determining serum vitamin B12 levels across different populations.

10.4.2 Folate

African Americans typically have lower serum and red blood cell (RBC) folate concentrations compared to other racial groups [69–71]. Several studies have identified genetic polymorphisms that influence folate metabolism and levels. One of the most researched polymorphisms is the methylenetetrahydrofolate reductase (MTHFR) 677C → T variant. This polymorphism is linked to lower plasma folate levels and elevated homocysteine levels, which can impact folate status [72, 73]. The prevalence of the MTHFR 677 T allele is lower in African populations compared to other racial and ethnic groups, which may suggest a different genetic influence on folate metabolism [74]. However, the presence of this polymorphism still significantly affects folate levels in those who carry it. For instance, individuals with the MTHFR 677TT genotype have been shown to have significantly lower serum folate levels than those with the CC genotype. Additionally, the MTHFR 677TT genotype is associated with a higher risk of folate deficiency-related conditions, such as neural tube defects during pregnancy and cardiovascular diseases [73].

10.4 Vitamin Blood Levels

10.4.3 Vitamin A

Vitamin A levels in African Americans are generally lower than in other ethnic groups, with a higher prevalence of marginal vitamin A status noted among African American women and children [75–77]. Hanson et al. found that African American women of childbearing age had significantly higher odds (3.1 times) of exhibiting serum retinol concentrations below 1.05 µmol/L compared to European American women, indicating a greater prevalence of marginal vitamin A status in this population [75]. Similarly, Ballew et al. reported that African American children and adults were more likely to have low serum retinol concentrations compared to their European American counterparts, even after adjusting for various covariates [76]. Additionally, Neuhouser et al. observed that African American adolescents had significantly lower serum retinol concentrations compared to European Americans, suggesting that racial differences in vitamin A levels exist from a young age [77].

10.4.4 Vitamin C

Vitamin C levels in African Americans have been examined in various contexts. According to data from the National Health and Nutrition Examination Surveys (NHANES) for 2003–2006, African Americans are among the groups significantly associated with insufficient plasma vitamin C levels [78]. Further analysis indicated that African Americans had lower mean plasma vitamin C concentrations compared to other ethnic groups [79]. Additionally, a study investigating racial differences in the relationship between vitamins and metabolic and inflammatory biomarkers found that lower vitamin C levels were linked to higher leukocyte counts in African Americans, suggesting a potential connection to inflammatory processes [80]. These findings imply that African Americans may face a higher risk for conditions related to vitamin C deficiency, such as impaired immune function and chronic inflammation.

One significant genetic factor linked to vitamin C deficiency is the polymorphism in the SLC23A1 gene, which encodes a sodium-dependent vitamin C transporter. Variations in this gene have been associated with differences in circulating concentrations of L-ascorbic acid (vitamin C) [81]. For instance, the rs33972313 variant in the SLC23A1 gene has been shown to reduce circulating vitamin C levels. Additionally, polymorphisms in genes related to antioxidant enzyme function, such as haptoglobin, glutathione-S-transferases, and manganese superoxide dismutase, can affect vitamin C levels by influencing its stability and oxidation in the body [82]. These genetic variations can lead to lower plasma vitamin C levels and increased susceptibility to deficiency, even with adequate dietary intake.

10.4.5 Vitamin E

Vitamin E levels in African Americans have been studied in various contexts. According to data from the Third National Health and Nutrition Examination Survey (NHANES III), African Americans have lower serum alpha-tocopherol concentrations compared to other racial groups [83]. Further studies, such as one by Talegawkar et al., show that despite the prevalent use of vitamin E supplements, a significant proportion of African Americans do not meet the Estimated Average Requirement (EAR) for vitamin E from food alone, with only 5.8% of men and 4.5% of women achieving the EAR through their diets [84]. This indicates that dietary intake alone is often insufficient for maintaining adequate vitamin E levels in this population. Additionally, Ford et al. reported that African Americans had significantly lower concentrations of serum alpha-tocopherol compared to European Americans, a finding consistent across various age groups and sexes [85]. Research has identified several genetic variations that influence vitamin E status. These variations can affect factors such as dietary vitamin E intake, absorption efficiency, and metabolism. For instance, Borel and Desmarchelier highlighted that single nucleotide polymorphisms in genes involved in vitamin E metabolism can significantly impact serum alpha-tocopherol levels [86]. Moreover, Schleicher et al. found that race-ethnicity strongly correlates with circulating fat-soluble nutrient concentrations, including vitamin E, even after adjusting for sociodemographic, lifestyle, and lipid-related variables [87]. This suggests that genetic factors, along with environmental and lifestyle influences, contribute to the observed differences in vitamin E levels among various racial groups. There is still controversy and no full agreement as to whether vitamin E supplementation causes more aggressive prostate cancer in African American men, as was suggested by a significant trial years ago [88–90]. Until this can be further investigated, caution your African American men approaching age 40 to consider this risk.

Clinicians have chosen to supplant these deficiencies with vitamin replacement, but that is not always the best answer. Given the nuanced nutritional needs of African Americans, multivitamins designed for people of European descent will not broadly meet their needs. Advising a combination of supplements designed to meet their needs will likely have more success.

Multiple investigations have tracked most of these low vitamin levels from childhood in African Americans, and while some believe this is linked to a lower socioeconomic status, larger studies have verified race/ethnicity as the strongest independent predictor [91]. Being deliberate about encouraging a vitamin-rich diet early in life is the best solution.

Vitamin Level Trends in African Americans	
Vitamin A	*Lower*
Vitamin B6	*Lower*
Vitamin B12	*Higher*
Vitamin C	*Lower*
Vitamin D	*Lower*
Vitamin E	*Lower*
Folate	*Lower*

10.5 Sickle Cell Disease

Sickle cell disease (SCD) is an inherited hemoglobinopathy and is the most common genetic blood disorder in the world. Sickled erythrocytes cause blood flow obstruction, hemolysis, and several hemostatic changes that promote coagulation. These events, in turn, induce chronic inflammation, which promote a hypercoagulable state, which can cause the downstream complications including end-organ compromise [92–94].

Like the protection afforded by apolipoprotein L1 gene (APOL1) to African sleeping sickness while conferring an increased risk for kidney failure, sickle cell anemia offered a survival advantage in African regions where malaria was prevalent. The exact process for how a sickle-shaped cell results in less malarial disease burden is still the topic of much debate, but there is no question that prior to the development of antimalarial medications, having sickle cell anemia afforded a competitive advantage to those individuals. After migration to the Americas, the selective advantage of sickle cell anemia was lost as the exposure to malaria was erased.

The Centers for Disease Control and Prevention (CDC) now estimates that sickle cell anemia occurs in 1 in 365 African American births. Sickle cell trait, the heterozygous presentation, affects 1 in 13 African Americans who usually have symptom-free lives. Emerging evidence, however, is pointing to an increased risk for kidney disease and a reduction in GFR in patients with sickle cell trait [95].

More than two million Americans are estimated to be either heterozygous or homozygous for sickle cell. Most of those affected are of African ancestry, but a minority are of Hispanic or Southern European, Middle Eastern, or Asian Indian descent.

Complications are common among those with sickle cell disease and occur throughout the lifespan. The sickle cell inflammatory response can cause occlusion of arterial vessels, which result in ischemia of the organs supplied. The ischemia leads to severe pain. These recurrent acute vaso-occlusive crises are the most common manifestation of sickle cell disease and the most common reason for hospital admission.

Chronic complications of sickle cell disease may occur as a result of repeated acute episodes. Several of the most common of the chronic complications like chronic pain, cognitive loss due to stroke, renal dysfunction, splenic infarction, pulmonary hypertension, and retinal problems cause a significant degree of suffering.

The hallmark of the successful management of any disease is the prevention of complications. In sickle cell disease, preventing infections is critical. All patients should be vaccinated against *Streptococcus pneumoniae* and should be instructed to seek immediate attention whenever an infection is likely (fever >101 F) [96, 97].

10.5.1 Renal Complications

Sickle cell disease can result in various renal complications, collectively known as sickle cell nephropathy. These complications arise from the distinct pathophysiology of SCD, which includes vaso-occlusive crisis and chronic hemolysis, potentially leading to impaired renal function. Such impairments may manifest in conditions like chronic kidney disease (CKD), hematuria, nephrotic syndrome, and renal tubular dysfunction [98, 99]. These deficits may begin with issues in urine concentration and acidification during early childhood, progressing with age to microalbuminuria, overt proteinuria, glomerulosclerosis, and, in some individuals, renal failure. It is critical to screen for albumin and protein in the urine to detect an early decline in function [100]. When albumin and protein suggest kidney function compromise in patients with sickle cell disease, angiotensin-converting enzyme (ACE) inhibitors or preferably angiotensin II receptor blockers (ARB), due to their better side effect profile in African Americans, have shown great value [100–104].

There are multiple genetic markers that play a role in SCD renal complications, including HMOX1, HBA1, HBA2, and APOL1 [98, 99, 105]. The APOL1 gene plays a significant role in renal complications associated with SCD. Variants of this gene, specifically the G1 and G2 alleles, are linked to an increased risk of CKD. The findings from genetic biomarkers underscore the importance of genetic screening for variants in managing renal complications. Individuals with APOL1 risk variants often develop albuminuria, an early marker of kidney damage. The presence of high-risk APOL1 genotypes significantly accelerates the progression of CKD in patients living with SCD. Lastly, APOL1 variants interact with the neighboring MYH9 gene, influencing proteinuria and the glomerular filtration rate [98, 99, 106].

In SCD, various biomarkers have been identified to assess renal complications, particularly for the early detection and monitoring of kidney damage. These biomarkers reflect the underlying pathophysiological processes such as inflammation, oxidative stress, and tubular injury. They include, but are not limited to, Kidney Injury Molecule-1 (KIM-1), Neutrophil Gelatinase-Associated Lipocalin (NGAL), Monocyte Chemoattractant Protein-1 (MCP-1), albuminuria, N-Acetyl-B-D-Glucosaminidase (NAG), Ceruloplasmin (CP), and Orosomucoid (ORM). These biomarkers are valuable for understanding the progression of sickle cell nephropathy and for initiating interventions [107–109].

10.5 Sickle Cell Disease

Renal medullary carcinoma (RMC) is a rare and aggressive form of kidney cancer that is strongly associated with sickle cell trait or disease. It predominantly affects young individuals of African descent. RMC is often diagnosed at an advanced stage due to its nonspecific symptoms, including hematuria, flank pain, and weight loss. Early detection and targeted therapies are crucial for improving outcomes in patients facing this challenging malignancy [110, 111].

Biomarker	Complication/implication
Kidney injury Molecule-1 (KIM-1)	Elevated in urine during kidney damage and may have role in early detection
Neutrophil gelatinase-associated Lipocallin (NGAL)	This biomarker is associated with acute kidney injury and chronic kidney disease (CKD). Elevated levels in urine or plasma indicate renal stress or damage
Monocyte chemoattractant Protein-1 (MCP-1)	Is linked to inflammation and is elevated in the urine in patients with SCD who have renal complications
Albuminuria	Persistent albumin in the urine is a hallmark of glomerular damage and is commonly used to monitor kidney function in SCD
N-acetyl-B-D-Glucosaminidase (NAG)	Marker of tubular injury and is elevated in the urine of patient with kidney damage
Ceruloplasmin (CP)	Reflecting iron homeostasis (CP levels are being explored as a potential biomarker for kidney injury)
Orosomucoid (ORM)	An inflammatory marker, which has shown promise in early identification of renal disease

10.5.2 Pulmonary Hypertension

Pulmonary hypertension (PH) is a significant and potentially life-threatening complication of sickle cell disease, and it is multifactorial, involving chronic hemolysis, vaso-occlusion, hypoxia, and thromboembolism. It is characterized by elevated pulmonary arterial pressure, which can lead to progressive heart and lung dysfunction due to several factors. In SCD, red blood cells break down more quickly than normal, releasing hemoglobin that reduces nitric oxide (NO), a molecule that helps blood vessels relax. Without sufficient NO, blood vessels constrict and become damaged. Additionally, sickled RBCs block small vessels in the lungs, leading to inflammation and decreased blood flow. Chronic low oxygen levels in SCD exacerbate the problem by increasing strain on the pulmonary vasculature. In some cases, thromboembolism may occur. Clinical features include shortness of breath, fatigue, chest pain, syncope, and signs of right heart failure, including peripheral edema and jugular vein distension [112–115].

The diagnosis consists of an echocardiogram and right heart catheterization (the gold standard). Some biomarkers include elevated levels of N-terminal pre-brain natriuretic peptide (NT-proBNP) and lactate dehydrogenase (LDH). Tricuspid regurgitation is more prevalent in sickle cell disease and is associated with increased mortality [116–119]. Pulmonary hypertension in SCD is associated with higher mortality rates, making early detection and intervention crucial. Hydroxyurea is often prescribed to prevent sickling; oxygen therapy improves oxygen levels in the body, and blood transfusions can increase the count of healthy RBCs.

10.5.3 Eye Complications

Sickle cell disease can lead to various eye complications, primarily due to the obstruction of small blood vessels by sickled red blood cells. These complications frequently impact the retina, the light-sensitive tissue at the back of the eye, resulting in a condition known as sickle cell retinopathy. This condition is classified into two stages: nonproliferative and proliferative. In the nonproliferative stage, patients may encounter retinal hemorrhages, microaneurysms, and areas of ischemia. These changes can cause visual disturbances, though they may initially be asymptomatic. If the condition advances to the proliferative stage, abnormal blood vessels develop in the retina in response to ischemia. These fragile vessels are susceptible to bleeding, which can lead to vitreous hemorrhage, retinal detachment, and permanent vision loss [120–122].

Proliferative sickle retinopathy and vitreous hemorrhage occur in up to 50% of patients [123].

10.5.4 Priapism

Priapism, the occurrence of painful erections lasting over 4 h, occurs in over a third of male patients with sickle cell disease, and most have their first occurrence before the age of 20 years [124]. This condition is characterized by prolonged erections that typically are not associated with sexual activity. Priapism can be classified into two types: stuttering priapism and major priapism. Stuttering priapism involves recurrent episodes of short duration, typically lasting less than 4 h, while major priapism refers to episodes lasting longer than 4 h, which can lead to permanent tissue damage and erectile dysfunction if not treated promptly. The pathophysiology of priapism in sickle cell disease is linked to chronic hemolysis, which reduces nitric oxide bioavailability, impairing vascular relaxation and increasing vascular resistance [125–127]. For a number of reasons, a much lower percentage goes to the hospital for the treatment of sickle cell-related priapism [128]. Associated conditions that predispose a sickle cell patient to priapism are fever, asplenia, sexual arousal, and dehydration [128]. The biomarkers in the table below summarize priapism-related considerations [129–131].

10.5 Sickle Cell Disease

Biomarker	Type	Role in priapism
Lactate dehydrogenase (LDH)	Biochemical	Elevated levels indicate hemolysis and tissue ischemia, contributing to priapism
Nitric oxide (NO) metabolites	Biochemical	Reduced NO bioavailability leads to impaired vascular relaxation and priapism
Hemoglobin concentration	Hematological	Low levels are associated with increased hemolysis and risk of priapism
Reticulocyte count	Hematological	Elevated counts reflect increased red blood cell turnover
Transforming growth factor-B receptor 3 (TGFBR3)	Genetic	Genetic polymorphism in TGFBR3 are associated with priapism risk
Klotho gene	Genetic	Variants in the klotho gene are linked to priapism susceptibility
Aspartate transaminase (AST)	Biochemical	Elevated levels indicate tissue damage
Platelet count	Hematological	Abnormal platelet count may contribute to thrombotic events

10.5.5 Stroke

Stroke, usually ischemic, occurs in up to 10% of children with sickle cell anemia and can cause weakness in the limbs, slurred speech, seizures, coma, and cognitive impairment. Recurrent strokes occur in a half to two-thirds of untreated patients [125, 132, 133]. "Silent" cerebral infarctions are a particular problem that often go unnoticed but can cause significant neurological damage and cognitive disability. There are estimates that these silent stokes are present in up to a third of children with sickle cell disease and represent the most common neurological complication [132–137]. The presence of these silent strokes is usually detected on magnetic resonance imaging (MRI) [138] or transcranial doppler [139], and may be prompted by poor academic performance, increasing cognitive deficits, or falling intelligence quotients (IQ) [136, 140]. The specific stroke trigger within a sickle cell patient population points to worsening anemia as a common cause. The anemia leads to increased cerebral demand for oxygen, and a cascade ending with infarction is the result. Given this rationale, transfusions are frequently the treatment for new strokes in sickle cell patients, and long-term repeated transfusions have been shown to be marginally effective in preventing recurrent strokes [141–144].

10.5.6 Aplastic Crisis

An aplastic crisis is a severe and potentially life-threatening complication of sickle cell disease, characterized by a sudden halt in the production of red blood cells by the bone marrow. This leads to acute profound anemia, which can manifest as extreme fatigue, pallor, dizziness, shortness of breath, and a rapid heart rate. The primary trigger for an aplastic crisis in SCD is an infection with parvovirus B19, a virus that targets and destroys erythroid progenitor cells in the bone marrow. These cells are responsible for producing new red blood cells, and their destruction results in a dramatic drop in hemoglobin levels. Individuals with SCD are particularly vulnerable to aplastic crises because their blood cells already have a shortened lifespan due to chronic hemolysis. Without adequate production of new red blood cells, the body cannot compensate for the ongoing destruction of sickled cells, leading to severe anemia. Aplastic crises are more common in children with SCD but can also occur in adults [112, 145, 146].

Sickle cell patients presenting with sudden pallor and weakness in conjunction with dropping hemoglobin levels are having an aplastic crisis. Thankfully, the infection is self-limited, typically lasting 7–10 days [147, 148].

Condition	Biomarkers	Children	Adults
Aplastic crisis	Reticulocyte count: low due to bone marrow suppression	More common in children; triggered by parvovirus B19 infection, leading to severe anemia	Less common; may present with similar biomarkers but often milder due to better immune response
	Hemoglobin: mildly decreased	Severe drop in hemoglobin levels, requiring transfusions	Hemoglobin drop may be less dramatic compared to children
	Hemoglobin drop may be less dramatic compared to children	High viral load often detected	Viral load may be lower or undetectable in adults

10.5.7 Acute Chest Syndrome

Acute chest syndrome—ischemia and hypoxia due to vaso-occlusion of the pulmonary microvasculature—is the leading cause of death in patients with sickle cell disease [149, 150]. It should be noted that an infection is the leading trigger of acute chest syndrome in children and adolescence, and bone marrow or fat embolism is the leading trigger in adults. Complications of infection in SCD include acute chest syndrome, acute pain crisis, meningitis, urinary tract infections, osteomyelitis, overwhelming sepsis, and death [151]. This is the most probable reason why this syndrome may have a more severe course and a higher mortality rate in adults [149]. Approximately 50% of patients with sickle cell will have an episode of acute chest syndrome in their lifetime. Although chest pain is the most frequent presenting symptom, this syndrome is frequently preceded or accompanied by vaso-occlusive pain crisis.

Acute chest syndrome is clinically defined as radiological evidence of a new pulmonary infiltrate, associated with one or more physical signs such as fever, chest pain, cough, tachypnea, or other signs of respiratory distress, including wheezing,

10.5 Sickle Cell Disease

rales, or hypoxia. Treatment goals involve managing the pain, alleviating the precipitating event (infection, dehydration, etc.) and anticipating and minimizing adverse sequelae. Emergent treatment includes intravenous fluid hydration, prophylactic antibiotics to address common organisms (Mycoplasma, Chlamydia, pneumococcus, *Haemophilus influenzae*), supplemental oxygen, and incentive spirometry. Simple or exchange transfusion can also be considered in moderate to severe acute chest syndrome. Patients with acute chest syndrome should also receive venous thromboembolism prophylaxis. Both hydroxyurea and chronic transfusion have been shown to reduce frequency of attacks [92]. Acute chest syndrome occurs with increased frequency in patients with a history of asthma or prior admission(s) for acute chest syndrome in the past [92, 112, 125, 152–154].

Condition	Biomarkers	Children	Adults
Acute chest syndrome	Secretory phospholipase A2 (sLAP2): Elevated in ACS episodes	Biomarkers like sPLA2 are useful for early detection in children	Similar biomarkers are elevated, but fat embolism is a more common trigger in adults
	Lactate dehydrogenase (LDH): Elevated due to hemolysis and tissue damage	High LDH levels indicate hemolysis and lung involvement	Elevated LDH levels are also observed, often linked to fat embolism or infection
	White blood cell (WBC) count: Elevated due to inflammation	WBC count is often higher in children due to infections triggering ACS	WBC elevation may be less pronounced unless infection is present

10.5.8 Splenic Sequestration

Splenic sequestration is a serious complication of SCD, characterized by the rapid trapping of a large number of sickled red blood cells in the spleen. This leads to splenic enlargement, a sudden drop in hemoglobin levels, and severe anemia. Splenic sequestration occurs most frequently in infants and young children before their spleen becomes nonfunctional due to repeated damage caused by the disease process (autosplenectomy). In addition to anemia, symptoms may include abdominal pain, pallor, and weakness. If untreated, the condition can progress rapidly to hypovolemic shock due to the pooling of blood within the spleen, which reduces circulating blood volume. Immediate treatment in critical cases typically includes blood transfusion to stabilize hemoglobin levels and improve oxygen delivery. Long-term management may involve splenectomy in patients with recurrent episodes to prevent future complications. Early recognition of splenic sequestration is essential, as delayed treatment can result in life-threatening outcomes [112, 125].

Condition	Biomarkers	Children	Adults
Splenic sequestration	Hemoglobin: decreased due to pooling of red blood cells in the spleen	More frequent in children; spleen enlargement is a key feature	Rare in adults due to autosplenectomy (loss of spleen function over time)
	Reticulocyte count: elevated as a compensatory response	High reticulocyte count due to increased red blood cell turnover	Reticulocyte response may be less pronounced in adults
	Platelet count: low due to sequestration in the spleen	Thrombocytopenia (low platelet) is a common finding	Platelet count changes are less significant in adults

10.5.9 Vaso-Occlusive Pain Management

Vaso-occlusive crisis (VOC) in sickle cell disease is a complex and multifaceted condition. It can occur anywhere in the body and causes cumulative damage to blood vessels and organs over a person's lifespan. It begins with the polymerization of deoxygenated sickle hemoglobin (HbS), which causes red blood cells to become rigid and take on a sickled shape. The sickled cells have reduced deformability, and the environment becomes sticky, leading to the cells' adherence to the endothelium of blood vessels, resulting in microvascular occlusion [97, 155]. This blockage restricts blood flow, leading to ischemia and severe pain. The pain can be sharp and intense, potentially causing emergency department visits and/or hospitalizations.

The pathophysiology of vaso-occlusive crisis (VOC) involves a cascade of events, including inflammation and the activation of various cellular and soluble elements. Leukocytes, platelets, and endothelial cells play significant roles in propagating the vaso-occlusive process [97]. The interaction between sickled red blood cells and these elements exacerbates occlusion and contributes to the severity of the crisis.

Recurrent episodes of VOC can lead to chronic complications, including osteonecrosis, retinopathy, renal failure, erectile dysfunction, cardiac conditions, hepatic conditions, leg ulcers, and an increased risk of stroke [155]. Hydroxyurea, a fetal hemoglobin-reactivating agent, is commonly used to reduce the frequency of VOC episodes [97].

There are three primary types of pain: nociceptive pain (arising from actual or potential damage to non-neuronal tissue and caused by the activation of nociceptors), neuropathic pain (resulting directly from a lesion or disease affecting the somatosensory system), and nociplastic pain (a long-term, complex pain that arises from altered perception without clear evidence of actual or threatened tissue damage) [156]. Each type of pain creates unique neurochemical signatures in both the peripheral and central nervous systems, requiring different methods for analgesic treatment. Understanding these mechanisms of pain is essential for creating effective pain management strategies.

10.5 Sickle Cell Disease

Pain is the most common reason patients with sickle cell disease seek medical attention. However, studies have shown healthcare providers tend to have a negative perception of an African American in pain that often interferes with conducting an adequate assessment and providing appropriate treatment [157–161]. The issues with the treatment of pain have worsened due to opioid restrictions imposed to address opioid abuse and overdose, yet the prevalence of opioid use disorders in patients with sickle cell is similar or lower than the general population [162]:

> with the exception of heart disease, the number of deaths due to opioid pain relievers in patients with sickle cell disease was less than other non-cancer pain conditions including fibromyalgia, low back pain, and migraine. Furthermore, the number of patients with sickle cell disease who died due to opioid pain relievers was significantly less than the total number of all patients with other diagnoses who died due to opioid pain relievers [162].

The goal standard of pain assessment is self-reporting, as other clinical parameters and laboratory tests do not correlate with pain severity [163].

Patients with sickle cell become well aware of their triggers of pain and can usually predict or identify their precipitating event (infection, dehydration, cold, stressful events) [162, 164]. A recent study looked at and confirmed that stress can act as a trigger for vaso-occlusive crises:

> Baseline anxiety had a significant effect on the vasoconstriction response in sickle cell subjects but not controls. In conclusion, mental stress causes vasoconstriction and autonomic nervous system reactivity in all subjects. Although the pattern of responses were not significantly different between two groups, the consequences of vasoconstriction can be quite significant in sickle cell disease because of the resultant entrapment of sickle cells in the microvasculature. This suggests that mental stress precipitates vaso-occlusive crisis in sickle cell disease by causing neural mediated vasoconstriction [164].

It is important for healthcare professionals to be familiar with possible triggers and to encourage patients to be aware as well, as this may reduce painful episodes. Chronic pain management should be individualized, which encourages self-management of pain and adequate step-up therapy with the inclusion of opioids [163]. Hydroxyurea has also been shown to reduce pain episodes [165, 166]:

> Although findings from the study of hydroxyurea in sickle cell disease indicate its beneficial effects in shortening the duration of crisis-related admissions and reducing the net dose of opioids, there have been concerns about its safety profile in pediatric sickle cell patients. Nevertheless, there is compelling evidence to support its use in patients as young as 9 months, given its reported ability to reduce the frequency of vaso-occlusive crises and acute chest syndrome with little or no adverse reactions. In fact, results from a protocol suggest minimal genotoxicity or carcinogenicity with long-term hydroxyurea exposure. A recent review further lends credence to its safety and efficacy in both pediatric and adult patients as there was no reported increase in the incidence of leukemia and teratogenicity [165].

Patrick McGann and Russell Ware from Cincinnati Children's Hospital Medical Center rendered an expert opinion that "hydroxyurea therapy should be considered standard-of-care for (sickle cell anemia), representing an essential component of patient management. Early initiation and broader use of hydroxyurea will alter the natural history of (sickle cell anemia), so affected children can live longer and healthier lives" [166].

Acute painful episodes that require hospital visits need prompt and adequate analgesia. Opioids are usually the recommended medication and are to be given IV within 30 min of presentation. Rapid and frequent reassessment of pain is advised to achieve pain control, with adequate acceleration of dosage as indicated. Patient-controlled analgesia (PCA) pumps may also be indicated in patients with difficult to control pain. A slow and closely monitored tapered therapy of opioids to the patient's baseline should be encouraged as a part of discharge care planning [165]. Despite advancements in treatment, a sickle cell vaso-occlusive crisis continues to be a significant cause of morbidity and healthcare utilization [155].

Pain Type and Its Relation to Sickle Cell Disease	
Pain type	Contribution to the overall pain experience in SCD
Nociceptive pain	Sickled red blood cells obstruct blood vessels, leading to ischemia and tissue damage. The resulting pain is nociceptive, as it is directly related to the activation of nociceptors due to tissue injury
Neuropathic pain	Repeated VOCs can lead to nerve damage, resulting in chronic neuropathic pain. This type of pain is often described as burning, tingling, or shooting and can be challenging to manage
Nociplastic pain	Recurrent VOCs can lead to a sustained noxious environment, causing acute pain to transition to chronic pain, further complicating their pain management

10.6 Thalassemia (Alpha and Beta)

The thalassemias are a group of inherited autosomal recessive blood disorders that disproportionately affect African Americans by impairing hemoglobin production. Hemoglobin is the oxygen-transporting protein of red blood cells and has a quaternary structure consisting of four polypeptide subunits: two alpha chains and two beta chains. Alpha and beta thalassemias are hereditary disorders characterized by reductions in the synthesis of these chains, causing reduced successful hemoglobin production. The lower hemoglobin content reduces both the overall red blood cell production and the quality of individual red blood cells and results in hypochromic microcytic anemia [167].

Alpha thalassemia is caused by reduced or absent synthesis of alpha-globin chains, and beta thalassemia is caused by reduced or absent synthesis of beta-globin chains. Because of the quaternary structure, imbalances of the alpha- or beta-globin chains disrupt overall production. The prevalence of thalassemia among African Americans is notable, with studies indicating that approximately 1.4% of African American males have heterozygous beta-thalassemia, while 5.7% possess the alpha-thalassemia trait [168, 169].

10.6 Thalassemia (Alpha and Beta)

Patients can be described as having the trait, intermedia, or major involvement. Patients with alpha or beta thalassemia trait are asymptomatic and require no treatment. Most persons with thalassemia trait are found incidentally when their blood count shows mild microcytic anemia. Another common classification separates transfusion dependent and non-transfusion dependent with African Americans comprising more non-transfusion-dependent patients [170].

In the intermedia or major thalassemia, the imbalance in the alpha- or beta-globin chain ratio leads to ineffective erythropoiesis, hemolytic anemia, hypercoagulability, and increased intestinal iron reabsorption. The body is retaining iron for red blood cell production, but because of the genetic imbalance, it cannot successfully complete the task. Anemia ensues, requiring transfusions and causing the iron body load to continue to rise. Transfusion-dependent patients will develop iron overload and require chelation therapy to remove the excess iron.

Thalassemia Minor: Minimal or no anemia (hemoglobin 9–12 g/dL); microcytosis; elevated RBC count.

Thalassemia Intermedia: Microcytic anemia with hemoglobin usually higher than 7 g/dL; growth failure; hepatosplenomegaly; hyperbilirubinemia; thalassemic facies (i.e., frontal bossing, mandibular malocclusion, prominent malar eminences due to extramedullary hematopoiesis) develop between the ages of 2 and 5 years.

Thalassemia Major (Cooley Anemia): Severe anemia (hemoglobin 1–6 g/dL) usually during the first year of life; hepatosplenomegaly; growth failure.

Thalassemia affects men and women equally. Alpha thalassemia occurs most often in persons of African and Southeast Asian descent, and beta thalassemia is most common in persons of Mediterranean, African, and Southeast Asian descent. Thalassemia trait affects 5–30% of persons in these ethnic groups [167].

Persons with beta thalassemia major are diagnosed during infancy. Pallor, irritability, growth retardation, abdominal swelling, and jaundice appear during the first years of life.

The complications that occur with beta thalassemia major or intermedia are related to overstimulation of the bone marrow, ineffective erythropoiesis, and iron overload from regular blood transfusions.

If you have a healthy African American male with mild anemia, microcytosis, and no other associated abnormalities, think of thalassemia trait as a potential cause.

The high prevalence of thalassemia among African Americans is partly due to the evolutionary advantage conferred by the carrier state against malaria, which is endemic in regions from which many African Americans descend. This evolutionary advantage arises because carriers of thalassemia traits are less susceptible to severe malaria. The altered hemoglobin in these individuals reduces the parasite's ability to thrive in red blood cells, offering a survival benefit in areas where malaria is common [171].

10.7 Glucose-6-Phosphate Dehydrogenase Deficiency (G6PD)

Glucose-6-phosphate dehydrogenase (G6PD) protects red blood cells from oxidative stress and hemolysis. G6PD deficiency is an inherited defect that makes red blood cells more susceptible to hemolysis. G6PD deficiency has a disproportionate occurrence among certain ethnic groups with approximately 12% prevalence in African Americans [172, 173]. This disorder, which is X-linked, usually presents with an acute hemolytic crisis that occurred after exposure to certain triggers, for example, the medication primaquine (an antimalarial medication). Patients are advised to stay away from such medications, fava beans, and chemicals such as henna and naphthalene, which are potential triggers. Affected individuals should also be aware that infections as well as poor control of diabetes (e.g., DKA) could be potential triggers.

John Thomas and colleagues found an association between G6PG deficiency and cardiovascular disease:

> Our study suggests 39.6% greater odds of identifying CVD (cardiovascular disease) in G6PD-deficient individuals. To our knowledge, ours is the largest study to show this association. Universal screening of G6PD status—already performed in U.S. military personnel—might prove useful in the general population, leading to earlier cardiovascular screening and therapeutic intervention in people with G6PD deficiency [174].

Treatment is aimed at supportive therapy for the acute hemolytic episode and the avoidance of triggers [175].

The genetic advantage of glucose-6-phosphate dehydrogenase deficiency in African Americans primarily relates to its protective effect against malaria. The protective mechanism involves the impaired ability of the malaria parasite, *Plasmodium falciparum*, to thrive in G6PD-deficient erythrocytes. Studies indicate that G6PD deficiency, particularly the A-variant, significantly reduces the risk of severe malaria, especially cerebral malaria, in hemizygous males and heterozygous females. This selective advantage has resulted in a higher prevalence of G6PD deficiency in malaria-endemic regions [176–178].

Important Differences in Hematology Results and Hematological Diseases

- African Americans may have significantly lower values in WBC, neutrophil count, monocyte count, and platelets.
- African Americans may have significantly lower values in hemoglobin (HGB), hematocrit (HCT), mean corpuscular hemoglobin (MCH), and mean corpuscular hemoglobin concentration (MCHC).
- Benign ethnic neutropenia (defined as between 1.0×10^9 cell/L and 1.5×10^9 cell/L) has increased prevalence in African American patients.
- When considering the general electrolytes, there are no significant differences in sodium, potassium, chloride, calcium, phosphorus, or magnesium between African Americans and European Americans.

(continued)

- African Americans may have lower TSH levels with a range of 0.37–3.46 mIU/L (compared to "overall" reference interval 0.512–5.22 mIU/L).
- The lipid profile in African Americans is generally more favorable with a higher HDL and lower total cholesterol, LDL, and triglycerides.
- The prostate-specific antigen (PSA) test is a better and more sensitive detector of prostate cancer in African Americans, and at any given PSA level are at a higher risk for prostate cancer than European Americans.
- African American women may have a CA-125 level that is significantly lower than that of European American women.
- African Americans are more likely to be CA 19-9 nonproducers, which results in an inability to synthesize CA 19-9 or detect pancreatic cancer with this test.
- Significant differences in serum vitamin levels exist across the population with lower levels of vitamin C, vitamin D, vitamin B6, vitamin E, and folate. African Americans tend to have higher vitamin B12 levels.
- Sickle cell anemia occurs in 1 in 365 African American births. Sickle cell trait affects 1 in 13 African Americans.
- Annual screening and treatment with angiotensin II receptor blockers (ARB) may delay renal disease progression in sickle cell disease.
- The spectrum of sickle hemoglobin-related nephropathy extends to sickle cell trait, with sickle cell trait conferring a twofold increased risk of chronic kidney disease.
- If African Americans with sickle cell disease have signs or symptoms suggestive of pulmonary hypertension, they should have echocardiography done (with particular attention to tricuspid regurgitation).
- End-stage renal disease is a rare complication but is associated with high mortality in sickle cell disease.
- Vision screening and ophthalmology evaluations should start early in sickle cell disease.
- Eye complications in sickle cell disease in the form of proliferative sickle retinopathy and vitreous hemorrhage occur in 50% of patients and can result in significant vision loss.
- Priapism is common, affecting 35% of boys and men with sickle cell disease.
- Acute chest syndrome—ischemia and hypoxia due to vaso-occlusion of the pulmonary microvasculature—is the leading cause of death in patients with sickle cell disease.
- Thalassemia is a hereditary disorder characterized by reduction in synthesis of globin chains (α or β), causing reduced hemoglobin synthesis and eventually hypochromic microcytic anemia.
- Thalassemia has microcytosis out of proportion to the degree of anemia.
- Thalassemia has abnormal RBC morphology with microcytes, hypochromia, acanthocytes, and target cells.

- Thalassemias are described as:
  - *Trait*, when there are laboratory features without clinical impact.
  - *Intermedia*, when there is an RBC transfusion requirement or other moderate clinical impacts.
  - *Major*, when the disorder is life-threatening.
- G6PD deficiency has a disproportionate occurrence with approximately 12% prevalence in African Americans.
- G6PD deficiency and Thalassemia both exist due to their protective effect against severe forms of malaria.

References

1. Harris K, Boyd JC. On dividing reference data into subgroups to produce separate reference ranges. Clin Chem. 1990;36(2):265–70.
2. Hsu CY, Yang W, Parikh RV, Anderson AH, Chen TK, Cohen DL, He J, Mohanty MJ, Lash JP, Mills KT, Muiru AN, Parsa A, Saunders MR, Shafi T, Townsend RR, Waikar SS, Wang J, Wolf M, Tan TC, Feldman HI, Go AS. Race genetic ancestry and estimating kidney function in CKD. N Engl J Med. 2021;385(19):1750–60. https://doi.org/10.1056/NEJMoa2103753.
3. Stevens PE, Ahmed SB, Carrero JJ, Foster B, Francis A, Hall RK, Herrington WG, Hill G, Inker LA, Kazancıoğlu R, Lamb E, et al. KDIGO 2024 clinical practice guideline for the evaluation and management of chronic kidney disease. Kidney Int. 2024;105(4):S117–314. https://doi.org/10.1016/j.kint.2023.10.018.
4. Inker LA, Eneanya ND, Coresh J, Tighiouart H, Wang D, Sang Y, Crews DC, Doria A, Estrella MM, Froissart M, Grams ME, Greene T, Grubb A, Gudnason V, Gutiérrez OM, Kalil R, Karger AB, Mauer M, Navis G, Nelson RG, Poggio ED, Rodby R, Rossing P, Rule AD, Selvin E, Seegmiller JC, Shlipak MG, Torres VE, Yang W, Ballew SH, Couture SJ, Powe NR, Levey AS. New creatinine- and cystatin C–based equations to estimate GFR without race. N Engl J Med. 2021;385(19):1737–49. https://doi.org/10.1056/NEJMoa2102953.
5. Silva AM, Shen W, Heo M, Gallagher D, Wang Z, Sardinha LB, Heymsfield SB. Ethnicity-related skeletal muscle differences across the lifespan. Am J Hum Biol. 2010;22(1):76–82. https://doi.org/10.1002/ajhb.20956.
6. Gbadegesin RA, Ulasi I, Ajayi S, Raji Y, Olanrewaju T, Osafo C, Ademola AD, Asinobi A, Winkler CA, Burke D, Arogundade F, Ekem I, Plange-Rhule J, Mamven M, Matekole M, Amodu O, Cooper R, Antwi S, Adeyemo AA, Ilori TO, Adabayeri V, Nyarko A, Ghansah A, Amira T, Solarin A, Awobusuyi O, Kimmel PL, Brosius FC, Makusidi M, Odenigbo U, Kretzler M, Hodgin JB, Pollak MR, Boima V, Freedman BI, Palmer ND, Collins B, Phadnis M, Smith J, Agwai CI, Okoye O, Abdu A, Wilson J, Williams W, Salako BL, Parekh RS, Tayo B, Adu D, Ojo A, H3Africa Kidney Disease Research Network. N Engl J Med. 2025;392(3):228–38. https://doi.org/10.1056/NEJMoa2404211.
7. Daneshpajouhnejad P, Kopp JB, Winkler CA, Rosenberg AZ. The evolving story of apolipoprotein L1 nephropathy: the end of the beginning. Nat Rev Nephrol. 2022;18(5):307–20. https://doi.org/10.1038/s41581-022-00538-3.
8. Grams ME, Rebholz CM, Chen Y, Rawlings AM, Estrella MM, Selvin E, Appel LJ, Tin A, Coresh J. Race APOL1 risk and eGFR decline in the general population. Clin J Am Soc Nephrol. 2016;27(9):2842–50. https://doi.org/10.1681/ASN.2015070763.
9. Mayo Clinic, Author. Medical Laboratory Sciences. 2015. [June 15, 2015]. http://www.mayo.edu/mshs/careers/laboratory-sciences.

10. Hickner J, Thompson PJ, Wilkinson T, et al. Primary care physicians' challenges in ordering clinical laboratory tests and interpreting results. J Am Board Fam Med. 2014;27(2):268–74.
11. Lim E, Miyamura J, Chen JJ. Racial/ethnic-specific reference intervals for common laboratory tests: a comparison among Asians, Blacks, Hispanics, and White. Hawaii J Med Public Health. 2015;74(9):302–10.
12. Beutler E, West C. Hematologic differences between African-Americans and whites: the roles of iron deficiency and α-thalassemia on hemoglobin levels and mean corpuscular volume. Blood. 2005;106(2):740–5. https://doi.org/10.1182/blood-2005-02-0713.
13. Bain BJ. Ethnic and sex differences in the total and differential white cell count and platelet count. J Clin Pathol. 1996;49(8):664–6.
14. Hsieh MM, Everhart JE, Byrd-Holt DD, et al. Prevalence of neutropenia in the U.S. population: age, sex, smoking status, and ethnic differences. Ann Intern Med. 2007;146(7):486–92.
15. Reed WW, Diehl LF. Leukopenia, neutropenia, and reduced hemoglobin levels in healthy American blacks. Arch Intern Med. 1991;151:501–5.
16. Freedman DS, Gates L, Flanders WD, et al. Black/white differences in leukocyte subpopulations in men. Int J Epidemiol. 1997;26:757–64.
17. Lim EM, Cembrowski G, Cembrowski M, Clarke G. Race-specific WBC and neutrophil count reference intervals. Int J Lab Hematol. 2010;32(6p2):590–7.
18. Reiner AP, Lettre G, Nalls MA, Ganesh SK, Mathias R, Austin MA, Dean E, Arepalli S, Britton A, Chen Z, Couper D, Curb JD, Eaton CB, Fornage M, Grant SF, Harris TB, Hernandez D, Kamatini N, Keating BJ, Kubo M, LaCroix A, Lange LA, Liu S, Lohman K, Meng Y, Mohler ER 3rd, Musani S, Nakamura Y, O'Donnell CJ, Okada Y, Palmer CD, Papanicolaou GJ, Patel KV, Singleton AB, Takahashi A, Tang H, Taylor HA Jr, Taylor K, Thomson C, Yanek LR, Yang L, Ziv E, Zonderman AB, Folsom AR, Evans MK, Liu Y, Becker DM, Snively BM, Wilson JG. Genome-wide association study of white blood cell count in 16388 African Americans: the continental origins and genetic epidemiology network (COGENT). PLoS Genet. 2011;7(6):e1002108. https://doi.org/10.1371/journal.pgen.1002108.
19. Reich D, Nalls MA, Kao WH, Akylbekova EL, Tandon A, Patterson N, Mullikin J, Hsueh WC, Cheng CY, Coresh J, Boerwinkle E, Li M, Waliszewska A, Neubauer J, Li R, Leak TS, Ekunwe L, Files JC, Hardy CL, Zmuda JM, Taylor HA, Ziv E, Harris TB, Wilson JG. Reduced neutrophil count in people of African descent is due to a regulatory variant in the Duffy antigen receptor for chemokines gene. PLoS Genet. 2009;5(1):e1000360. https://doi.org/10.1371/journal.pgen.1000360.
20. Lee S, Ong CM, Zhang Y, AHB W. Narrowed reference intervals for complete blood count in a multiethnic population. Clin Chem Lab Med. 2019;57(9):1382–7. https://doi.org/10.1515/cclm-2018-1263.
21. Omuse G, Maina D, Mwangi J, Wambua C, Radia K, Kanyua A, Kagotho E, Hoffman M, Ojwang P, Premji Z, Ichihara K, Erasmus R. Complete blood count reference intervals from a healthy adult urban population in Kenya. PLoS One. 2018;13(6):e0198444. https://doi.org/10.1371/journal.pone.0198444.
22. Palmblad J, Hoglund P. Ethnic benign neutropenia: a phenomenon finds an explanation. Pediatr Blood Cancer. 2018;65(12):e27361. https://doi.org/10.1002/pbc.27361.
23. Lakhotia R, Aggarwal A, Link ME, et al. Natural history of benign ethnic neutropenia in individuals of African ancestry. Blood Cells Mol Dis. 2019;77:12–6.
24. Charles BA, Hsieh MM, Adeyemo AA, Shriner D, Ramos E, Chin K, Srivastava K, Zakai NA, Cushman M, LA MC, Howard V, Flegel WA, Rotimi CN, Rodgers GP. Analyses of genome wide association data cytokines and gene expression in African-Americans with benign ethnic neutropenia. PLoS One. 2018;13(3):e0194400. https://doi.org/10.1371/journal.pone.0194400.
25. Liu JM, Luo HR. Novel neutrophil biology insights underlying atypical chemokine receptor-1/Duffy antigen receptor of chemokines-associated neutropenia. Curr Opin Hematol. 2024;31(6):302–6. https://doi.org/10.1097/MOH.0000000000000834.

26. Denic S, Narchi H, Mekaini A, et al. Prevalence of neutropenia in children by nationality. BMC Hematol. 2016;16:15.
27. Thobakgale CF, Ndung'u T. Neutrophil counts in persons of African origin. Curr Opin Hematol. 2014;21:50–7.
28. Hershman D, Weinberg M, Rosner Z, et al. Ethnic neutropenia and treatment delay in African American women undergoing chemotherapy for early-stage breast cancer. J Natl Cancer Inst. 2003;95:1545–8.
29. Merz LE, Achebe M. When non-whiteness becomes a condition. Blood. 2021;137(1):13–5. https://doi.org/10.1182/blood.2020008600.
30. Tahmasebi H, Trajcevski K, Higgins V, Adeli K. Influence of ethnicity on population reference values for biochemical markers. Crit Rev Clin Lab Sci. 2018;55(5):359–75. https://doi.org/10.1080/10408363.2018.1476455. Epub 2018 Jun 6
31. CLSI. Defining, establishing, and verifying reference intervals in the clinical laboratory; approved guideline, CLSI document EP28-A3c, vol. 28, No. 30. 3rd ed. Wayne: Clinical and Laboratory Standards Institute; 2008.
32. Garber JR, Cobin RH, Gharib H, Hennessey JV, Klein I, Mechanick JI, Pessah-Pollack R, Singer PA, Woeber KA. Clinical practice guidelines for hypothyroidism in adults: cosponsored by the American Association of Clinical Endocrinologists and the American Thyroid Association. Endocr Pract. 2012;18(6):988–1028. https://doi.org/10.4158/EP12280.GL.
33. Hollowell JG, Staehling NW, Flanders WD, Hannon WH, Gunter EW, Spencer CA, Braverman LE. J Clin Endocrinol Metab. 2002;87(2):489–99. https://doi.org/10.1210/jcem.87.2.8182.
34. Wade AN, Guare L, Hayat M, Straub P, Gao Z, Medici M, Teumer A, Davis LK, Ramsay M, Ritchie MD, PM BB, Cappola AR. Strength of genetic associations with thyrotropin values differs between populations with similarity to African and European reference populations. Thyroid®. 2025;35(2):131–42. https://doi.org/10.1089/thy.2024.0525.
35. Malinowski JR, Denny JC, Bielinski SJ, Basford MA, Bradford Y, Peissig PL, Carrell D, Crosslin DR, Pathak J, Rasmussen L, Pacheco J, Kho A, Newton KM, Li R, Kullo IJ, Chute CG, Chisholm RL, Jarvik GP, Larson EB, CA MC, Masys DR, Roden DM, de Andrade M, Ritchie MD, Crawford DC. Genetic variants associated with serum Thyroid Stimulating Hormone (TSH) levels in European Americans and African Americans from the eMERGE network. PLoS One. 2014;9(12):e111301. https://doi.org/10.1371/journal.pone.0111301.
36. Boucai L, Hollowell JG, Surks MI. An approach for development of age-, gender-, and ethnicity-specific thyrotropin reference limits. Thyroid. 2011;21(1):5–11. https://doi.org/10.1089/thy.2010.0092. Epub 2010 Nov 8
37. Bentley AR, Rotimi CN. Interethnic differences in serum lipids and implications for cardiometabolic disease risk in African ancestry populations. Glob Heart. 2017;12(2):141–50.
38. Grundy SM, Stone NJ, Bailey AL, Beam C, Birtcher KK, Blumenthal RS, Braun LT, de Ferranti S, Faiella-Tommasino J, Forman DE, Goldberg R, Heidenreich PA, Hlatky MA, Jones DW, Lloyd-Jones D, Lopez-Pajares N, Ndumele CE, Orringer CE, Peralta CA, Saseen JJ, Smith SC Jr, Sperling L, Virani SS, Yeboah J. AHA/ACC/AACVPR/AAPA/ABC/ACPM/ADA/AGS/APhA/ASPC/NLA/PCNA guideline on the management of blood cholesterol: a report of the American College of Cardiology/American Heart Association Task Force on Clinical Practice Guidelines. Circulation. 2018;139(25):e1082. https://doi.org/10.1161/CIR.0000000000000625.
39. Bays HE, Jones PH, Brown WV, Jacobson TA. National lipid association annual summary of clinical lipidology 2015. J Clin Lipidol. 2014;8(6):S1–S36. https://doi.org/10.1016/j.jacl.2014.10.002.
40. Jacobson TA, Maki KC, Orringer CE, Jones PH, Kris-Etherton P, Sikand G, La Forge R, Daniels SR, Wilson DP, Morris PB, Wild RA, Grundy SM, Daviglus M, Ferdinand KC, Vijayaraghavan K, Deedwania PC, Aberg JA, Liao KP, McKenney JM, Ross JL, Braun LT, Ito MK, Bays HE, Brown WV, Underberg JA. National lipid association recommendations for patient-centered management of dyslipidemia: Part 2. J Clin Lipidol. 2015;9(6):S1–S122.e1. https://doi.org/10.1016/j.jacl.2015.09.002.

41. Bentley AR, Chen G, Shriner D, Doumatey AP, Zhou J, Huang H, Mullikin JC, Blakesley RW, Hansen NF, Bouffard GG, Cherukuri PF, Maskeri B, Young AC, Adeyemo A, Rotimi CN. Gene-based sequencing identifies lipid-influencing variants with ethnicity-specific effects in African Americans. PLoS Genet. 2014;10(3):e1004190. https://doi.org/10.1371/journal.pgen.1004190.
42. Basu A, Tang H, Lewis CE, North K, Curb JD, Quertermous T, Mosley TH, Boerwinkle E, Zhu X, Risch NJ. Admixture mapping of quantitative trait loci for blood lipids in African-Americans. Hum Mol Genet. 2009;18(11):2091–8. https://doi.org/10.1093/hmg/ddp122.
43. Tang P, Du W, Xie K, et al. Characteristics of baseline PSA and PSA velocity in young men without prostate cancer: racial differences. Prostate. 2012;72:173–80.
44. Saraiya M, Kottiri BJ, Leadbetter S, et al. Total and percent free prostate-specific antigen levels among U.S. men, 2001–2002. Cancer Epidemiol Biomarkers Prev. 2005;14:2178–82.
45. Giri VH, Egleston B, Ruth K, et al. Race, genetic West African ancestry, and prostate cancer prediction by PSA in prospectively screened high-risk men. Cancer Prev Res (Phila). 2009;2(3):244–50.
46. Kallingal GJ, Walker MR, Musser JE, et al. Impact of race in using PSA velocity to predict for prostate cancer. Mil Med. 2014;179(3):329–32.
47. D'Amico AV, Chen MH, Roehl KA, et al. Preoperative PSA velocity and the risk of death from prostate cancer after radical prostatectomy. N Engl J Med. 2004;351:125–35.
48. Hoffmann TJ, Graff RE, Madduri RK, Rodriguez AA, Cario CL, Feng K, Jiang Y, Wang A, Klein RJ, Pierce BL, Eggener S, Tong L, Blot W, Long J, Goss LB, Darst BF, Rebbeck T, Lachance J, Andrews C, Adebiyi AO, Adusei B, Aisuodionoe-Shadrach OI, Fernandez PW, Jalloh M, Janivara R, Chen WC, Mensah JE, Agalliu I, Berndt SI, Shelley JP, Schaffer K, Machiela MJ, Freedman ND, Huang WY, Li SA, Goodman PJ, Till C, Thompson I, Lilja H, Ranatunga DK, Presti J, Van Den Eeden SK, Chanock SJ, Mosley JD, Conti DV, Haiman CA, Justice AC, Kachuri L, Witte JS. Genome-wide association study of prostate-specific antigen levels in 392522 men identifies new loci and improves prediction across ancestry groups. Nat Genet. 2025;57(2):334–44. https://doi.org/10.1038/s41588-024-02068-z.
49. Wei JT, Barocas D, Carlsson S, Coakley F, Eggener S, Etzioni R, Fine SW, Han M, Kim SK, Kirkby E, Konety BR, Miner M, Moses K, Nissenberg MG, Pinto PA, Salami SS, Souter L, Thompson IM, Lin DW. Early detection of prostate cancer: AUA/SUO guideline Part I: prostate cancer screening. J Urol. 2023;210(1):46–53. https://doi.org/10.1097/JU.0000000000003491.
50. Kensler KH, Johnson R, Morley F, Albrair M, Dickerman BA, Gulati R, Holt SK, Iyer HS, Kibel AS, Lee JR, Preston MA, Vassy JL, Wolff EM, Nyame YA, Etzioni R, Rebbeck TR. Prostate cancer screening in African American men: a review of the evidence. JNCI J Natl Cancer Inst. 2023;116(1):34–52. https://doi.org/10.1093/jnci/djad193.
51. Garraway IP, Carlsson SV, Nyame YA, Vassy JL, Chilov M, Fleming M, Frencher SK, George DJ, Kibel AS, King SA, Kittles R, Mahal BA, Pettaway CA, Rebbeck T, Rose B, Vince R, Winn RA, Yamoah K, Oh WK. Prostate cancer foundation screening guidelines for black Men in the United States. NEJM Evid. 2024;3(5):EVIDoa2300289. https://doi.org/10.1056/EVIDoa2300289.
52. Sasamoto N, Vitonis AF, Fichorova RN, Yamamoto HS, Terry KL, Cramer DW. Racial/ethnic differences in average CA125 and CA15.3 values and its correlates among postmenopausal women in the USA. Cancer Causes Control. 2021;32(3):299–309. https://doi.org/10.1007/s10552-020-01384-z.
53. AJB S, Gleason E, Kadiyala S, Wang X, Howell EA, McCarthy AM. Cancer antigen 125 levels at time of ovarian cancer diagnosis by race and ethnicity. JAMA Netw Open. 2025;8(3):e251292. https://doi.org/10.1001/jamanetworkopen.2025.1292.
54. Smith AJB, Gleason E, Kadiyala S, Wang X, Howell EA, McCarthy AM. Current diagnostic guidelines and perpetuation of inequities in ovarian cancer: a national cancer database study. J Clin Oncol. 2024;42(16_suppl):11027. https://doi.org/10.1200/JCO.2024.42.16_suppl.11027.

55. Wu G, Wu J, Pan X, Liu B, Yao Z, Guo Y, Shi X, Ding Y. Racial disparities in alpha-fetoprotein testing and alpha-fetoprotein status associated with the diagnosis and outcome of hepatocellular carcinoma patients. Cancer Med. 2019;8(15):6614–23. https://doi.org/10.1002/cam4.2549.
56. Nguyen MH, Garcia RT, Simpson PW, Wright TL, Keeffe EB. Racial differences in effectiveness of α-fetoprotein for diagnosis of hepatocellular carcinoma in hepatitis C virus cirrhosis. Hepatology. 2002;36(2):410–7. https://doi.org/10.1053/jhep.2002.34744.
57. Omore I, Gandhi S, Wu L, Cohen DJ. Exploring racial disparities and tumor characteristics of CA19-9 producer and non-producer among patients with advanced pancreatic ductal adenocarcinoma (PDAC): implications for survival and personalized treatment strategies. J Clin Oncol. 2024;42(16_suppl):e16309. https://doi.org/10.1200/JCO.2024.42.16_suppl.e16309.
58. Martos MP, Dickey EM, Yanala UR, Abdilleh K, Ogobuiro I, Box EW, Ahmad SA, Maithel SK, Hammill CW, Kim HJJ, Abbott DE, Kooby DA, Parikh AA, Hosein PJ, Merchant NB, Datta J, Hester CA. Association of race and CA 19-9 nonproduction with limited pathologic response to neoadjuvant chemotherapy in patients with localized pancreatic cancer. J Clin Oncol. 2024;42(3_suppl):609. https://doi.org/10.1200/JCO.2024.42.3_suppl.609.
59. Parra-Robert M, Santos VM, Canis SM, Pla XF, JMA F, Porto RM. Relationship between CA 19.9 and the lewis phenotype: options to improve diagnostic efficiency. Anticancer Res. 2018;38(10):5883–8. https://doi.org/10.21873/anticanres.12931.
60. Libon F, Cavalier E, Nikkels AF. Skin color is relevant to vitamin D synthesis. Dermatology (Basel). 2013;227:250–4.
61. Nessvi S, Johansson L, Jopson J, et al. Association of 25-hydroxyvitamin D3 levels in adult New Zealanders with ethnicity, skin color and self-reported skin sensitivity to sun exposure. Photochem Photobiol. 2011;87:1173–8.
62. Gozdzik A, Barta JL, Wu H, et al. Low wintertime vitamin D levels in a sample of healthy young adults of diverse ancestry living in the Toronto area: associations with vitamin D intake and skin pigmentation. BMC Public Health. 2008;8:336.
63. Kant AK, Graubard BI. Race-ethnic, family income, and education differentials in nutritional and lipid biomarkers in US children and adolescents: NHANES 2003–2006. Am J Clin Nutr. 2012;96:601–12.
64. Morris MS, Picciano MF, Jacques PF, Selhub J. Plasma pyridoxal 5′-phosphate in the US population: the national health and nutrition examination survey 2003–2004. Am J Clin Nutr. 2008;87(5):1446–54. https://doi.org/10.1093/ajcn/87.5.1446.
65. O'Logbon J, Crook M, Steed D, Harrington DJ, Sobczyńska-Malefora A. J Clin Pathol. 2022;75(9):598–604. https://doi.org/10.1136/jclinpath-2021-207519.
66. Sobczyńska-Malefora A, Katayev A, Steed D, O'Logbon J, Crook M, Harrington DJ. Age- and ethnicity-related reference intervals for serum vitamin B12. Clin Biochem. 2023;111:66–71. https://doi.org/10.1016/j.clinbiochem.2022.10.007.
67. Hinds HE, Johnson AA, Webb MC, Graham AP. Iron folate and vitamin B12 status in the elderly by gender and ethnicity. J Natl Med Assoc. 2011;103(9–10):870–8. https://doi.org/10.1016/S0027-9684(15)30442-9.
68. Bowen Raffick AR, Wong Betty YL, Cole David EC. Population-based differences in frequency of the transcobalamin II Pro259Arg polymorphism. Clin Biochem. 2004;37(2):128–33. https://doi.org/10.1016/j.clinbiochem.2003.09.001.
69. Ford ES, Bowman BA. Serum and red blood cell folate concentrations race and education: findings from the third National Health and Nutrition Examination Survey. Am J Clin Nutr. 1999;69(3):476–81. https://doi.org/10.1093/ajcn/69.3.476.
70. Pfeiffer CM, Sternberg MR, Zhang M, Fazili Z, Storandt RJ, Crider KS, Yamini S, Gahche JJ, Juan W, Wang CY, Potischman N, Williams J, LaVoie DJ. Folate status in the US population 20 y after the introduction of folic acid fortification. Am J Clin Nutr. 2019;110(5):1088–97. https://doi.org/10.1093/ajcn/nqz184.
71. Fazili Z, Sternberg MR, Potischman N, Wang CY, Storandt RJ, Yeung L, Yamini S, Gahche JJ, Juan W, Qi YP, Paladugula N, Gabey G, Pfeiffer CM. Demographic physiologic and lifestyle

characteristics observed with serum total folate differ among folate forms: Cross-sectional data from fasting samples in the NHANES 2011–2016. J Nutr. 2020;150(4):851–60. https://doi.org/10.1093/jn/nxz278.

72. Guéant-Rodriguez RM, Guéant JL, Debard R, Thirion S, Hong LX, Bronowicki JP, Namour F, Chabi NW, Sanni A, Anello G, Bosco P, Romano C, Amouzou E, Arrieta HR, Sánchez BE, Romano A, Herbeth B, Guilland JC, Mutchinick OM. Prevalence of methylenetetrahydrofolate reductase 677T and 1298C alleles and folate status: a comparative study in Mexican West African and European populations. Am J Clin Nutr. 2006;83(3):701–7. https://doi.org/10.1093/ajcn.83.3.701.

73. Yang QH, Botto LD, Gallagher M, Friedman JM, Sanders CL, Koontz D, Nikolova S, Erickson JD, Steinberg K. Prevalence and effects of gene-gene and gene-nutrient interactions on serum folate and serum total homocysteine concentrations in the United States: findings from the third National Health and Nutrition Examination Survey DNA Bank. Am J Clin Nutr. 2008;88(1):232–46. https://doi.org/10.1093/ajcn/88.1.232.

74. Cheng TD, Ilozumba MN, Balavarca Y, Neuhouser ML, Miller JW, SAA B, Zheng Y, Song X, Duggan DJ, Toriola AT, Bailey LB, Green R, Caudill MA, Ulrich CM. Associations between genetic variants and blood biomarkers of one-carbon metabolism in postmenopausal women from the Women's Health Initiative observational study. J Nutr. 2022;152(4):1099–106. https://doi.org/10.1093/jn/nxab444.

75. Hanson C, Lyden E, Abresch C, Anderson-Berry A. Serum retinol concentrations race and socioeconomic status in of women of childbearing age in the United States. Nutrients. 2016;8(8):508. https://doi.org/10.3390/nu8080508.

76. Ballew C, Bowman BA, Sowell AL, Gillespie C. Serum retinol distributions in residents of the United States: third national health and nutrition examination survey 1988–1994. Am J Clin Nutr. 2001;73(3):586–93. https://doi.org/10.1093/ajcn/73.3.586.

77. Neuhouser ML, Rock CL, Eldridge AL, Kristal AR, Patterson RE, Cooper DA, Neumark-Sztainer D, Cheskin LJ, Thornquist MD. Serum concentrations of retinol α-tocopherol and the carotenoids are influenced by diet race and obesity in a sample of healthy adolescents. J Nutr. 2001;131(8):2184–91. https://doi.org/10.1093/jn/131.8.2184.

78. Crook J, Horgas A, Yoon SJ, Grundmann O, Johnson-Mallard V. Insufficient vitamin C levels among adults in the United States: results from the NHANES surveys 2003–2006. Nutrients. 2021;13(11):3910. https://doi.org/10.3390/nu13113910.

79. Schleicher RL, Carroll MD, Ford ES, Lacher DA. Serum vitamin C and the prevalence of vitamin C deficiency in the United States: 2003–2004 National Health and Nutrition Examination Survey (NHANES). Am J Clin Nutr. 2009;90(5):1252–63. https://doi.org/10.3945/ajcn.2008.27016.

80. Suarez EC, Schramm-Sapyta NL. Race differences in the relation of vitamins A C E and β-carotene to metabolic and inflammatory biomarkers. Nutr Res. 2014;34(1):1–10. https://doi.org/10.1016/j.nutres.2013.10.001.

81. Timpson NJ, Forouhi NG, Brion MJ, Harbord RM, Cook DG, Johnson P, McConnachie A, Morris RW, Rodriguez S, Luan J, Ebrahim S, Padmanabhan S, Watt G, Bruckdorfer KR, Wareham NJ, Whincup PH, Chanock S, Sattar N, Lawlor DA, Davey Smith G. Genetic variation at the SLC23A1 locus is associated with circulating concentrations of l-ascorbic acid (vitamin C): evidence from 5 independent studies with >15000 participants. Am J Clin Nutr. 2010;92(2):375–82. https://doi.org/10.3945/ajcn.2010.29438.

82. Michels AJ, Hagen TM, Frei B. Human genetic variation influences vitamin C homeostasis by altering vitamin C transport and antioxidant enzyme function. Annu Rev Nutr. 2013;33(1):45–70. https://doi.org/10.1146/annurev-nutr-071812-161246.

83. Ford ES, Sowell A. Serun-tecopherol status in the United States population: findings from the third national health and nutrition examination survey. Am J Epidemiol. 1999;150(3):290–300. https://doi.org/10.1093/oxfordjournals.aje.a010001.

84. Talegawkar SA, Johnson EJ, Carithers T, Taylor HA Jr, Bogle ML, Tucker KL. Total α-tocopherol intakes are associated with serum α-tocopherol concentrations in african american adults. J Nutr. 2007;137(10):2297–303. https://doi.org/10.1093/jn/137.10.2297.
85. Ford ES, Schleicher RL, Mokdad AH, Ajani UA, Liu S. Distribution of serum concentrations of α-tocopherol and γ-tocopherol in the US population 1–3. AmJ. Clin Nutr. 2006;84(2):375–83. https://doi.org/10.1093/ajcn/84.1.375.
86. Borel P, Desmarchelier C. Genetic variations involved in vitamin E status. Int J Mol Sci. 2016;17(12):2094. https://doi.org/10.3390/ijms17122094.
87. Schleicher RL, Sternberg MR, Pfeiffer CM. Race-ethnicity is a strong correlate of circulating fat-soluble nutrient concentrations in a representative sample of the U.S. population. J Nutr. 2013;143(6):966S–76S. https://doi.org/10.3945/jn.112.172965.
88. Lippman SM, Klein EA, Goodman PJ, Lucia MS, Thompson IM, Ford LG, Parnes HL, Minasian LM, Gaziano JM, Hartline JA, Parsons JK, Bearden JD 3rd, Crawford ED, Goodman GE, Claudio J, Winquist E, Cook ED, Karp DD, Walther P, Lieber MM, Kristal AR, Darke AK, Arnold KB, Ganz PA, Santella RM, Albanes D, Taylor PR, Probstfield JL, Jagpal TJ, Crowley JJ, Meyskens FL Jr, Baker LH, Coltman CA Jr. Effect of selenium and vitamin E on risk of prostate cancer and other cancers. JAMA. 2009;301(1):39. https://doi.org/10.1001/jama.2008.864.
89. Klein EA, Thompson IM Jr, Tangen CM, Crowley JJ, Lucia MS, Goodman PJ, Minasian LM, Ford LG, Parnes HL, Gaziano JM, Karp DD, Lieber MM, Walther PJ, Klotz L, Parsons JK, Chin JL, Darke AK, Lippman SM, Goodman GE, Meyskens FL Jr, Baker LH. Vitamin E and the risk of prostate cancer. JAMA. 2011;306(14):1549. https://doi.org/10.1001/jama.2011.1437.
90. Loh WQ, Youn J, Seow WJ. Vitamin E intake and risk of prostate cancer: a meta-analysis. Nutrients. 2023;15(1):14. https://doi.org/10.3390/nu15010014.
91. Carmel R. Ethnic and racial factors in cobalamin metabolism and its disorders. Semin Hematol. 1999;36:88–100.
92. Yawn BP, Buchanan GR, Afenyi-Annan AN, et al. Management of sickle cell disease: summary of the 2014 evidence-based report by expert panel members. JAMA. 2014;312(10):1033–48.
93. Elendu C, Amaechi DC, Alakwe-Ojimba CE, Elendu TC, Elendu RC, Ayabazu CP, Aina TO, Aborisade O, Adenikinju JS. Understanding sickle cell disease: causes symptoms and treatment options. Medicine. 2023;102(38):e35237. https://doi.org/10.1097/MD.0000000000035237.
94. The Lancet Haematology. Sickle cell disease: a year in review. Lancet Haematol. 2022;9(6):e385. https://doi.org/10.1016/S2352-3026(22)00144-2.
95. Sickle Cell Disease|CDC. Retrieved from https://www.cdc.gov/ncbddd/sicklecell/facts.html.
96. Noronha SA, Sadremeli SC, Strouse JJ. Management of sickle cell disease in children. South Med J. 2016;109(9):495–502.
97. Darbari DS, Sheehan VA, Ballas SK. The vaso-occlusive pain crisis in sickle cell disease: Definition pathophysiology and management. Eur J Haematol. 2020;105(3):237–46. https://doi.org/10.1111/ejh.13430.
98. Ataga KI, Saraf SL, Derebail VK. The nephropathy of sickle cell trait and sickle cell disease. Nat Rev Nephrol. 2022;18(6):361–77. https://doi.org/10.1038/s41581-022-00540-9.
99. Zahr RS, Saraf SL. Sickle cell disease and CKD: an update. Am J Nephrol. 2024;55(1):56–71. https://doi.org/10.1159/000534865.
100. Naik RP, Derebail VK, Grams ME, et al. Association of sickle cell trait with chronic kidney disease and albuminuria in African Americans. JAMA. 2014;312:2115–25.
101. Liem RI, Lanzkron S, D Coates T, DeCastro L, Desai AA, Ataga KI, Cohen RT, Haynes J, Osunkwo I, Lebensburger JD, Lash JP, Wun T, Verhovsek M, Ontala E, Blaylark R, Alahdab F, Katabi A, Mustafa RA, American Society of Hematology. Guidelines for sickle cell disease: cardiopulmonary and kidney disease. Blood Adv. 2019;3(23):3867–97. https://doi.org/10.1182/bloodadvances.2019000916.

102. Quinn CT, Saraf SL, Gordeuk VR, Fitzhugh CD, Creary SE, Bodas P, George A, Raj AB, Nero AC, Terrell CE, McCord L, Lane A, Ackerman HC, Yang Y, Niss O, Taylor MD, Devarajan P, Malik P. Losartan for the nephropathy of sickle cell anemia: a phase-2 multicenter trial. Am J Hematol. 2017;92(9):E520. https://doi.org/10.1002/ajh.24810.
103. Yee ME, Lane PA, Archer DR, Joiner CH, Eckman JR, Guasch A. Losartan therapy decreases albuminuria with stable glomerular filtration and permselectivity in sickle cell anemia. Blood Cells Mol Dis. 2018;69:65–70. https://doi.org/10.1016/j.bcmd.2017.09.006.
104. Amarapurkar P, Roberts L, Navarrete J, El Rassi F. Sickle cell disease and kidney. Adv Chronic Kidney Dis. 2022;29(2):141–148.e1. https://doi.org/10.1053/j.ackd.2022.03.004.
105. Pincez T, Ashley-Koch AE, Lettre G, Telen MJ. Genetic modifiers of sickle cell disease. Hematol Oncol Clin North Am. 2022;36(6):1097–124. https://doi.org/10.1016/j.hoc.2022.06.006.
106. Young BA, Wilson JG, Reiner A, Kestenbaum B, Franceschini N, Bansal N, Correa A, Himmelfarb J, Katz R. APOL1 sickle cell trait and CKD in the Jackson Heart Study. Kidney Med. 2021;3(6):962–973.e1. https://doi.org/10.1016/j.xkme.2021.05.004.
107. Safdar OY, Baghdadi RM, Alahmadi SA, Fakieh BE, Algaydi AM. Sickle cell nephropathy: a review of novel biomarkers and their potential roles in early detection of renal involvement. World J Clin Pediatr. 2022;11(1):14–26. https://doi.org/10.5409/wjcp.v11.i1.14.
108. Laurentino MR, SLA PF, LLC P, da Silva Júnior GB, Daher EF, RPG L. Non-invasive urinary biomarkers of renal function in sickle cell disease: an overview. Ann Hematol. 2019;98(12):2653–60. https://doi.org/10.1007/s00277-019-03813-9.
109. Lemes RPG, Rocha Laurentino M, Castelo LR, Silva Junior G. Sickle cell disease and the kidney: pathophysiology and novel biomarkers. Contrib Nephrol. 2021;199:114–21. https://doi.org/10.1159/000517703. Epub 2021 Aug 3
110. Elliott A, Bruner E. Renal medullary carcinoma. Arch Pathol Lab Med. 2019;143(12):1556–61. https://doi.org/10.5858/arpa.2017-0492-RS.
111. Vokshi BH, Davidson G, Tawanaie Pour Sedehi N, Helleux A, Rippinger M, Haller AR, Gantzer J, Thouvenin J, Baltzinger P, Bouarich R, Manriquez V, Zaidi S, Rao P, Msaouel P, Su X, Lang H, Tricard T, Lindner V, Surdez D, Kurtz JE, Bourdeaut F, Tannir NM, Davidson I, Malouf GG. SMARCB1 regulates a TFCP2L1-MYC transcriptional switch promoting renal medullary carcinoma transformation and ferroptosis resistance. Nature Communications. 2023;14(1):3034. https://doi.org/10.1038/s41467-023-38472-y.
112. Bender MA, Carlberg K. Sickle cell disease. 2003 Sept 15 [updated 2025 Feb 13]. In: Adam MP, Feldman J, Mirzaa GM, Pagon RA, Wallace SE, Amemiya a, editors. GeneReviews® [internet]. Seattle: University of Washington, Seattle; 1993–2025.
113. Al Kahf S, Roche A, Baron A, Chantalat-Auger C, Savale L. Pulmonary hypertension in sickle cell disease. Prensa Med. 2023;52(4):104209. https://doi.org/10.1016/j.lpm.2023.104209.
114. Sachdev V, Rosing DR, Thein SL. Cardiovascular complications of sickle cell disease. Trends Cardiovasc Med. 2021;31(3):187–93. https://doi.org/10.1016/j.tcm.2020.02.002.
115. Sheikh AB, Nasrullah A, Lopez ED, Tanveer Ud Din M, Sagheer S, Shah I, Javed N, Shekhar R. Sickle cell disease-induced pulmonary hypertension: a review of pathophysiology management and current literature. Pulse. 2021;9(3–4):57–63. https://doi.org/10.1159/000519101.
116. Naik RP, Derebail VK. The spectrum of sickle hemoglobin-related nephropathy: from sickle cell disease to sickle trait. Expert Rev Hematol. 2017;10(12):1087–94.
117. Fonseca GH, Salemi VC, Gualandro DM, Jardim C, Sousa R, Gualandro SF. Diagnosis of pulmonary hypertension in adults with sickle cell disease. Eur Heart J. 2010;31:759.
118. Liem RI, Nevin MA, Prestridge A, Young LT, Thompson AA. Tricuspid regurgitant jet velocity elevation and its relationship to lung function in pediatric sickle cell disease. Pediatr Pulmonol. 2009;44(3):281–9.
119. Arslankoylu AE, Halioglu O, Yilgor E, Duzovali O. Assessment of cardiac functions in sickle cell anemia with Doppler myocardial performance index. J Trop Pediatr. 2010;56(3):195–7. https://www.cdc.gov/NCBDDD/sicklecell/data.html

120. Hicks RE, Alsabri M, Peichev M, Kusum V. More than meets the eye: orbital swelling in an adolescent with sickle cell disease. Int J Hematol-Oncol Stem Cell Res. 2023;17(1):56. https://doi.org/10.18502/ijhoscr.v17i1.11714.
121. AlRyalat SA, Nawaiseh M, Aladwan B, Roto A, Alessa Z, Al-Omar A. Ocular manifestations of sickle cell disease: signs symptoms and complications. Ophthalmic Epidemiol. 2020;27(4):259–64. https://doi.org/10.1080/09286586.2020.1723114.
122. AlRyalat SA, BAM J, Alzarea AA, Alzarea AA, Alosaimi WA, Al Saad M. Ocular manifestations of sickle cell disease in different genotypes. Ophthalmic Epidemiol. 2021;28(3):185–90. https://doi.org/10.1080/09286586.2020.1801762.
123. Bachmeier I, Blecha C, Föll J, Wolff D, Jägle H. Makulopathie bei Sichelzellerkrankung. Maculopathy in sickle cell disease. Der Ophthalmologe. 2021;118(10):1013–23. https://doi.org/10.1007/s00347-020-01319-8.
124. Adeyoju AB, Olujohungbe AB, Morris J, et al. Priapism in sickle-cell disease; incidence, risk factors and complications—an international multicentre study. BJU Int. 2002;90:898–902.
125. Kavanagh PL, Fasipe TA, Wun T. Sickle cell disease. JAMA. 2022;328(1):57. https://doi.org/10.1001/jama.2022.10233.
126. Idris IM, Burnett AL, MR DB. Epidemiology and treatment of priapism in sickle cell disease. Hematology. 2022;2022(1):450–8. https://doi.org/10.1182/hematology.2022000380.
127. Ahuja G, Ibecheozor C, Okorie NC, Jain AJ, Coleman PW, Metwalli AR, Tonkin JB. Priapism and sickle cell disease: special considerations in etiology management and prevention. Urology. 2021;156:e40–7. https://doi.org/10.1016/j.urology.2021.06.010.
128. Dupervil B, Grosse S, Burnett A, Parker C. Emergency department visits and inpatient admissions associated with priapism among males with sickle cell disease in the United States, 2006–2010. PLoS One. 2016;11(4):e0153257.
129. Adesanya O, Burnett AL. Priapism-related biomarkers in sickle cell disease: a systematic review. Sex Med Rev. 2025;13:246. https://doi.org/10.1093/sxmrev/qeaf004.
130. CVB F, Santiago RP, da Guarda CC, Oliveira RM, Fiuza LM, SCMA Y, Carvalho SP, JSDS N, AMJ O, Fonseca CA, VML N, Lyra IM, Aleluia MM, Goncalves MS. Priapism in sickle cell disease: associations between NOS3 and EDN1 genetic polymorphisms and laboratory biomarkers. PLoS One. 2021;16(2):e0246067. https://doi.org/10.1371/journal.pone.0246067.
131. Pereira DA, Calmasini FB, Costa FF, Burnett AL, Silva FH. Nitric oxide resistance in priapism associated with sickle cell disease: mechanisms therapeutic challenges and future directions. J Pharmacol Exp Ther. 2024;390(2):203–12. https://doi.org/10.1124/jpet.123.001962.
132. Ohene-Frempong K, Weiner SJ, Sleeper LA, Miller ST, Embury S, Moohr JW, et al. Cerebrovascular accidents in sickle cell disease: rates and risk factors. Blood. 1998;91(1):288–94.
133. Kirkham FJ, Lagunju IA. Epidemiology of stroke in sickle cell disease. J Clin Med. 2021;10(18):4232. https://doi.org/10.3390/jcm10184232.
134. Parikh T, Goti A, Yashi K, Gopalakrishnan Ravikumar NP, Parmar N, Dankhara N, Satodiya V. Pediatric sickle cell disease and stroke: a literature review. Cureus. 2023;15:e34003. https://doi.org/10.7759/cureus.34003.
135. DeBaun MR, Jordan LC, King AA, Schatz J, Vichinsky E, Fox CK, McKinstry RC, Telfer P, Kraut MA, Daraz L, Kirkham FJ, Murad MH, American Society of Hematology. Guidelines for sickle cell disease: prevention diagnosis and treatment of cerebrovascular disease in children and adults. Blood Adv. 2020;4(8):1554–88. https://doi.org/10.1182/bloodadvances.2019001142.
136. Alakbarzade V, Maduakor C, Khan U, Khandanpour N, Rhodes E, Pereira AC. Cerebrovascular disease in sickle cell disease. Pract Neurol. 2023;23(2):131–8. https://doi.org/10.1136/pn-2022-003440.
137. Ghafuri DL, Abdullahi SU, Dambatta AH, Galadanci J, Tabari MA, Bello-Manga H, Idris N, Inuwa H, Tijjani A, Suleiman AA, Jibir BW, Gambo S, Gambo AI, Khalifa Y, Haliru L, Abdulrasheed S, Zakari MA, Greene BC, Trevathan E, Jordan LC, Aliyu MH, Baumann AA, DeBaun MR. Establishing sickle cell disease stroke prevention teams in Africa is fea-

sible: program evaluation using the RE-AIM framework. Am J Pediatr Hematol Oncol. 2022;44(1):e56–61. https://doi.org/10.1097/MPH.0000000000002179.
138. Mallon D, Doig D, Dixon L, Gontsarova A, Jan W, Tona F. Neuroimaging in sickle cell disease: a review. J Neuroimaging. 2020;30(6):725–35. https://doi.org/10.1111/jon.12766.
139. Abdullahi SU, Sunusi S, Aminu H, Umar R, Abba MS, Jibir BW, Sani S, Gambo S, Bello-Manga H, Galadanci NA, Covert Greene B, Kassim AA, Jordan LC, Aliyu MH, Rodeghier M, DeBaun MR, Volanakis EJ. Transcranial doppler velocity in iron-deficient Nigerian children with sickle cell anemia. Am J Hematol. 2024;99(4):797–9. https://doi.org/10.1002/ajh.27230.
140. Sahu T, Pande B, Sinha M, Sinha R, Verma HK. Neurocognitive changes in sickle cell disease: a comprehensive review. Ann Neurosci. 2022;29(4):255–68.
141. Fortin PM, Hopewell S, Estcourt LJ. Red blood cell transfusion to treat or prevent complications in sickle cell disease: an overview of cochrane reviews. Cochrane Database Syst Rev. 2018;(8):CD012082.
142. Estcourt LJ, Fortin PM, Hopewell S, et al. Blood transfusion for preventing primary and secondary stroke in people with sickle cell disease. Cochrane Database Syst Rev. 2013;(11):CD003146.
143. Abboud MR. Cerebral vasculopathy in patients with sickle cell disease and stroke: now you see it now you don't. Haematologica. 2024;109(10):3108–9. https://doi.org/10.3324/haematol.2024.285383.
144. Sparkenbaugh EM, Henderson MW, Miller-Awe M, Abrams C, Ilich A, Trebak F, Ramadas N, Vital S, Bohinc D, Bane KL, Chen C, Patel M, Wallisch M, Renné T, Gruber A, Cooley B, Gailani D, Kasztan M, Vercellotti GM, Belcher JD, Gavins FE, Stavrou EX, Key NS, Pawlinski R. Factor XII contributes to thrombotic complications and vaso-occlusion in sickle cell disease. Blood. 2023;141(15):1871–83. https://doi.org/10.1182/blood.2022017074.
145. Serjeant BE, Mason K, Reid M, Hambleton I, Serjeant GR. The aplastic crisis in HbSS: observations from the jamaican birth cohort. Hemoglobin. 2024;48(4):274–9. https://doi.org/10.1080/03630269.2024.2407633.
146. Borhade MB, Patel P, Kondamudi NP. Sickle cell crisis. 2024 Feb 25. In: StatPearls [Internet]. Treasure Island: StatPearls Publishing; 2025.
147. Hankins JS, Penkert RR, Lavoie P, et al. Original research: parvovirus B19 infection in children with sickle cell disease in the hydroxyurea era. Exp Biol Med (Maywood). 2016;241(7):749–54.
148. Shaik L, Ranjha S, Katta RR, Shah R, Nelekar S. Parvovirus infection and thrombotic thrombocytopenic purpura in an adult patient with sickle cell beta-thalassemia. Cureus. 2021;13:e16173. https://doi.org/10.7759/cureus.16173.
149. Dastgiri S, Dolatkhah R. Blood transfusions for treating acute chest syndrome in people with sickle cell disease. Cochrane Database Syst Rev. 2016;(8):CD007843. https://doi.org/10.1002/14651858.CD007843.pub3.
150. Meloy P, Rutz DR, Bhambri A. Acute chest syndrome. J Educ Teach Emerg Med. 2023;8(1):O1–O23. https://doi.org/10.21980/J80S8J. PMID: 37465032; PMCID: PMC10332774
151. Scourfield Lily EA, Nardo-Marino A, Williams Thomas N, Rees DC. Infections in sickle cell disease. Haematologica. 2020;110:546. https://doi.org/10.3324/haematol.2024.285066.
152. Ogu UO, Badamosi NU, Camacho PE, Freire AX, Adams-Graves P. Management of sickle cell disease complications beyond acute chest syndrome. J Blood Med. 2021;12:101–14. https://doi.org/10.2147/JBM.S291394.
153. Koehl JL, Koyfman A, Hayes BD, Long B. High risk and low prevalence diseases: acute chest syndrome in sickle cell disease. Am J Emerg Med. 2022;58:235–44. https://doi.org/10.1016/j.ajem.2022.06.018.
154. Bhasin N, Sarode R. Acute chest syndrome in sickle cell disease. Transfus Med Rev. 2023;37(3):150755. https://doi.org/10.1016/j.tmrv.2023.150755.

155. Jang T, Poplawska M, Cimpeanu E, Mo G, Dutta D, Lim SH. Vaso-occlusive crisis in sickle cell disease: a vicious cycle of secondary events. J Transl Med. 2021;19(1):397. https://doi.org/10.1186/s12967-021-03074-z.
156. TJP M, Dirckx M, FJPM H. Different types of pain in complex regional pain syndrome require a personalized treatment strategy. J Pain Res. 2023;16:4379–91. https://doi.org/10.2147/JPR.S432209.
157. Haywood C, Diener-West M, Strouse J, et al. Perceived discrimination in health care is associated with a greater burden of pain in sickle cell disease. J Pain Symptom Manag. 2014;48(5):934–43.
158. Green CR, Anderson KO, Baker TA, et al. The unequal burden of pain: confronting racial and ethnic disparities in pain. Pain Med. 2003;4:277–94.
159. Burgess DJ, Grill J, Noorbaloochi S, et al. The effect of perceived racial discrimination on bodily pain among older African American men. Pain Med. 2009;10:1341–52.
160. Eltorki M, Hall M, Ramgopal S, Chaudhari PP, Badaki-Makun O, Rees CA, Bergmann KR, Shapiro DJ, Gonzalez F, Phamduy T, Neuman MI. Trends and hospital practice variation for analgesia for children with sickle cell disease with vaso-occlusive pain episodes: an 11-year analysis. Am J Emerg Med. 2024;86:129–34. https://doi.org/10.1016/j.ajem.2024.10.028.
161. Admiraal M, van Daalen J, MWJ R, Dekker J, CFJ v T, Nur E, Hollmann MW, Hermanns H, Hermanides J, Biemond BJ. A multimodal pain protocol for treatment of vaso-occlusive crisis in patients with sickle cell disease: implementation and evaluation. Eur J Haematol. 2023;111(3):382–90. https://doi.org/10.1111/ejh.14017.
162. Ruta NS, Ballas SK. The opioid drug epidemic and sickle cell disease: guilt by association. Pain Med. 2016;17(10):1793–8.
163. Chou R, Fanciullo GJ, Fine PG, et al. Clinical guidelines for the use of chronic opioid therapy in chronic noncancer pain. J Pain. 2009;10(2):113–30.
164. Shah P, Khaleel M, Thuptimdang W, et al. Mental stress causes vasoconstriction in sickle cell disease and normal controls. Haematologica. 2019;Pii:haematol 2018.211391.
165. Uwaezuoke SN, Ayuk AC, Ndu IK, et al. Vaso-occlusive crisis in sickle cell disease: current paradigm on pain management. J Pain Res. 2018;11:3141–50.
166. McGann PT, Ware RE. Hydroxyurea therapy for sickle cell anemia. Expert Opin Drug Saf. 2015;14(11):1749–58.
167. Muncie HL, Campbell J. Alpha and beta thalassemia. Am Fam Physician. 2009;80(4):339–44.
168. Pierce HI, Kurachi S, Sofroniadou K, Stamatoyannopoulos G. Frequencies of thalassemia in American blacks. Blood. 1977 Jun;49(6):981–6.
169. Baird DC, Batten SH, Sparks SK. Alpha- and beta-thalassemia: rapid evidence review. Am Fam Physician. 2022;105(3):272–80.
170. Vichinsky E, Cohen A, Thompson AA, et al. Epidemiologic and clinical characteristics of nontransfusion-dependent thalassemia in the United States. Pediatr Blood Cancer. 2018;65(7):e27067. https://doi.org/10.1002/pbc.27067. Epub 2018 Apr 10
171. Taher AT, Musallam KM, Cappellini MD. β-thalassemias. N Engl J Med. 2021;384(8):727–43. https://doi.org/10.1056/NEJMra2021838.
172. Nkhoma ET, Poole C, Vannappagari V, et al. The global prevalence of glucose-6-phosphate dehydrogenase deficiency: a systematic review and meta-analysis. Blood Cells Mol Dis. 2009;42:267–78.
173. Chinevere TD, Murry CK, Grant E, et al. Prevalence of glucose-6-phosphate dehydrogenase deficiency in U.S. Army personnel. Mil Med. 2006;17(9):905–7.
174. Thomas JE, Kang S, Wyatt CJ, et al. Glucose-6-phosphate dehydrogenase deficiency is associated with cardiovascular disease in U.S. military centers. Tex Heart Inst J. 2018;45(3):144–50.
175. Belfield KD, Tichy EM. Review and drug therapy implications of glucose-6-phosphate dehydrogenase deficiency. Am J Health Syst Pharm. 2018;75(3):97–104.
176. Luzzatto L, Ally M, Notaro R. Glucose-6-phosphate dehydrogenase deficiency. Blood. 2020;136(11):1225–40. https://doi.org/10.1182/blood.2019000944.

177. Mbanefo EC, Ahmed AM, Titouna A, Elmaraezy A, Trang NT, Phuoc Long N, Hoang Anh N, Diem Nghi T, The Hung B, Van Hieu M, Ky Anh N, Huy NT, Hirayama K. Association of glucose-6-phosphate dehydrogenase deficiency and malaria: a systematic review and meta-analysis. Sci Rep. 2017;7(1):45963. https://doi.org/10.1038/srep45963.
178. Clarke GM, Rockett K, Kivinen K, Hubbart C, Jeffreys AE, Rowlands K, Jallow M, Conway DJ, Bojang KA, Pinder M, Usen S, Sisay-Joof F, Sirugo G, Toure O, Thera MA, Konate S, Sissoko S, Niangaly A, Poudiougou B, Mangano VD, Bougouma EC, Sirima SB, Modiano D, Amenga-Etego LN, Ghansah A, Koram KA, Wilson MD, Enimil A, Evans J, Amodu OK, Olaniyan S, Apinjoh T, Mugri R, Ndi A, Ndila CM, Uyoga S, Macharia A, Peshu N, Williams TN, Manjurano A, Sepúlveda N, Clark TG, Riley E, Drakeley C, Reyburn H, Nyirongo V, Kachala D, Molyneux M, Dunstan SJ, Phu NH, Quyen NN, Thai CQ, Hien TT, Manning L, Laman M, Siba P, Karunajeewa H, Allen S, Allen A, Davis TM, Michon P, Mueller I, Molloy SF, Campino S, Kerasidou A, Cornelius VJ, Hart L, Shah SS, Band G, Spencer CC, Agbenyega T, Achidi E, Doumbo OK, Farrar J, Marsh K, Taylor T, Kwiatkowski DP, MalariaGEN Consortium. Characterisation of the opposing effects of G6PD deficiency on cerebral malaria and severe malarial anaemia. eLife. 2017;6:e15085. https://doi.org/10.7554/eLife.15085.

Chapter 11
A Precision Medicine Approach to Gastrointestinal and Hepatic Diseases in African Americans

Contents

11.1	Hepatitis B.	220
11.2	Hepatitis C.	222
11.3	Hepatocellular Carcinoma.	225
11.4	Inflammatory Bowel Diseases.	227
	11.4.1 Crohn's Disease and Ulcerative Colitis.	227
11.5	GERD.	229
11.6	Barrett's Esophagus.	230
11.7	Helicobacter Pylori.	231
11.8	Gallbladder Disease.	232
References.		234

Health disparities in gastroenterology among African Americans are well-documented and multifactorial. African Americans have higher incidence and mortality rates for several gastrointestinal cancers, including colorectal cancer, pancreatic cancer, and liver cancer, compared to other racial/ethnic groups [1–4]. For instance, the American Gastroenterological Association notes that African American men and women have 24% and 19% higher colorectal cancer incidence rates, respectively, compared to European Americans, and stage-adjusted colorectal cancer mortality rates are 47% higher in African American men and 34% higher in African American women [1]. Disparities in colorectal cancer screening are significant contributors to these outcomes. African Americans are less likely to undergo screening, which is associated with higher mortality rates. In the context of inflammatory bowel disease (IBD) including Crohn's disease and ulcerative colitis, African Americans are more likely to experience severe disease phenotypes and complications, and they have higher rates of emergency department visits and hospitalizations [5, 6]. They are more likely to experience perianal disease, fistulizing disease, and fibrostenotic disease and have higher rates of IBD-related surgeries and complications [6, 7]. They are also less likely to receive specialist care and advanced therapies like biologics [8]. Surgical outcomes for GI cancers also show disparities. African Americans are less likely to receive surgery for GI cancers, contributing to lower survival rates. They also experience higher postoperative complications and longer hospital stays [9]. The American College of Gastroenterology (ACG) guidelines also highlight that the *Helicobacter pylori* burden is disproportionately higher in non-Hispanic Black individuals, with a prevalence of 40.2% compared to 20.1% in non-Hispanic Whites [10, 11]. This increased prevalence is associated with higher rates of *H. pylori*-related complications, such as peptic ulcer disease and gastric cancer, in this population. Health disparities related to hepatitis among African Americans are significant and multifaceted as well. African Americans have a higher prevalence of both hepatitis B virus (HBV) and hepatitis C virus (HCV) infections compared to other racial groups. Here are more details related to the most dramatic differences.

11.1 Hepatitis B

African Americans have the highest rate of acute hepatitis B infections of all racial groups in the USA with a two- to threefold higher prevalence of chronic hepatitis B infection [12–16]. Chronic hepatitis B is frequently asymptomatic, but long-term infection can lead to cirrhosis and/or hepatocellular carcinoma. Since the initiation of universal vaccination of newborn babies and catch-up vaccination of children and adolescents began in 1991, a steady and dramatic decline in hepatitis B infections has continued [17].

The principal modes of hepatitis B transmission across all US populations include IV drug users, the incarcerated/institutionalized, healthcare personnel, those needing multiple transfusions, organ transplant patients, those with multiple sex partners, and newborns to mothers with hepatitis B [13–15, 18, 19].

Hepatitis B infections are common among patients and staff of hemodialysis units. Up to half of the renal dialysis patients who contract hepatitis B become chronic carriers of the hepatitis B antigen allowing for multiple exposures to dialysis staff, transportation personnel, and close family contacts [20]. The hepatitis B virus can remain viable on environmental surfaces for a week [21].

Kimberly Forde at the University of Pennsylvania reviewed ethnic disparities in chronic hepatitis B infections and reported the following [22]:

> Though there has been a decline in infection rates for all racial and ethnic groups from 2000–2014, African Americans continue to have the highest rate of new infections. New infections among African Americans were most often reported in patients who were male, 30–39 years of age, and those who engaged in high-risk behaviors that increase risk of transmission of hepatitis B infection, particularly use of intravenous (IV) drugs, men who have sex with men (MSM), and having two or more sexual partners [22]

Some of the persisting amplified risk in African Americans is the increased occurrence of hepatitis B and other sexually transmitted diseases (STD) in incarcerated and previously incarcerated African Americans. Information regarding exact numbers of infections in this population has been elusive but most report twice the occurrence [23] of hepatitis B and other STDs when compared to never incarcerated. It has been well established that African Americans compose a startling and disproportionate percentage of the incarcerated with the most recent percentage nationally of 37% compared to a 13% US population [24]. The increased incidence in this population leads to excess exposure to the communities in which they reside after release [25].

Thirty percent of people reporting an acute hepatitis B infection have been incarcerated at some point prior [23, 25]. In addition, repeated incarcerations increase the risk for hepatitis B directly [23]. The highest prevalence of chronic hepatitis B was in HIV-positive populations [23, 26].

In terms of testing and treatment for hepatitis B patients without immunity from vaccination, an analysis by Hu et al. at the National Center for HIV, Viral Hepatitis, STDs, and TB Prevention looked at data for US ethnic minorities and found "more than half of racial/ethnic minority persons in these communities had not been tested for hepatitis B, and only about one-half of those who tested positive had ever received treatment" [27].

The major goal of hepatitis B therapy is to prevent the development of cirrhosis/liver failure and/or prevent hepatocellular carcinoma and its sequelae. Evidence of its benefit is presumed due to lower viral DNA [28]. For African Americans, who have a higher prevalence of chronic Hepatitis B, achieving durable suppression of HBV DNA is essential to reduce the risk of liver complications and improve overall outcomes. The American Association for the Study of Liver Diseases (AASLD) emphasizes that the goal of therapy is to prevent liver-related morbidity and mortality by suppressing HBV replication, which in turn reduces histological activity and the risk of disease progression [29]. Because the time it takes to progress from active infection to chronic infection to end-stage event takes many years, tracking this population over decades can be challenging.

Finally, the clinical course and consequences of hepatitis B infection are influenced by several factors including viral load, host immune status, environment, and viral genotypes (A–H). Different HBV genotypes are associated with different regions in the world [30–32].

> Genotype A is widespread in sub-Saharan Africa, Northern Europe, and Western Africa; genotypes B and C are common in Asia; genotype C is primarily observed in Southeast Asia; genotype D is dominant in Africa, Europe, Mediterranean countries, and India; genotype G is reported in France, Germany, and the United States; and genotype H is commonly encountered in Central and South America [30]

HBV genotypes are closely related with optimal treatment strategies for chronic hepatitis B patients. Genotype A HBV, which is more prevalent in people of sub-Saharan African descent, is associated with a more chronic and long-standing infection. Genotype A is also more responsive to accepted treatments like interferon-based therapy [30].

Class II HLA alleles play a significant role in HBV infection persistence. A study by Thio et al. found that in African Americans, HBV persistence was significantly associated with the HLA class II alleles DQA1*0501 and DQB1*0301, as well as the two-locus haplotype consisting of these alleles and the three-locus haplotype DQA1*0501*, DQB1*0301, and DRB1*1102. These alleles are involved in the immune response, and their presence may affect the ability to clear the virus, leading to chronic infection [33]. Additionally, a novel variant in the HLA-DPB1 3′ untranslated region (3′UTR), specifically rs9277534, has been identified as significantly associated with HBV recovery in African Americans. This variant distinguishes the protective HLA-DPB1*04:01 allele from the more susceptible HLA-DPB1*01:01 allele, suggesting that differences in HLA-DP expression levels may influence the risk of persistent HBV infection [34]. These genetic predispositions underscore the importance of the HLA-mediated immune response in the persistence and clearance of HBV infection among African Americans, contributing to the observed health disparities in this population.

African Americans are at significant risk of hepatocellular carcinoma (HCC). Studies have shown that African Americans with chronic HBV infection have a higher risk of developing HCC than other racial groups [35]. This increased risk is attributed to higher HBV DNA levels and the prevalence of genotype A. This genotype is associated with a higher likelihood of HCC development [35]. Additionally, factors such as delayed diagnosis, lower antiviral treatment rates, and socioeconomic disparities contribute to the increased incidence and poorer outcomes of HCC in this population. Unfortunately, this more indolent and long-term presence is also associated with a four- to fivefold increased risk for hepatocellular carcinoma [22]. Screen your older African Americans for hepatitis B, and then refer them for risk stratification and treatment.

11.2 Hepatitis C

African Americans are disproportionately infected by hepatitis C and represent 23% of the estimated 3.2 million people in the USA who are believed to be infected [36–38]. Younger African Americans are 1.6 times more likely to be chronically infected, and those over age 60 are ten times more likely to have the infection [36]. These rates are likely underestimated as hepatitis prevalence studies often exclude vulnerable populations including African Americans [37]. It is also well established that African Americans have a lower response rate to current treatments [39]. Increased prevalence coupled with lower response to treatment makes for a dismal outlook, but there are interventions that clinicians can make that will have a very positive impact.

Overall, hepatitis C virus (HCV) infections are the leading cause of cirrhosis and hepatocellular carcinoma and the most common cause for liver transplantation [38, 40]. Before the more widespread availability of newer direct-acting antiviral agents that "cure" hepatitis C, many African Americans were considered ineligible for treatment with interferon-based medications due to comorbidity contraindications that included seizures, cardiac diseases, hemoglobinopathies (sickle cell, thalassemia, etc.), bipolar disorder, and depression [41, 42].

11.2 Hepatitis C

Screen for Hepatitis C
- Current or prior IV drug users
- Transfusions prior to 1987
- Hemodialysis patients
- Persistently high ALT (alanine aminotransferase) levels
- HIV infection
- Organ transplant before 1992
- Blood exposure to someone with hepatitis C
- Children born to mothers with hepatitis C
- Patients with unlicensed or noncommercially obtained tattoos
- History of homelessness or incarceration

Aside from comorbidities that are contraindications to treatment with interferon-based therapies, African Americans disproportionately get infected with a hepatitis C virus with a genotype (currently there are 6 major genotypes and more than 50 subtypes) that is more difficult to treat (genotype 1) [43]. Genotype 1 of the hepatitis C virus is the most prevalent genotype impacting African Americans with studies showing that 85–90% of African Americans with HCV are infected with genotype 1, with a significant proportion being subtype 1b. This high prevalence of genotype 1 among African Americans is notable because genotype 1 has historically been associated with lower response rates to interferon-based therapies. However, the advent of direct-acting antivirals has significantly improved treatment outcomes across all genotypes [38, 43].

The economic burden of hepatitis C extends deeply into hospitalization costs. Teshale, Xing, and colleagues at the Division of Viral Hepatitis at the Centers for Disease Control and Prevention found that African Americans had substantially higher hospital admission rates and length of stay [44].

Similar to other health conditions, despite the higher occurrence, African Americans tend to be screened less often for hepatitis C than European Americans and once diagnosed are referred for specialty care less often [45, 46]. Tran and colleagues discussed this curious disparity:

> The quality of HCV care differed by patient race/ethnicity. This result is consistent with previous studies, which showed that patients of minority race/ethnicity were less likely to receive recommended HCV care and treatment. Patients in racial minority groups had a lower probability of receiving pre- and post-treatment testing than whites. In addition, the odds of undergoing HCC screening every 6 months were lower among African-American patients, while Hispanics had higher odds, compared to whites [46]

These studies also showed a significant referral bias against minorities. While 71% of European Americans with hepatitis C were referred for specialty care, only 32% of African Americans had evidence of a referral [45]. In contrast, studies have also shown that African Americans are more prone to decline interferon-based therapy after discussion with a specialist [47, 48]. Between lower referral rates and decreased acceptance on the patient's part, hepatitis C has been woefully addressed in African Americans.

Spontaneous clearance of hepatitis C occurs in up to half of acute infections overall, but studies involving African Americans show a much lower clearance incidence of closer to 10% [49, 50]. Researchers suspect that the overall higher prevalence in African Americans may be due to the lower clearance after the acute infection.

Despite the increased occurrence and lower clearance of hepatitis C in African Americans, there is a curious decrease in fibrosis and piecemeal necrosis of the liver [51]. Researchers suggest that the progression of hepatitis C may be slower in African Americans. This slower progression manifests itself as less hepatic necrosis, less liver fibrosis, and lower liver function tests, particularly ALT levels when compared to European American patients [52].

Several studies have identified genetic factors that may play a role in the progression of liver fibrosis in African Americans with HCV. For instance, admixture mapping has identified specific genomic regions associated with cirrhosis risk in African Americans, such as loci on chromosomes 2q21.1 and 6p21.2 [53]. These findings suggest that genetic ancestry may influence the risk of developing advanced liver disease. Additionally, polymorphisms in genes related to immune response, such as myxovirus resistance-1 (Mx1) and protein kinase (PKR), have been associated with less severe hepatic fibrosis in African Americans [54]. These genetic variations may contribute to this population's milder liver necroinflammation and fibrosis. Furthermore, studies have shown that African Americans with HCV have lower levels of liver inflammation and fibrosis compared to European Americans, which genetic differences may partially explain. Multistate model analyses have supported the protective effect of African American race on fibrosis progression [55].

Direct-acting antiviral agents (DAAs) for hepatitis C are much more efficacious and have improved tolerability in all populations including African Americans; however, getting access to these medications has shown a significant disparity. Julia Marcus and colleagues looked at the initiation of these medications among Kaiser Permanente members (all insured) and found that racial/ethnic minorities (and persons of lower socioeconomic status) were much less likely to be prescribed these curative medicines [56]. They also found that reporting drug abuse, alcohol use, and/or smoking was also associated with a lower likelihood of being prescribed direct-acting antiviral agents. Omar Sims and researchers at the University of Alabama found a similar trend [57]:

> Though DAAs have eliminated many historically, long-standing medical barriers to HCV treatment, several racial, psychological and socioeconomic barriers, and disparities remain. Consequently, patients who are African American, uninsured, and actively use drugs and alcohol will suffer from increased HCV-related morbidity and mortality in the coming years if deliberate public health and clinical efforts are not made to facilitate access to DAAs [57]

While there are a number of challenges with African Americans and hepatitis C, thanks to newer medications, the future is bright. As clinicians properly profile, screen, and treat African Americans with hepatitis C, the overall burden of this disease will fade. Kendall Beck and colleagues at the University of California confirmed that [58]:

> despite the known medical and psychosocial challenges faced by underserved (African American) populations, the availability of DAA-based therapies has significantly improved treatment eligibility, treatment initiation, treatment success, as well as adherence to HCV care compared to pre-DAA era therapies. DAA access appears to be the single most important factor influencing engagement with HCV care among the underserved African American population. Thus, eliminating the barrier of access to DAA regimens will likely significantly reduce hepatitis C disparities, a public health priority, in this underserved population [58]

11.3 Hepatocellular Carcinoma

Because hepatocellular carcinoma (HCC) is so frequently a result of long-standing hepatitis B and C infection in African Americans, it is better reviewed in close conjunction with these infections (rather than in Chap. 6).

Hepatocellular carcinoma, the most common type of liver cancer, has significant implications for African American populations. Several factors contribute to this disparity, including a higher prevalence of chronic liver diseases such as hepatitis C virus (HCV) infection, nonalcoholic fatty liver disease (NAFLD), and cirrhosis, which are prevalent in African American communities [59]. Additionally, lifestyle factors like obesity, diabetes, and alcohol consumption exacerbate the risk of developing HCC [59]. African Americans are also more likely to present with advanced disease compared to European Americans [60, 61]. They are less likely to be diagnosed at an early stage and less likely to receive curative treatments such as liver transplantation or surgical resection [62, 63]. This disparity in early detection and treatment contributes to poorer survival outcomes for African Americans with HCC. Socioeconomic factors exacerbate these disparities, including lower household income and geographic location, particularly in more rural areas. African Americans from small to medium metro areas have a higher mortality risk compared to those from large metro areas [64]. Additionally, African Americans with HCC are more likely to have larger tumors and more aggressive tumor characteristics, such as poor differentiation and microvascular invasion [64]. These characteristics further contribute to less favorable prognoses.

Yu and colleagues at the University of Maryland looked at the incidence of hepatocellular carcinoma and found dramatically increased rate in African Americans and the patients were "much younger" than European American patients [65]. They noted a median age with HCC of 53 in African Americans compared to 67 in European Americans. They also found an increased occurrence of hepatitis B, hepatitis C, co-occurring hepatitis B and C, and hepatitis B and C with diabetes. Finally, there was a twofold decreased occurrence of alcoholic liver disease in African Americans [65].

Hepatitis C is the most common risk factor for hepatocellular carcinoma and is found in 25% of cases. The hepatitis C cases were also associated with younger age and therefore earlier infection. Concurrent hepatitis B and C infections increased the risk for hepatocellular carcinoma by 2–20 times compared with hepatitis B alone, and alcoholic liver disease plus hepatitis C was associated with a 200–400% increase risk compared with hepatitis C alone.

Diabetes increased the relative risk of hepatocellular carcinoma by 60–500% in individuals with hepatitis B, hepatitis C, and alcoholic liver disease. Hepatitis B and C were twice as prevalent among African American than European American patients, and those two infections comprised half of the hepatocellular carcinomas in African American patients [65].

Like other cancers, early detection is the key to improved prognosis in hepatocellular carcinoma. Amy Kim and Amit Singal looked at health disparities in the early detection of hepatocellular carcinoma [66]:

> Guidelines from the American Association for the Study of Liver Diseases (AASLD) recommend HCC surveillance in patients with cirrhosis and/or chronic HBV using ultrasound every 6 months. Surveillance is efficacious for early stage detection and is associated with higher rates of curative treatment and improved survival in at-risk patients. However, despite a strong evidence base and guideline recommendations, less than 20% of patients with cirrhosis currently receive surveillance. Underuse of surveillance may be mediated by patient-level factors (e.g., nonadherence), provider-level factors (e.g., lack of knowledge or disbelief regarding benefits of HCC surveillance), and/or system-level factors (e.g., lack of access to medical care) [66].

In the Surveillance Epidemiology and End Results (SEER)-Medicare database, African Americans had the lowest screening rate for hepatocellular carcinoma at 12%, European Americans were 15%, Hispanic/Latino were 17%, and Asian Americans had the highest screening rate at 28%. Overall, patients with the higher median income and/or educational levels were more likely to be screened [67].

The 5-year survival rate for patients diagnosed with hepatocellular carcinoma varies significantly based on the stage at diagnosis and the treatment modalities employed. According to the National Cancer Institute's SEER database, the overall 5-year survival rate for HCC in the USA is approximately 19.6% [68]. However, survival rates can be much higher for patients diagnosed at an early stage who undergo curative treatments such as surgical resection, liver transplantation, or ablation. For instance, patients who receive curative intent treatments have a significantly better prognosis, with some studies reporting 5-year survival rates exceeding 50% in these cases [69, 70]. Conversely, for patients with advanced or metastatic disease, the 5-year survival rate can be as low as 2.5% [68].

11.4 Inflammatory Bowel Diseases

Inflammatory bowel diseases (IBD), which primarily include Crohn's disease and ulcerative colitis, have been increasingly recognized in African American populations, showing unique patterns and challenges [71, 72]. While historically, IBD was perceived as predominantly affecting European Americans, recent studies indicate that African Americans experience a rising incidence of these conditions [73]. As with a number of other conditions, this community often presents with more severe disease at diagnosis, leading to higher rates of complications and hospitalizations. Factors contributing to these disparities include genetic predispositions, socioeconomic variables, and access to healthcare. Genetic studies have identified African-specific susceptibility loci for IBD, such as SNPs at HLA-DRB1, ZNF649, and LSAMP for ulcerative colitis, and USP25 for IBD [74, 75]. Management of IBD in African Americans requires a culturally sensitive approach, recognizing the unique social determinants affecting this population. Enhancing awareness and education about IBD, improving access to healthcare, and promoting early detection are crucial steps in addressing these disparities. Furthermore, ongoing research into the genetic and environmental factors specific to African Americans will help tailor more effective treatment strategies, ultimately improving patient outcomes in this group.

11.4.1 Crohn's Disease and Ulcerative Colitis

Crohn's disease is a chronic inflammatory bowel disease that primarily affects the gastrointestinal tract, causing inflammation that can occur anywhere from the mouth to the anus [76]. However, it most commonly impacts the terminal ileum and the proximal aspect of the colon. Symptoms vary widely among individuals but typically include abdominal pain and cramping, chronic diarrhea (which may contain blood or mucus), fatigue, weight loss, fever, and mouth sores [77]. The exact cause of Crohn's disease remains unclear; however, factors such as genetics, immune system dysfunction, and environmental influences like diet and smoking are believed to contribute to its development [7, 76]. Crohn's disease in African Americans has distinct characteristics and outcomes compared to other racial groups. Studies indicate that African Americans with Crohn's disease are more likely to experience severe disease phenotypes, including perianal disease, fistulizing disease, and fibrostenotic disease [7, 78]. They also have higher rates of IBD-related surgeries and complications [79]. African Americans are more likely to have colonic involvement and less likely to have ileal disease compared to European American patients [78, 80]. They also have higher rates of extraintestinal manifestations such as uveitis and sacroiliitis. Additionally, African Americans with Crohn's disease are more likely to develop complications such as abscesses and require antitumor necrosis factor therapy [80] and have increased rates of extraintestinal manifestations such as arthralgias and ankylosing spondylitis/sacroiliitis [7]. Socioeconomic factors and healthcare access disparities contribute to worse outcomes in African American Crohn's disease patients. They are more likely to use emergency departments and have higher hospitalization rates [81]. Despite these challenges, medication utilization patterns are generally similar between African American and white patients [80]. Cigarette smoking has a significant negative impact on the course of Crohn's disease, particularly in African American patients who already experience severe disease phenotypes and complications. Smoking is associated with increased disease activity, higher flare rates, and an increased need for surgical interventions [82]. A meta-analysis by To et al. found that smokers with Crohn's disease have a 56% higher risk of disease flares and a twofold increased risk of flares after surgery compared to nonsmokers [82]. The American Gastroenterological Association guidelines emphasize that smoking exacerbates disease activity and accelerates disease recurrence, recommending smoking cessation for all Crohn's disease patients [83]. For African American patients, who are more prone to severe disease phenotypes anyway, smoking can further complicate disease management. Smoking has been shown to increase the need for biologic drugs and maintenance treatments, and it is an independent predictor of a stenosing disease phenotype [84]. Additionally, smoking adversely affects the response to anti-TNF therapy, with smokers being less likely to respond to treatments like infliximab [84].

Ulcerative colitis (UC) is a chronic inflammatory bowel disease that primarily affects the colon and rectum, leading to inflammation and ulceration of the intestinal lining. Symptoms typically include abdominal pain, diarrhea (often with blood or mucus), urgency to have bowel movements, and fatigue [73]. Ulcerative colitis in African American patients exhibits distinct characteristics and outcomes compared to other racial groups. African Americans with UC tend to have more severe disease at presentation and worse clinical outcomes, including higher rates of colon cancer [73, 85]. They are more likely to experience increased mortality, higher rates of emergency department visits, and hospitalizations compared to white patients [73]. African American UC patients are often diagnosed at an older age and, like Crohn's disease, have higher rates of extraintestinal manifestations such as arthralgias and ankylosing spondylitis/sacroiliitis. They also tend to have more distal disease involvement, with a higher prevalence of proctitis compared to European American patients [86, 87]. Despite these severe presentations, African Americans are less likely to receive advanced therapies, including corticosteroids and immunomodulators, which contributes in some part to their worse outcomes [86]. There are specific genetic markers associated with ulcerative colitis in African American patients. Genome-wide association studies (GWAS) have identified several significant loci in this population. Single-nucleotide polymorphisms (SNPs) at HLA-DRB1, ZNF649, and LSAMP have been associated with UC in African Americans [74]. The KCNQ2 gene, located near TNFRSF6B, has also been implicated in UC in this population [74]. Further studies have highlighted the role of the HLA region, particularly HLA-DRB1 alleles, which show both shared and ethnicity-specific associations with UC across different populations, including African Americans. The IL-18 gene polymorphisms, such as rs1946518, rs187238, and rs360718, have also been associated with an increased risk of UC among African Americans [88, 89]. These genetic markers contribute to the distinct disease characteristics, higher rates of extraintestinal manifestations, and worse clinical outcomes observed in African American UC patients.

A racial disparity in specialty referrals, emergency department use, and higher-end medical therapies was found in patients with Crohn's and ulcerative colitis by Geoffrey Nguyen and colleagues at John Hopkins University [5]:

> Our study provides additional evidence of racial disparities in the field of IBD (inflammatory bowel disease) that may impact the overall effectiveness of medical therapy. Clinical trials tout the potent efficacy of biologics, but these results were derived under ideal study conditions, in which minorities are underrepresented. The relatively lower utilization of specialist care and anti-TNF agents among (African Americans) outside of a protocol-driven milieu may generate racial differences in how well the efficacy of clinical trials is translated into real-world effectiveness. [5]

Surgical interventions were reviewed by Eliot Arsoniadis and colleagues at the University of Minnesota and Isabel Dos Santos Marques at the University of Alabama and found that African Americans had a greater number of postoperative complications [90, 91]. For Crohn's disease, these include increased rates of sepsis, surgical site infections, and overall postoperative morbidity. Specifically, African American patients have a higher incidence of postoperative sepsis (10.9% vs. 6.6%) and surgical site infections (17.6% vs. 14.8%) compared to non-African American patients. Additionally, they are more likely to require blood transfusions and experience renal insufficiency postoperatively [90, 91]. For ulcerative colitis, African American patients have higher rates of composite postoperative morbidity (CPM) at 26.1% compared to other racial groups. This includes complications such as bleeding requiring transfusions, sepsis, and extended hospital stays [92]. The odds of experiencing these complications are significantly higher for African American patients even after adjusting for other risk factors.

11.5 GERD

Gastroesophageal reflux disease (GERD) is a chronic digestive condition characterized by the backflow of stomach acid into the esophagus, leading to symptoms such as heartburn, regurgitation, and difficulty swallowing. In the African American population, GERD prevalence and severity is influenced by various factors including diet, lifestyle, and socioeconomic status. Studies indicate that African Americans have a similar prevalence of GERD symptoms compared to other racial groups in the USA, but they tend to have a lower prevalence of complications such as erosive esophagitis and Barrett's esophagus [93–95]. For instance, El-Serag et al. found that while the prevalence of GERD symptoms was similar among different racial groups, African Americans had a significantly lower prevalence of erosive esophagitis compared to European Americans (24% vs. 50%) [93]. Additionally, Vega et al. reported that Barrett's esophagus was less common in African Americans compared to non-Hispanic whites (4.5% vs. 15.8%) [95].

Type 2 diabetes (DM2) has been identified as an independent risk factor for GERD among urban African Americans, with a higher prevalence of GERD in those with DM2 (41.5%) compared to those without DM2 (20.6%) [96]. This association appears to be stronger in men than in women. Furthermore, lifestyle factors such as body mass index, smoking, a higher consumption of fried foods, spicy dishes, carbonated beverages, and alcohol consumption are also associated with an increased prevalence of GERD symptoms in African Americans [97]. GERD significantly increases the risk of esophageal adenocarcinoma, esophageal squamous cell carcinoma, laryngeal squamous cell carcinoma, thyroid cancer, and oral cavity and pharyngeal cancers [98–100]. Effective management of GERD in this population often requires a comprehensive approach, including lifestyle modifications, dietary changes, and, when necessary, medical interventions.

11.6 Barrett's Esophagus

While gastroesophageal reflux disease prevalence seems to be the same across races, Barrett's esophagus also has a curiously decreased prevalence in African Americans [101, 102]. Ahmad Alkaddour and colleagues at the University of Florida looked at over 15,000 endoscopies and found a confirmed decreased occurrence of mucosal changes consistent with Barrett's esophagus in African Americans [101]. This decreased occurrence was despite similarities in GERD history, cigarette/alcohol use, medications prescribed, and body mass index. There is also a decreased risk for Barrett's esophagus following erosive esophagitis formation in African Americans [102–104].

These findings have significant implications for clinical practice. African Americans with GERD are less likely to develop Barrett's esophagus and its complications, such as dysplasia and esophageal adenocarcinoma. This suggests that the risk stratification and screening guidelines for Barrett's esophagus may need to be tailored to account for racial differences. The American Society for Gastrointestinal Endoscopy notes that European descent is a significant risk factor for Barrett's esophagus and esophageal adenocarcinoma. Current guidelines support screening primarily in European American men aged over 50 with chronic GERD symptoms [104–106]. Research has identified specific genetic factors that may contribute to this disparity. A study by Sun et al. used admixture mapping to investigate the genetic differences between African Americans and European Americans with Barrett's esophagus and esophageal adenocarcinoma [107]. The study found that African Americans with Barrett's esophagus or esophageal adenocarcinoma had regions of excess European ancestry on chromosomes 11p and 8q, suggesting that genetic susceptibility to Barrett's esophagus and esophageal adenocarcinoma is higher in individuals with European ancestry [107]. Additionally, Ferrer-Torres et al. identified that African Americans have constitutively higher levels of glutathione S-transferase theta 2 in their esophageal tissues. This enzyme protects cells against DNA damage from genotoxic stress, which may reduce the risk of GERD-induced damage and subsequent development of Barrett's esophagus and esophageal adenocarcinoma [108].

11.7 Helicobacter Pylori

The overall prevalence of *Helicobacter pylori* infections in the USA has declined over the past 60 years as the availability of antibiotics and acid blockers has increased [109–111]. Unfortunately, the prevalence has not declined in African Americans as distinctly as in European Americans [109, 111]. Theresa Nguyen and colleagues looked at the prevalence of *H. pylori* in 1200 veterans in Texas and found over half of the African American men were positive for *H. pylori* compared to under 10% of European Americans [112]. Shah and colleagues replicated that study and again confirmed this dramatic disparity [111]. Some of the increased *H. pylori* risk was related to socioeconomic factors, but these did not account for all of the differences [109, 112].

Genetic factors significantly impact the prevalence and severity of *H. pylori* infections. Studies have shown that African Americans with higher proportions of African ancestry have increased odds of *H. pylori* seropositivity, particularly to virulent strains such as CagA-positive *H. pylori*. For example, individuals with high African ancestry ($\geq 95\%$) have a 13.1-fold increased odds of being seropositive for CagA compared to those with lower African ancestry [11, 113]. Genetic variants associated with African ancestry may also contribute to the higher prevalence of *H. pylori* infection. A study in a Latin American urban center found that each 10% increase in African ancestry was associated with a 22% increase in the odds of *H. pylori* infection, independent of socio-environmental factors [114]. This suggests that genetic predisposition plays a significant role in the higher infection rates observed in African Americans. Moreover, African American strains of *H. pylori* often retain genetic markers from African origins, such as the ins180 insertion, which may influence the bacterium's virulence and the host's immune response [113]. These genetic factors contribute to the higher prevalence and potentially more severe outcomes of *H. pylori* infections in African American populations, including an increased risk of gastric cancer. The increased prevalence of *H. pylori* infection among African Americans, particularly with virulent strains, contributes to the higher incidence of gastric cancer observed in that community. Given these disparities, targeted screening and eradication strategies for *H. pylori* in high-risk populations, including African Americans, would be beneficial. The American Society for Gastrointestinal Endoscopy (ASGE) suggests that such strategies could potentially reduce the risk of gastric cancer in these groups [115, 116].

11.8 Gallbladder Disease

The prevalence of gallbladder disease in African Americans is lower compared to other ethnic groups. According to a study using data from the National Health and Nutrition Examination Survey (NHANES), the age-standardized prevalence of gallbladder disease among African American men was 5.3%, which is lower than that of European American men (8.6%) and Mexican American men (8.9%). Among women, the age-adjusted prevalence was 13.9% for African American women, which is lower than that for Mexican American women (26.7%) and European American women (16.6%) [117, 118]. The impact of gallbladder disease on African Americans includes disparities in healthcare utilization and outcomes. African American patients with symptomatic cholelithiasis have higher odds of emergency department revisits compared to other racial groups, indicating potential disparities in follow-up care and management [118]. Additionally, African American patients have been found to have lower rates of cholecystectomy during hospitalizations for acute gallstone pancreatitis compared to European American patients, which may contribute to worse outcomes [119]. Furthermore, the incidence of gallbladder cancer among African Americans has been increasing, with a notable rise in rates among successive birth cohorts [120]. This trend contrasts with the overall decline in gallbladder cancer incidence in other racial/ethnic groups, highlighting a unique and concerning pattern among non-Hispanic Blacks.

Despite the higher risk of gallbladder disease with increasing obesity rates, there is a slightly decreased risk for gallstone formation and subsequent disease in African Americans [121, 122].

Recent research has identified several genetic loci associated with gallstone disease, including the hepatic cholesterol transporter ABCG8, TM4SF4, SULT2A1, glucokinase regulatory protein, and CYP7A1. These loci have been shown to influence cholesterol metabolism and bile acid synthesis, which are critical in gallstone formation. Specifically, the ABCG8 locus variants (rs11887534 and rs4245791) have been positively associated with gallstone disease risk in African American populations [123]. Additionally, a study examining the relationship between ethnic admixture and gallbladder surgery found that African admixture was marginally associated with decreased gallbladder surgery in African Americans, suggesting a protective genetic component [124]. This protective effect may contribute to the lower prevalence of gallbladder disease observed in this population.

Sickle cell disease is associated with the formation of gallstones that frequently progress to cholecystitis. Because a sickle cell crisis may present with similar symptoms, prophylactic cholecystectomy should be strongly considered when stones are noted [122]. Complications from surgery, whether planned or emergent, are significant [122].

A Precision Medicine Approach to Gastrointestinal and Hepatic Diseases in African Americans
- African Americans have the highest rate of acute hepatitis B virus (HBV) infections of all racial groups in the USA with a two- to threefold higher prevalence.
- African Americans with a history of incarceration have a greatly increased risk for hepatitis B, hepatitis C, and other sexually transmitted diseases.
- HBV genotypes are closely related with optimal treatment strategies for chronic hepatitis B patients, and type A is most frequent in African Americans and more responsive to interferon-based therapy.
- While African Americans comprise approximately 13% of the US population, they make up approximately 25% of the hepatitis C population.
- African Americans disproportionately get infected with a hepatitis C virus with a genotype that is more difficult to treat.
- African Americans' clearance of hepatitis C after acute infection occurs at a much lower rate and accounts for some of the increased overall prevalence.
- Despite the increased occurrence and lower clearance of hepatitis C in African Americans, there is a curious decrease in fibrosis and piecemeal necrosis of the liver upon biopsy.
- Despite the higher occurrence of both hepatitis B and C, African Americans tend to be screened less often and once diagnosed are referred for specialty care less often.
- The availability of DAA-based therapies for HCV cure has significantly improved treatment eligibility, treatment initiation, and treatment successes in African American patients.
- African Americans have increased risk for hepatocellular carcinoma and the related mortality, and it occurs at a significantly earlier age (age 53 vs. 67 in European Americans).
- African Americans have the lowest screening rate for hepatocellular carcinoma despite the increased risk.
- Once diagnosed with HCC, African Americans are less likely to be referred for resection, ablation, or liver transplantation.
- Inflammatory bowel diseases occur disproportionately less often in African Americans.
- African Americans with Crohn's disease have more prominent joint symptoms and possibly more perianal disease.
- Stressing smoking cessation in patients with Crohn's disease is critical.
- African Americans requiring surgery for Crohn's disease have a greater number of postoperative complications.
- GERD has a similar occurrence in African Americans when compared to European Americans but has a much lower transformation to esophagitis or adenocarcinoma.

(continued)

- Barrett's esophagus has a decreased prevalence in African Americans.
- There is a higher prevalence of *Helicobacter pylori* infections in African Americans.
- There is a marginally decreased risk for gallbladder disease in African Americans when compared to European Americans.
- Sickle cell disease is associated with the formation of gallstones that frequently progress to cholecystitis. Because a sickle cell crisis may present with similar symptoms, prophylactic cholecystectomy should be strongly considered when stones are noted.

References

1. Shaukat A, Kahi CJ, Burke CA, Rabeneck L, Sauer BG, Rex DK. ACG clinical guidelines: colorectal cancer screening 2021. Am J Gastroenterol. 2021;116(3):458–79. https://doi.org/10.14309/ajg.0000000000001122.
2. Bliton JN, et al. Understanding racial disparities in gastrointestinal cancer outcomes: lack of surgery contributes to lower survival in African American patients. Cancer Epidemiol Biomarkers Prev. 2021;30(3):529–38. https://doi.org/10.1158/1055-9965.EPI-20-0950.
3. Bui A, Yang L, Soroudi C, May FP. Racial and ethnic disparities in incidence and mortality for the five most common gastrointestinal cancers in the United States. J Natl Med Assoc. 2022;114(4):426–9.
4. Ouni A, Cardiel Nunez K, Garrett A, Heckman M, Brahmbhatt B, Woodward TA. Disparities in colorectal cancer: trends of reduced screening among minority populations. J Clin Oncol. 2023;41(4_suppl):18. https://doi.org/10.1200/JCO.2023.41.4_suppl.18.
5. Nguyen GC, LaVeist TA, Harris ML, et al. Racial disparities in utilization of specialist care and medications in inflammatory bowel disease. Am J Gastroenterol. 2010;105(10):2202–8.
6. Booth A, Keller E, Forster E, Axon R, Magwood G, Curran T. P068 Racial and Socioeconomic Disparities in Acute Care Utilization in a National Cohort of Veterans With IBD. J Am J Gastroenterol. 2021;116(1):S18. https://doi.org/10.14309/01.ajg.0000798872.15657.44.
7. Burstiner LS, Owings AH, Tacy C, Perez M, Royer A, Hreish Y, Johnson J, Barr M, Laird H, Tarugu S, et al. A focused retrospective study on differences in IBD characteristics between black and white patients in the south. Am J Med Sci. 2023;365(6):488–95.
8. Frieder JS, Montorfano L, De Stefano F, Ortiz Gomez C, Ferri F, Liang H, Gilshtein H, Rosenthal RJ, Wexner SD, Sharp SP. A national inpatient sample analysis of racial disparities after segmental colectomy for inflammatory colorectal diseases. Am Surg. 2023;89(12):5131–9.
9. Bakkila BF, Kerekes D, Nunez-Smith M, Billingsley KG, Ahuja N, Wang K, Oladele C, Johnson CH, Khan SA. Evaluation of racial disparities in quality of care for patients with gastrointestinal tract cancer treated with surgery. JAMA Netw Open. 2022;5(4):e225664.
10. Chey WD, Leontiadis GI, Howden CW, Moss SF. ACG clinical guideline: treatment of helicobacter pylori infection. Am J Gastroenterol. 2017;119(9):1730–53. https://doi.org/10.14309/ajg.0000000000002968.
11. Epplein M, Signorello LB, Zheng W, Peek RM Jr, Michel A, Williams SM, Pawlita M, Correa P, Cai Q, Blot WJ. Race, African ancestry, and helicobacter pylori infection in a low-income United States population. Cancer Epidemiol Biomarkers Prev. 2011;20(5):826–34.

12. Forde KA, Tanapanpanit O, Reddy KR. Hepatitis B and C in African Americans: current status and continued challenges. Clin Gastroenterol Hepatol. 2014;12(5):738–48.
13. Kim HS, Rotundo L, Yang JD, Kim D, Kothari N, Feurdean M, Ruhl C, Unalp-arida A. Racial/ethnic disparities in the prevalence and awareness of hepatitis B virus infection and immunity in the United States. J Viral Hepat. 2017;24(11):1052–66.
14. Jones P, Soler J, Solle NS, Martin P, Kobetz E. A mixed-methods approach to understanding perceptions of hepatitis B and hepatocellular carcinoma among ethnically diverse black communities in South Florida. Cancer Causes Control. 2020;31:1079–91.
15. Weng MK, et al. Universal Hepatitis B vaccination in adults aged 19–59 years: updated recommendations of the advisory committee on immunization practices – United States 2022. MMWR. 2022;71(13):477–83. https://doi.org/10.15585/mmwr.mm7113a1.
16. Liu JK, Kam LY, Huang DQ, Henry L, Cheung R, Nguyen MH. Racial and ethnic disparities in characteristics and care patterns of chronic hepatitis B patients in the United States. Clin Gastroenterol Hepatol. 2023;21(10):2606–15.
17. Wasley A, Kruszon-Moran D, Kuhnert W, Simard EP, Finelli L, McQuillan G, et al. The prevalence of hepatitis B virus infection in the United States in the era of vaccination. J Infect Dis. 2010;202(2):192–201.
18. Carroll KC, Hobden JA, Miller S, Morse SA, Mietzner TA, Detrick B, Mitchell TG, JH MK, Sakanari JA, editors. Hepatitis viruses. In: Jawetz, Melnick, & Adelberg's medical microbiology. New York: McGraw-Hill. p. 27.
19. Khalili M, Leonard KR, Ghany MG, Hassan M, Roberts LR, Sterling RK, Belle SH, Lok AS, Lau DT, Chung RT, Di Bisceglie AM. Racial disparities in treatment initiation and outcomes of chronic hepatitis B virus infection in North America. JAMA Netw Open. 2023;6(4):e237018.
20. Khalesi Z, Razizadeh MH, Javadi M, Bahavar A, Keyvanlou Z, Saadati H, Letafati A, Khatami A, Kachooei A, Khales P, Alborzi E. Global epidemiology of HBV infection among hemodialysis patients: a systematic review and meta-analysis. Microb Pathog. 2023;179:106080.
21. Hepatitis B. Questions and Answers for the Public. Centers for Disease Control and Prevention. https://www.cdc.gov/hepatitis/hbv/bfaq.htm. Accessed 12 May 2019.
22. Forde F. Ethnic disparities in chronic hepatitis B infection: African American and Hispanic Americans. Curr Hepatol Rep. 2017,16(2).105–12.
23. Hennessey KA, Kim AA, Griffin V, et al. Prevalence of infection with hepatitis B and C viruses and co-infection with HIV in three jails: a case for viral hepatitis prevention in jails in the United States. J Urban Health. 2009;86(1):93–105.
24. Statistics Inmate Race. Federal Bureau of Prisons. 2019. https://www.bop.gov/about/statistics/statistics_inmate_race.jsp . Accessed 12 May 2019.
25. Gupta S, Altice FL. Hepatitis B virus infection in US correctional facilities: a review of diagnosis, management, and public health implications. J Urban Health. 2009;86(2):263–79.
26. Leumi S, Bigna JJ, Amougou MA, Ngouo A, Nyaga UF, Noubiap JJ. Global burden of hepatitis B infection in people living with human immunodeficiency virus: a systematic review and meta-analysis. Clin Infect Dis. 2020;71(11):2799–806.
27. Hu DJ, Xing J, Tohme RA, Liao Y, Pollack H, Ward JW, et al. Hepatitis B testing and access to care among racial and ethnic minorities in selected communities across the United States, 2009–2010. Hepatology. 2013;58(3):856–62.
28. Sorrell MF, Belongia EA, Costa J, et al. National institutes of health consensus development conference of hepatitis B. Ann Intern Med. 2009;150(2):104–10.
29. Terrault NA, Bzowej NH, Chang KM, Hwang JP, Jonas MM, Murad MH. A ASLD guidelines for treatment of chronic hepatitis B. Hepatology. 2016;63(1):261–83.
30. Sunbul M. Hepatitis B virus genotypes: global distribution and clinical importance. World J Gastroenterol. 2014;20(18):5427–34.
31. DiBisceglie AM, King WC, Lisker-Melman M, et al. Age, race and viral genotype are associated with the prevalence of hepatitis B antigen in children and adults with chronic hepatitis. J Viral Hepat. 2019;26:856. https://doi.org/10.1111/jvh.13104.

32. Hassan MA, Kim WR, Li R, Smith CI, Fried MW, Sterling RK, Ghany MG, Wahed AS, Ganova-Raeva LM, Roberts LR, Lok AS. Characteristics of US-born versus foreign-born Americans of African descent with chronic hepatitis B. Am J Epidemiol. 2017;186(3):356–66.
33. Thio CL, Carrington M, Marti D, O'Brien SJ, Vlahov D, Nelson KE, Astemborski J, Thomas DL. Class II HLA alleles and hepatitis B virus persistence in African Americans. J Infect Dis. 1999;179(4):1004–6.
34. Thomas R, Thio CL, Apps R, Qi Y, Gao X, Marti D, Stein JL, Soderberg KA, Moody MA, Goedert JJ, Kirk GD. A novel variant marking HLA-DP expression levels predicts recovery from hepatitis B virus infection. J Virol. 2012;86(12):6979–85.
35. Mittal S, Kramer JR, Omino R, Chayanupatkul M, Richardson PA, El-Serag HB, Kanwal F. Role of age and race in the risk of hepatocellular carcinoma in veterans with hepatitis B virus infection. Clin Gastroenterol Hepatol. 2018;16(2):252–9.
36. Denniston MM, Jiles RB, Drobeniuc J, et al. Hepatitis C virus infection in the United States, national health and nutrition examination survey 2003 to 2010. Ann Intern Med. 2014;160(5):293–300.
37. Wilder J, Saraswathula A, Hasselblad V, Muir A. A systematic review of race and ethnicity in hepatitis C clinical trial enrollment. J Natl Med Assoc. 2016;108(1):24–9.
38. Falade-Nwulia O, Kelly SM, Amanor-Boadu S, Nnodum BN, Lim JK, Sulkowski M. Hepatitis C in black individuals in the US: a review. JAMA. 2023;330(22):2200–8.
39. Conjeevaram HS, Fried MW, Jeffers LJ, et al. Peginterferon and ribavirin treatment in African American and Caucasian American patients with hepatitis C genotype 1. Gastroenterology. 2006;131(2):470–7.
40. Saab S, Jackson C, Nieto J, Francois F. Hepatitis C in African Americans. Am J Gastroenterol. 2014;109(10):1576–84.
41. Talal AH, LaFleur J, Hoop R, et al. Absolute and relative contraindications to pegylated-interferon or ribavirin in the US general patient population with chronic hepatitis C: results from a US database of over 45 000 HCV-infected, evaluated patients. Aliment Pharmacol Ther. 2013;37(4):473–81.
42. Rowan PJ, Tabasi S, Abdul-Latif M, et al. Psychosocial factors are the most common contraindications for antiviral therapy at initial evaluation in veterans with chronic hepatitis C. J Clin Gastroenterol. 2004;38:530–4.
43. Gordon SC, Trudeau S, Li J, Zhou Y, Rupp LB, Holmberg SD, Moorman AC, Spradling PR, Teshale EH, Boscarino JA, Daida YG. Race, age, and geography impact hepatitis C genotype distribution in the United States. J Clin Gastroenterol. 2019;53(1):40–50.
44. Teshale EH, Xing J, Moorman A, et al. Higher all-cause hospitalization among patients with chronic hepatitis C: the chronic Hepatitis C cohort study (CHeCS), 2006–2013. J Viral Hepat. 2016;23(10):748–54.
45. Trooskin SB, Navarro VJ, Winn RJ, et al. Hepatitis C risk assessment, testing and referral for treatment in urban primary care: role of race ethnicity. World J Gastroenterol. 2007;13(7):1074–8.
46. Tran L, Jung J, Feldman R, Riley T III. Disparities in the quality of care for chronic hepatitis C among Medicare beneficiaries. PLoS One. 2022;17(3):e0263913.
47. Khokhar OS, Lewis JH. Reasons why patients infected with chronic hepatitis C virus choose to defer treatment: do they alter their decision with time? Dig Dis Sci. 2007;52(5):1168–76.
48. Borum ML, Igiehon E, Shafa S, et al. African Americans may differ in their reasons for declining hepatitis C therapy compared to non-African Americans. Dig Dis Sci. 2009;54:1604–5.
49. Thomas DL, Astemborski J, Rai RM, et al. The natural history of hepatitis c virus infection: host, viral, and environmental factors. JAMA. 2000;284:450–6.
50. Mir HM, Stepanova M, Afendy M, et al. African Americans are less likely to have clearance of hepatitis C virus infection: the findings from recent U.S. population data. J Clin Gastroenterol. 2012;46(8):e62–5.

51. Sterling RK, Stravitz RT, Luketic VA, et al. A comparison of the spectrum of chronic hepatitis C virus between Caucasians and African Americans. Clin Gastroenterol Hepatol. 2004;2(6):469–73.
52. Crosse K, Umeadi OG, Anania FA, et al. Racial difference in liver inflammation and fibrosis related to chronic hepatitis C. Clin Gastroenterol Hepatol. 2004;2(6):463–8.
53. Kim HS, Shetty PB, Tsavachidis S, Dong J, Amos CI, El-Serag HB, Thrift AP. Admixture mapping in African Americans identifies new risk loci for HCV-related cirrhosis. Clin Gastroenterol Hepatol. 2023;21(4):1023–30.
54. Yee LJ, Tang YM, Kleiner DE, Wang D, Im K, Wahed A, Tong X, Rhodes S, Su X, Whelan RM, Fontana RJ. Myxovirus-1 and protein kinase haplotypes and fibrosis in chronic hepatitis C virus. Hepatology. 2007;46(1):74–83.
55. Bacchetti P, Boylan R, Astemborski J, Shen H, Mehta SH, Thomas DL, Terrault NA, Monto A. Progression of biopsy-measured liver fibrosis in untreated patients with hepatitis C infection: non-Markov multistate model analysis. PLoS One. 2011;6(5):e20104.
56. Marcus JL, Hurley LB, Chamberland S. Disparities in initiation of direct-acting antiviral agents for hepatitis C virus infection in an insured population. Public Health Rep. 2018;133(4):452–60.
57. Sims OT, Guo Y, Shoreibah MG, et al. Short article: alcohol and substance use, race, and insurance status predict nontreatment for hepatitis C virus in the era of direct acting antivirals: a retrospective study in a large urban tertiary center. Eur J Gastroenterol Hepatol. 2017;29(11):12191222.
58. Beck KR, Kim NJ, Khalili M. Direct acting antivirals improve HCV treatment initiation and adherence among underserved African Americans. Ann Hepatol. 2018;17(3):413–8.
59. Estevez J, Yang JD, Leong J, Nguyen P, Giama NH, Zhang N, Ali HA, Lee MH, Cheung R, Roberts L, Schwartz M. Clinical features associated with survival outcome in African-American patients with hepatocellular carcinoma. J Am College Gastroenterol. 2019;114(1):80–8.
60. Rich NE, Carr C, Yopp AC, Marrero JA, Singal AG. Racial and ethnic disparities in survival among patients with hepatocellular carcinoma in the United States: a systematic review and meta-analysis. Clin Gastroenterol Hepatol. 2022;20(2):e267–88.
61. Chikovsky L, Kutuk T, Rubens M, Balda AN, Appel H, Chuong MD, Kaiser A, Hall MD, Contreras J, Mehta MP, Kotecha R. Racial disparities in clinical presentation, surgical procedures, and hospital outcomes among patients with hepatocellular carcinoma in the United States. Cancer Epidemiol. 2023;82:102317.
62. Wagle NS, Park S, Washburn D, Ohsfeldt R, Kum HC, Singal AG. Racial and ethnic disparities in hepatocellular carcinoma treatment receipt in the United States: a systematic review and meta-analysis. Cancer Epidemiol Biomarkers Prev. 2024;33(4):463–70.
63. Patel S, Khalili M, Singal AG, Pinheiro PS, Jones PD, Kim RG, Kode V, Thiemann A, Zhang W, Cheung R, Wong RJ. Significant disparities in hepatocellular carcinoma outcomes by race/ethnicity and sociodemographic factors. Cancer Epidemiol Biomarkers Prev. 2025;34(2):355–65.
64. Franco RA, Fan Y, Jarosek S, Bae S, Galbraith J. Racial and geographic disparities in hepatocellular carcinoma outcomes. Am J Prev Med. 2018;55(5):S40–8.
65. Yu L, Sloane DA, Guo C, Howell CD. Risk factors for primary hepatocellular carcinoma in black and white Americans in 2000. Clin Gastroenterol Hepatol. 2006;4(3):355–60.
66. Kim AK, Singal AG. Health disparities in diagnosis and treatment of hepatocellular carcinoma. Clin Liver Dis (Hoboken). 2015;4(6):143–5.
67. Davila JA, Morgan RO, Richardson PA, et al. Use of surveillance for hepatocellular carcinoma among patients with cirrhosis in the United States. Hepatology. 2010;52:132–41.
68. Chidambaranathan-Reghupaty S, Fisher PB, Sarkar D. Hepatocellular carcinoma (HCC): epidemiology, etiology and molecular classification. Adv Cancer Res. 2021;149:1–61.
69. Shah MM, Meyer BI, Rhee K, NeMoyer RE, Lin Y, Tzeng CW, Jabbour SK, Kennedy TJ, Nosher JL, Kooby DA, Maithel SK. Conditional survival analysis of hepatocellular carcinoma. J Surg Oncol. 2020;122(4):684–90.

70. Longo DL, Augusto V. Hepatocellular Carcinoma. N Engl J Med. 2016;380(15):1450–62. https://doi.org/10.1056/NEJMra1713263.
71. Xu F, et al. Prevalence of inflammatory bowel disease among medicare fee-for-service beneficiaries – United States 2001–2018. MMWR. 2021;70(19):698–701. https://doi.org/10.15585/mmwr.mm7019a2.
72. Aniwan S, Harmsen WS, Tremaine WJ, et al. Incidence of inflammatory bowel disease by race and ethnicity in a population-based inception cohort from 1970 through 2010. Ther Adv Gastroenterol. 2019;12:1756284819827692.
73. Sofia MA, Rubin DT, Hou N, Pekow J. Clinical presentation and disease course of inflammatory bowel disease differs by race in a large tertiary care hospital. Dig Dis Sci. 2014;59(9):2228–35.
74. Brant SR, Okou DT, Simpson CL, Cutler DJ, Haritunians T, Bradfield JP, Chopra P, Prince J, Begum F, Kumar A, Huang C. Genome-wide association study identifies African-specific susceptibility loci in African Americans with inflammatory bowel disease. Gastroenterology. 2017;152(1):206–17.
75. Cordero RY, Cordero JB, Stiemke AB, Datta LW, Buyske S, Kugathasan S, McGovern DP, Brant SR, Simpson CL. Trans-ancestry, Bayesian meta-analysis discovers 20 novel risk loci for inflammatory bowel disease in an African American, east Asian and European cohort. Hum Mol Genet. 2023;32(5):873–82.
76. McQuaid KR. Gastrointestinal disorders. In: Papadakis MA, McPhee SJ, Rabow MW, editors. Current medical diagnosis & treatment. New York: McGraw-Hill; 2019.
77. Bertha M, Vasantharoopan A, Kumar A, et al. IBD serology and disease outcomes in African Americans with Crohn's disease. Inflamm Bowel Dis. 2018;24(1):209–16.
78. Nguyen GC, Torres EA, Regueiro M, et al. Inflammatory bowel disease characteristics among African Americans, Hispanics, and non-Hispanic whites: characterization of a large north American cohort. Am J Gastroenterol. 2006;101(5):1012–23.
79. Jackson JF III, Dhere T, Sitaraman S, Repaka A, Shaukat A. Crohn's disease in an African-American population. Am J Med Sci. 2008;336(5):389–92.
80. Barnes EL, Kochar B, Long MD, Pekow J, Ananthakrishnan A, Anyane-Yeboa A, Martin C, Galanko J, Herfarth HH, Kappelman MD, Sandler RS. Lack of difference in treatment patterns and clinical outcomes between black and white patients with inflammatory bowel disease. Inflamm Bowel Dis. 2018;24(12):2634–40.
81. Walker C, Allamneni C, Orr J, Yun H, Fitzmorris P, Xie F, Malik TA. Socioeconomic status and race are both independently associated with increased hospitalization rate among Crohn's disease patients. Sci Rep. 2018;8(1):4028.
82. To N, Gracie DJ, Ford AC. Systematic review with meta-analysis: the adverse effects of tobacco smoking on the natural history of Crohn's disease. Aliment Pharmacol Ther. 2016;43(5):549–61.
83. Lichtenstein GR, Loftus EV, Isaacs KL, Regueiro MD, Gerson LB, Sands BE. ACG clinical guideline: management of Crohn's disease in adults. J Am College Gastroenterol. 2018;113(4):481–517.
84. Farraye FA, Melmed GY, Lichtenstein GR, Kane SV. ACG clinical guideline: preventive care in inflammatory bowel disease. J Am College Gastroenterol. 2017;112(2):241–58.
85. McFalls C, Chaaban L, Melia J. Black race is associated with decreased exposure to advanced therapies and worse outcomes in individuals with ulcerative colitis. Aliment Pharmacol Ther. 2025;61(3):513–23.
86. Moore L, Gaffney K, Lopez R, Shen B. Comparison of the natural history of ulcerative colitis in African Americans and non-Hispanic Caucasians: a historical cohort study. Inflamm Bowel Dis. 2012;18(4):743–9.
87. Booth A, Keller E, Forster E, Axon R, Magwood G, Curran T. P068 racial and socioeconomic disparities in acute care utilization in a national cohort of veterans with IBD. J Am College Gastroenterol. 2021;116:S18.

88. Degenhardt F, Mayr G, Wendorff M, Boucher G, Ellinghaus E, Ellinghaus D, ElAbd H, Rosati E, Hübenthal M, Juzenas S, Abedian S. Transethnic analysis of the human leukocyte antigen region for ulcerative colitis reveals not only shared but also ethnicity-specific disease associations. Hum Mol Genet. 2021;30(5):356–69.
89. Wang Y, Tong J, Chang B, Wang BF, Zhang D, Wang BY. Genetic polymorphisms in the IL-18 gene and ulcerative colitis risk: a meta-analysis. DNA Cell Biol. 2014;33(7):438–47.
90. Arsoniadis EG, Ho YY, Melton GB, Madoff RD, et al. African Americans and short-term outcomes after surgery for Crohn's disease: an ACS-NSQIP analysis. J Crohns Colitis. 2017;11(4):468–73.
91. Marques IC, Theiss LM, Wood LN, Gunnells DJ, Hollis RH, Hardiman KM, Cannon JA, Morris MS, Kennedy GD, Chu DI. Racial disparities exist in surgical outcomes for patients with inflammatory bowel disease. Am J Surg. 2021;221(4):668–74.
92. Ore AS, Vigna C, Fabrizio A, Messaris E. Evaluation of racial/ethnic disparities in the surgical management of inflammatory bowel disease. J Gastrointest Surg. 2022;26(12):2559–68.
93. El-Serag HB, Petersen NJ, Carter J, et al. Gastroesophageal reflux among different racial groups in the United States. Gastroenterology. 2004;126(7):1692–9.
94. Sharma P, Wani S, Romero Y, Johnson D, Hamilton F. Racial and geographic issues in gastroesophageal reflux disease. J Am College Gastroenterol. 2008;103(11):2669–80.
95. Vega KJ, Chisholm S, Jamal MM. Comparison of reflux esophagitis and its complications between African Americans and non-Hispanic whites. World J Gastroenterol. 2009;15(23):2878.
96. Natalini J, Palit A, Sankineni A, Friedenberg FK. Diabetes mellitus is an independent risk for gastroesophageal reflux disease among urban African Americans. Dis Esophagus. 2015;28(5):405–11.
97. Friedenberg FK, Makipour K, Palit A, Shah S, Vanar V, Richter JE. Population-based assessment of heartburn in urban Black Americans. Dis Esophagus. 2013;26(6):561–9.
98. Rustgi AK, El-Serag HB. Esophageal carcinoma. N Engl J Med. 2014;371(26):2499–509.
99. Wang SM, Freedman ND, Katki HA, Matthews C, Graubard BI, Kahle LL, Abnet CC. Gastroesophageal reflux disease: a risk factor for laryngeal squamous cell carcinoma and esophageal squamous cell carcinoma in the NIH-AARP Diet and Health Study cohort. Cancer. 2021;127(11):1871–9.
100. Wu G, Liu Y, Ning D, Zhao M, Li X, Chang L, Hu Q, Li Y, Cheng L, Huang Y. Unraveling the causality between gastroesophageal reflux disease and increased cancer risk: evidence from the UK biobank and GWAS consortia. BMC Med. 2024;22(1):323.
101. Alkaddour A, McGaw C, Hritani R, et al. Protective propensity of race or environmental features in the development of Barrett's esophagus in African Americans – a single center pilot study. J Natl Med Assoc. 2019;111(2):198–201.
102. Nguyen TH, Thrift AP, Ramsey D, Green L, Shaib YH, Graham DY, El-Serag HB. Risk factors for Barrett's esophagus compared between African Americans and non-Hispanic whites. J Am College Gastroenterol. 2014;109(12):1870–80.
103. Alkaddour A, McGaw C, Hritani R, et al. African American ethnicity is not associated with development of Barrett's esophagus after erosive esophagitis. Dig Liver Dis. 2015;47(10):853–6.
104. Wang A, Shaukat A, Acosta RD, Bruining DH, Chandrasekhara V, Chathadi KV, Eloubeidi MA, Fanelli RD, Faulx AL, Fonkalsrud L, Gurudu SR. Race and ethnicity considerations in GI endoscopy. Gastrointest Endosc. 2015;82(4):593–9.
105. Qumseya B, Sultan S, Bain P, Jamil L, Jacobson B, Anandasabapathy S, Agrawal D, Buxbaum JL, Fishman DS, Gurudu SR, Jue TL. ASGE guideline on screening and surveillance of Barrett's esophagus. Gastrointest Endosc. 2019;90(3):335–59.
106. Rubenstein JH, Omidvari AH, Lauren BN, Hazelton WD, Lim F, Tan SX, Kong CY, Lee M, Ali A, Hur C, Inadomi JM. Endoscopic screening program for control of esophageal adenocarcinoma in varied populations: a comparative cost-effectiveness analysis. Gastroenterology. 2022;163(1):163–73.

107. Sun X, Chandar AK, Canto MI, Thota PN, Brock M, Shaheen NJ, Beer DG, Wang JS, Falk GW, Iyer PG, Abrams JA. Genomic regions associated with susceptibility to Barrett's esophagus and esophageal adenocarcinoma in African Americans: the cross BETRNet admixture study. PLoS One. 2017;12(10):e0184962.
108. Ferrer-Torres D, Nancarrow DJ, Steinberg H, Wang Z, Kuick R, Weh KM, Mills RE, Ray D, Ray P, Lin J, Chang AC. Constitutively higher level of GSTT2 in esophageal tissues from African Americans protects cells against DNA damage. Gastroenterology. 2019;156(5):1404–15.
109. Grad Y, Lipsitch M, Aiello AE. Secular trends in *helicobacter pylori* seroprevalence in adults in the United States: evidence for sustained race/ethnic disparities. Am J Epidemiol. 2012;175(1):54–9.
110. Parsonnet J. The incidence of *helicobacter pylori* infection. Aliment Pharmacol Ther. 1995;9(suppl 2):45–51.
111. Shah SC, Halvorson AE, Lee D, Bustamante R, McBay B, Gupta R, Denton J, Dorn C, Wilson O, Peek R Jr, Gupta S. Helicobacter pylori burden in the United States according to individual demographics and geography: a nationwide analysis of the veterans healthcare system. Clin Gastroenterol Hepatol. 2024;22(1):42–50.
112. Nguyen T, Ramsey D, Graham D, et al. The prevalence of *helicobacter pylori* remains high in African Americans and Hispanic veterans. Helicobacter. 2015;20(4):305–15.
113. McNulty SL, Mole BM, Dailidiene D, Segal I, Ally R, Mistry R, Secka O, Adegbola RA, Thomas JE, Lenarcic EM, Peek RM Jr. Novel 180-and 480-base-pair insertions in African and African-American strains of helicobacter pylori. J Clin Microbiol. 2004;42(12):5658–63.
114. de Sena-Reis JS, Bezerra DD, Figueiredo CA, Barreto ML, Alcântara-Neves NM, da Silva TM. Relationship between African biogeographical ancestry and helicobacter pylori infection in children of a large Latin American urban center. Helicobacter. 2019;24(6):e12662.
115. Chey WD, Leontiadis GI, Howden CW, Moss SF. ACG clinical guideline: treatment of helicobacter pylori infection. J Am College Gastroenterol. 2017;112(2):212–39.
116. Kumar S, Metz DC, Ellenberg S, Kaplan DE, Goldberg DS. Risk factors and incidence of gastric cancer after detection of helicobacter pylori infection: a large cohort study. Gastroenterology. 2020;158(3):527–36.
117. Everhart JE, Khare M, Hill M, Maurer KR. Prevalence and ethnic differences in gallbladder disease in the United States. Gastroenterology. 1999;117(3):632–9.
118. Shenoy R, Kirkland P, Jackson N, DeVirgilio M, Zingmond D, Russell MM, Maggard-Gibbons M. Identifying vulnerable populations with symptomatic cholelithiasis at risk for increased health care utilization. J Trauma Acute Care Surg. 2022;93(6):863–71.
119. Nguyen GC, Tuskey A, Jagannath SB. Racial disparities in cholecystectomy rates during hospitalizations for acute gallstone pancreatitis: a national survey. J Am College Gastroenterol. 2008;103(9):2301–7.
120. Raza SA, da Costa WL, Thrift AP. Increasing incidence of gallbladder cancer among non-Hispanic blacks in the United States: a birth cohort phenomenon. Cancer Epidemiol Biomarkers Prev. 2022;31(7):1410–7.
121. Stinton LM, Shaffer EA. Epidemiology of gallbladder disease: cholelithiasis and cancer. Gut Liver. 2012;6(2):172–87.
122. Figueiredo JC, Haiman C, Porcel J, et al. Sex and ethnic/racial-specific risk factors for gallbladder disease. BMC Gastroenterol. 2017;17(1):153.
123. Joshi AD, Andersson C, Buch S, Stender S, Noordam R, Weng LC, Weeke PE, Auer PL, Boehm B, Chen C, Choi H, et al. Four susceptibility loci for gallstone disease identified in a meta-analysis of genome-wide association studies. Gastroenterology. 2016;151(2):351–63.
124. Nassir R, Qi L, Kosoy R, Garcia L, Robbins J, Seldin MF. Relationship between gallbladder surgery and ethnic admixture in African American and Hispanic American women. J Am College Gastroenterol. 2012;107(6):932–40.

Chapter 12
Stress, Mental Illness, Sleep, and Substance Abuse in African Americans

Contents

12.1	Stress		241
	12.1.1	Less Educational Opportunities	242
	12.1.2	More Unemployment	242
	12.1.3	Less Household Income	243
	12.1.4	Systemic Pressure	243
	12.1.5	Stress-Induced Inflammation	243
	12.1.6	Stress Leads to Obesity	244
	12.1.7	Stress and Cancer	244
	12.1.8	Stress and Cardiometabolic Disease	245
12.2	Mental Illness		245
	12.2.1	Depression	247
	12.2.2	Biased Mental Health Diagnoses	250
	12.2.3	Heart Rate Variability, Mental Illness and Stress	251
12.3	Increased Exposure to Death		252
12.4	Sleep Differences		253
12.5	Alcohol and Drug Use		254
References			256

12.1 Stress

Stress is a state of mental or emotional strain or tension resulting from adverse or demanding circumstances. It can manifest physically, emotionally, and behaviorally, affecting overall well-being. Stress significantly impacts the health of African Americans, deeply intertwined with various socioeconomic and environmental factors. Chronic stressors such as racial discrimination, economic disparity, and community violence contribute to heightened psychological and physical health issues within this community [1, 2]. For instance, experiences of systemic racism can lead to increased rates of anxiety and depression, while financial insecurity results in chronic stress that exacerbates health conditions like hypertension and cardiovascular disease, which already disproportionately affect African Americans. Additionally, these stressors can lead to unhealthy coping mechanisms, such as substance abuse or avoidance behaviors, further deteriorating health outcomes. Access to healthcare also poses a challenge, as economic barriers and a history of distrust in the medical system can limit the ability to seek timely care for stress-related conditions [3–5].

12.1.1 Less Educational Opportunities

Educational attainment and labor force participation significantly contribute to the stress experienced by African Americans, with systemic barriers exacerbating these challenges [6–8]. Many African Americans face inequities in access to quality education, resulting in lower high school graduation rates and underrepresentation in higher education institutions compared to the majority population. This educational gap limits job opportunities and career advancement, leading to financial stress as individuals often struggle to secure stable, well-paying jobs. In the labor market, African Americans encounter discrimination that affects hiring and promotional prospects, with studies indicating that resumes with traditionally African American-sounding names receive fewer callbacks, despite equivalent qualifications [9]. This systemic bias contributes to higher unemployment rates and job insecurity within the community. Many African Americans are employed in low-wage positions that lack benefits and protections, creating additional economic pressures, insecurity, and chronic stress [10]. The cumulative effect of these educational and employment challenges not only impacts financial stability but also heightens the occurrence of both mental and physical health issues.

12.1.2 More Unemployment

Unemployment rates among African Americans consistently exceed those of other racial/ethnic groups, reflecting a complex web of systemic barriers and economic challenges. For instance, as of 2023, the unemployment rate for African Americans was approximately 6.4%, compared to a national average of around 3.7% [10]. Young African Americans face even steeper obstacles, with youth unemployment rates often exceeding 30% [11]. Additionally, educational disparities play a crucial role, as many African Americans attend underfunded schools that limit access to quality education and higher-paying job opportunities. Economic downturns, such as those experienced during the COVID-19 pandemic, disproportionately impact African American communities, leading to higher rates of unemployment and slower recovery. The consequences of this persistent unemployment include economic instability, housing and food insecurity, and increased mental health challenges.

12.1.3 Less Household Income

African American households often experience lower income levels, with the median income around $56,000 compared to the national median of approximately $80,000, reflecting systemic barriers such as discrimination in hiring and limited access to quality education [12]. This financial disparity is further exacerbated by the high prevalence of single-parent households within the African American community, where over 64% of African American children live with single parents [13]. The economic challenges faced by these single parents, who typically rely on a single income, can lead to chronic financial stress, making it difficult to meet basic needs like housing, healthcare, and education. This constant strain can result in illness, both mental and physical.

12.1.4 Systemic Pressure

Arrest rates in the USA reveal significant disparities that contribute to heightened stress levels among African Americans. Despite making up approximately 13% of the US population, African Americans account for a disproportionately high percentage of arrests, particularly for drug-related offenses and violent crimes [14–16]. For example, African Americans are arrested at rates nearly three times higher than their European American counterparts [15]. This systemic over-policing not only leads to higher incarceration rates but also perpetuates a cycle of stress and trauma within the community. The constant threat of arrest, along with negative interactions with law enforcement, fosters an environment of fear and anxiety, which can exacerbate mental health issues [16]. Furthermore, the stigma associated with arrest and incarceration can lead to social isolation, economic instability, and diminished opportunities for employment and education, compounding the stress experienced by individuals and families. The psychological toll of living under such conditions can manifest in chronic stress, contributing to various physical health issues, such as hypertension and heart disease.

12.1.5 Stress-Induced Inflammation

Stress-induced inflammation in African Americans is influenced by a complex interplay of genetic predispositions, epigenetic modifications, and social stressors, which collectively heighten the risk of inflammation-related diseases. Research indicates that certain genetic factors may predispose individuals to inflammatory responses, making them more susceptible to the health impacts of chronic stress [2, 3]. Moreover, epigenetic modifications—changes in gene expression triggered by environmental factors—can occur in response to prolonged stress, further exacerbating inflammation. Social stressors, such as racial discrimination, economic hardship, and community violence, contribute significantly to this inflammatory response by activating the body's stress response systems. For instance, experiences of systemic racism can lead to chronic psychological stress, which is linked to the release of pro-inflammatory cytokines in the body [4, 5]. Chronic stress triggers the activation of the hypothalamic-pituitary-adrenal (HPA) axis and the sympathetic-adrenal-medullary (SAM) axis, resulting in the release of key hormones such as glucocorticoids and catecholamines. These hormones play a crucial role in the body's stress response, modulating various physiological functions, including immune function. However, prolonged exposure to elevated levels of these hormones can lead to glucocorticoid receptor resistance (GCR), which impairs the body's ability to effectively regulate inflammation [2]. This dysregulation creates a persistent pro-inflammatory state, whereby the immune system remains in a heightened state of alertness. This heightened inflammatory state is associated with an increased prevalence of conditions such as hypertension, diabetes, and cardiovascular diseases, as well as the exacerbation of asthma, rheumatic diseases, inflammatory bowel disease, and more [1, 17–19].

12.1.6 Stress Leads to Obesity

The relationship between stress and obesity is particularly pronounced among African Americans, where systemic factors contribute to both chronic stress and higher obesity rates [2, 20]. African Americans often face multiple stressors, including economic disparities, racial discrimination, and community violence, which can lead to emotional eating and unhealthy coping mechanisms [21]. For instance, individuals may turn to high-calorie comfort foods as a way to manage stress, which can contribute to weight gain over time. Additionally, the stress hormone cortisol is linked to increased fat accumulation, particularly in the abdominal area, exacerbating obesity-related health issues such as diabetes and cardiovascular disease, which disproportionately affect this community [2]. Socioeconomic factors also play a role; many African Americans reside in food deserts with limited access to healthy food options, making it challenging to maintain a balanced diet. Furthermore, cultural perceptions of body image influence health behaviors, with some individuals viewing higher body weight as acceptable or even desirable [22].

12.1.7 Stress and Cancer

Stress is increasingly recognized as a potential factor related to both cancer risk and recurrence, although it is not a direct cause of cancer. Research suggests that chronic stress can influence biological processes that may contribute to cancer development and progression [23–26]. For instance, prolonged stress can weaken the immune system, making it less effective at detecting and eliminating cancer cells, which increases the likelihood of cancer recurrence after treatment [23]. Additionally, stress is associated with elevated levels of inflammation in the body, which has been linked to tumor growth and metastasis. Psychological factors play a significant role as well; individuals experiencing high levels of stress may engage in unhealthy coping behaviors, such as poor diet, inactivity, and substance abuse, which can adversely affect overall health and treatment outcomes. Studies have shown that cancer survivors with heightened stress or anxiety may face a greater risk of recurrence, particularly in cases like breast and colorectal cancer [23, 25].

12.1.8 Stress and Cardiometabolic Disease

Last but certainly not least, stress is a significant contributing factor to the prevalence of cardiometabolic conditions among African Americans, who experience higher rates of hypertension, diabetes, and cardiovascular disease compared to other racial groups. Chronic stress activates the hypothalamic-pituitary-adrenal (HPA) axis and the sympathetic nervous system, leading to elevated levels of cortisol and catecholamines. This persistent activation results in increased blood pressure and vascular resistance, contributing to the development of hypertension [2]. Additionally, the cumulative effects of stress can lead to a pro-inflammatory state, which is associated with the onset of conditions like atherosclerosis and metabolic syndrome [2, 3]. The stress-induced activation of the HPA axis and the sympathetic nervous system also affects glucose metabolism. Elevated cortisol levels promote gluconeogenesis and insulin resistance, increasing the risk of type 2 diabetes [2, 27, 28]. Additionally, chronic stress can lead to unhealthy behaviors such as poor diet and physical inactivity, further exacerbating diabetes risk [27, 28]. Given these interconnections, effective stress management strategies are crucial in addressing the cardiometabolic health disparities faced by African Americans. By tackling the root causes of stress and promoting healthier behaviors, it is possible to improve health outcomes and reduce the burden of cardiometabolic diseases within this community. Furthermore, fostering a sense of community and belonging can enhance mental well-being, which in turn positively impacts physical health. By addressing the social determinants of health and implementing targeted interventions, we can work toward a more equitable and healthier future for African Americans.

12.2 Mental Illness

The mental health outcomes by race/ethnicity would suggest that African Americans have fewer overall. But this assertion, particularly in terms of anxiety, depression, and suicide, is a complex issue that warrants careful consideration. Research indicates that African Americans report lower rates of certain mental health disorders, including major depressive disorder and anxiety, than their European American counterparts [29]. However, these statistics can be misleading due to a variety of factors. Cultural perceptions surrounding mental health play a significant role; in many African American communities, there is a stigma attached to mental illness, which can lead to underreporting and reluctance to seek help. Additionally, access to mental health services is often limited for African Americans due to socioeconomic barriers, lack of insurance, and a scarcity of culturally congruent providers in their communities [30, 31]. This results in untreated mental health issues that may not be reflected in prevalence data. Stigma can significantly deter individuals from seeking mental health treatment, as they may fear being judged or misunderstood. This fear is often compounded by concerns over confidentiality and the belief that mental health issues should be managed privately or within the family. Consequently, many African Americans might choose to endure their struggles in silence rather than accessing professional help, perpetuating a cycle of untreated mental health conditions. Figure 12.1 shows the most recent data for major depressive disorder by race/ethnicity [32].

African American men are less likely to seek the help of a psychiatric professional than European American men, and their presentation can be different. Sidney Hankerson at Columbia University looked at treatment disparities among African American men and made the following observations:

> Racial and gender differences in depressive symptomatology may contribute to the misdiagnosis of depression among African American men. The core symptoms of MDD (major depressive disorder) are remarkably consistent across cultures, however, African Americans with MDD are more likely to have somatic symptoms (e.g., sleep disturbance or pain)

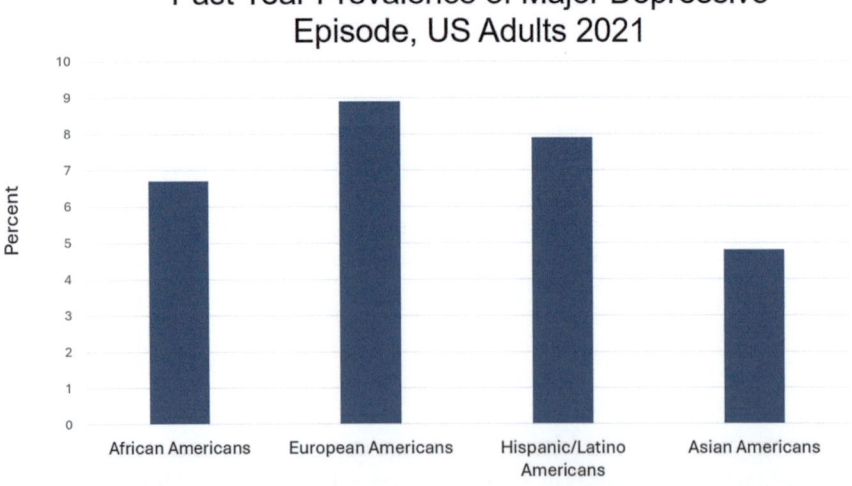

Fig. 12.1 Prevalence of major depression in US adults by race/ethnicity. National Institute of Mental Health https://www.nimh.nih.gov/health/statistics/major-depression

compared to (European) Americans with MDD. African Americans' somatization of emotional problems may make it difficult for primary care physicians to detect clinical depression. Researchers have increasingly studied a "male depressive syndrome" to describe how men experience and express depression. Depressed men, compared with women, are more likely to exhibit irritability, anger attacks, and abusive behavior. Men may be more likely to engage in externalizing behaviors, such as substance abuse and over-working, as a way to cope with depressive episodes. These gender differences in symptom presentation may lead to under-detection and misdiagnosis. [33]

12.2.1 Depression

Depression can frequently lead to suicide, and Fig. 12.2 shows a surprising disparity with African Americans showing a much lower overall rate. Statistical data indicates that while the overall suicide rate for African Americans has historically been lower—approximately 6.9 per 100,000 in 2020 compared to 14.1 per 100,000 for European Americans—this gap has begun to narrow in recent years [34]. Several factors contribute to this lower risk, including strong cultural and community ties, which provide essential support through extended families and religious organizations. These connections foster resilience and a sense of belonging, acting as protective factors against suicidal ideation [35, 36]. Additionally, African Americans often employ unique coping strategies, such as relying on spirituality and community engagement, which can help mitigate feelings of isolation and despair [35, 37, 38]. However, it is important to recognize that the stigma surrounding mental health can lead to the underreporting of suicidal thoughts, potentially resulting in lower recorded rates. Emerging trends indicate a concerning rise in suicide rates among

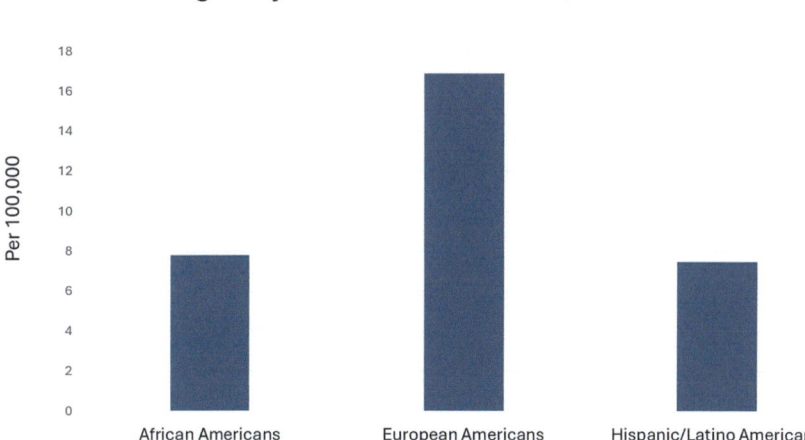

Fig. 12.2 Suicide rates by race/ethnicity. (National Center for Health Statistics, https://www.cdc.gov/nchs/products/databriefs/db450.htm [34])

young African Americans, particularly adolescents, highlighting the urgent need for targeted mental health interventions.

Socioeconomic status (SES) significantly affects the prevalence of major depressive disorder among different races and ethnicities. Lower SES, characterized by lower income, education, and fewer assets, is associated with higher rates of depression across all racial and ethnic groups [39, 40]. African Americans generally have fewer socioeconomic assets compared to European Americans, which contributes to higher unadjusted rates of depression. However, when SES factors are controlled, African Americans exhibit lower odds of probable depression. This suggests that SES disparities play a crucial role in the observed differences in depression rates [39, 41, 42]. Education, income, and employment status are key SES markers that influence depression prevalence. For instance, lower income and fewer years worked are strongly associated with higher depressive symptoms among African Americans. Additionally, neighborhood SES impacts depression rates, with lower neighborhood SES correlating with higher depressive symptoms among African Americans [39, 41, 42]. The interaction between race/ethnicity and SES is complex. For example, European Americans with lower SES exhibit higher rates of depression compared to their higher SES counterparts, while the protective effect of higher SES is more pronounced among African Americans [39, 41, 42].

Some of the "under-detection" of depression and other mood disorders is provider-driven and has its roots in bias. African Americans are disproportionately more diagnosed with schizophrenia and other psychotic disorders while less often diagnosed with mood disorders like depression and anxiety [33]. Cultural mistrust of medical providers is frequently attributed to paranoia rather than a variation in perspective [43]. Derek Suite and colleagues wrote about this phenomenon:

> ... it may not be readily apparent to the treatment provider who interacts with a person of color that more than 200 years' worth of anecdotal and documentary evidence on racism in medicine and mental health cuts across age, gender and different racial/ethnic groups, leading to a high degree of vigilance, mistrust and disdain towards the medical establishment in general and mental health in particular. [44]

Arthur Whaley looked at the impact of gender- and race-matching patients and providers and found increased diagnostic accuracy when an African American male provider assessed an African American male patient with a strong racial identity [43]. The shared history (and reality) between race-matched providers and patients allowed for improved connections.

Researchers also noted that African Americans have higher stress levels than European Americans [45]. Having higher stress levels yet lower major depressive episodes forms the basis for another racial paradox:

> Major epidemiologic studies in the US reveal a consistent "paradox" by which psychiatric outcomes such as major depressive disorder (MDD) are less prevalent among (African Americans) relative to (European Americans), despite greater exposure to social and economic stressors and worse physical health outcomes. A second paradox, which has received less attention and has never been systematically documented, is the discrepancy between these patterns and (African American-European American) comparisons in psychological distress, which reveal consistently higher levels among (African Americans). [45]

12.2 Mental Illness

As scholars try to understand why African Americans, with all of the increased disease and premature death, would have a lower psychiatric burden, an array of theories have been proposed. Keep in mind that these theories are merely hypotheses that have yet to be confirmed or refuted. Like anything in medicine, sometimes the best answer is "it is what it is" … just as African Americans bear an increased burden in the kidney and cardiovascular disease, they show an overall decreased burden psychiatrically. Since other theories were advanced for why other disease burdens exist, it is also fair to look at postulates here.

Jackson and colleagues at the University of Michigan proposed that increased stress leads to unhealthy coping mechanisms (like drug use) that protect against severe mental illness but adds to morbidity and premature mortality [46]:

> Thus, we hypothesize that when individuals are chronically confronted with stressful conditions in daily life (e.g., poverty, crime, poor housing), they will engage in unhealthy behaviors (e.g., smoking, alcohol use and abuse, drug use, and overeating, especially of comfort foods) that help to alleviate the resulting symptoms of stress. However, these same behaviors silently contribute to physical health morbidities and early mortality. [46]

Their hypothesis suggests that by activating the hypothalamic axis through alcohol, smoking, pleasure foods, illegal stimulants, and other illicit drugs, African Americans directly alleviate the symptoms of the stressor but also do irreparable damage to their long-term physical health:

> (African) American women show heightened rates of obesity over the life course. Overeating is an effective, early, well-learned response to chronic environmental stressors that only strengthens over the life course. In contrast, for a variety of social and cultural reasons, (African) American men's coping choices and trajectories are different from that of (African American) women's. Early in life, (African American) men tend to lead active, athletic lives, but in middle age the viability and effectiveness of this dopamine-producing coping strategy is reduced because of physical deterioration. It is at middle age that (African American) men begin to show increased rates of smoking, alcohol consumption, and illicit drug use. [47]

Other studies relating to mental health in African Americans confirm the increased incidence of having concurrent chronic physical health conditions (cardiovascular disease or diabetes) in addition to existing mood or anxiety disorders. African Americans have increased comorbidities, so it is also understandable that if there is mental illness, comorbidities would coexist as well.

The legitimacy of Jackson's theory would hold better if there were confirmed higher substance use and abuse in African Americans, but there is not [48–50]. Leah Wilty at Northwestern University looked at drug and alcohol use disorders in youths over a 12-year period:

> We found striking racial/ethnic differences. Contrary to popular stereotypes of African Americans, the prevalence of drug-use disorders such as cocaine and hallucinogen or PCP was lowest among African Americans, followed by Hispanics, then non-Hispanic Whites. For example, non-Hispanic Whites had more than 30 times the odds of having cocaine-use disorder than African Americans. [51]

The disparities in illicit drug use shrink as African Americans age, but related suicides and personal impact from drugs remain higher in European Americans.

Despite the lower prevalence of depression in African Americans, there are still significant areas of concern. When African Americans have depression, the symptoms are more severe and persistent and usually go untreated [52]. Williams and colleagues at the Institute for Social Research at the University of Michigan looked at depression in African Americans, Caribbean-born African Americans, and European Americans and summarized their findings:

> We found that both black populations with MDD (major depressive disorder) were overrepresented among persons with very severe impairment, with African Americans having higher levels than Caribbean blacks on some indicators of impairment. Blacks with severe impairment, irrespective of ethnicity, reported substantially more days out of role than the national average for persons with MDD. These data suggest that when blacks develop MDD, it is likely debilitating in impact and persistent in its course. It is important to find out why blacks who develop this illness have a poorer prognosis than their white counterparts. These findings also emphasize the need for the treatment of blacks with MDD. In the United States, 57% of adults with MDD receive treatment, but we found that most blacks with MDD, irrespective of ethnicity, do not receive treatment. Only 48% of African Americans and 22% of Caribbean blacks with severe symptoms received treatment. [53]

As providers, remember to keep depression in mind as a driver for a number of other complaints that African American patients may report. Suggest that insomnia, fatigue, overeating, and an array of other complaints may be a manifestation of depression. Trust, time, and education will help them agree to treatment.

12.2.2 Biased Mental Health Diagnoses

As alluded to earlier, African Americans are much more likely to be diagnosed with a schizophrenia-spectrum diagnosis (psychoses) than an affective diagnosis (depression, bipolar, anxiety) when compared to European Americans [54–56]. Schizophrenia is a chronic and severe mental health disorder characterized by disruptions in thought processes, perceptions, emotional responsiveness, and social interactions. Individuals with schizophrenia may experience a range of symptoms, including hallucinations (often hearing voices), delusions (firmly held false beliefs), disorganized thinking, and impaired functioning in daily life [57]. Schwartz and colleagues explored two possibilities as the cause: epigenetic differences by race or a systematic and consistent error or bias in the diagnostic process:

> The present study found that African Americans were diagnosed with a schizophrenia-spectrum diagnosis at a higher rate than (European American) individuals, which was also evident in the rate of (European American) individuals diagnosed with an affective disorder compared with African Americans. More important, no differences in symptoms were found. [55]

The authors proposed that making a diagnosis is based on a constellation of symptoms, and while the symptoms might be the same between an African American and a European American patient, the final diagnosis involves a "higher level" of reasoning. Diagnoses, they suggest, "reflect a global, overall impression, that includes multiple streams of information including behavioral observation but also historical information and collateral report" [55]. These added "considerations" lead to skewed diagnostic outcomes and lasting stigmatization. These overdiagnosed patients carry the added burden of the diagnosis and the side-effect profile of whatever antipsychotic medication was started.

Your approach to a new patient with a history of schizophrenia may be different from an approach to the same patient with a history of depression; if the patient is African American, consider overdiagnosis as a possibility.

12.2.3 Heart Rate Variability, Mental Illness and Stress

One final hypothesis for dealing with system stressors and mental health challenges is that African Americans employ a "culturally compelled coping" style. Briana Brownlow and colleagues explain:

> The inescapability of structural racism has informed how Black people have historically and presently learned to cope with pervasive racialized stress. Although Black Americans and their experiences are not homogenous, Black individuals are often compelled by the culture of racism inherent in this society to engage in persistent and effortful coping styles, emphasizing inhibition, restraint, and vigilance. In fact, this regulatory style is reflected in other culturally based coping styles (e.g., John Henryism, Superwoman Schema). Both John Henryism and Superwoman Schema emphasize the use of high inhibitory control, emotional and behavioral restraint, and high distress tolerance as a means of navigating a racialized world. Taken at face value, many of the ways that Black Americans cope with racialized stress appear to fit within an "overcontrolled" framework of coping. [58]

This approach to life has mental and physiological implications. "Vigilance and restraint are associated with greater depressive symptoms" as well as increased "heart rate variability" [58].

Heart rate variability (HRV) is an important physiological measure that reflects the body's ability to respond to stress, and it can vary significantly among different populations, including African Americans. Heart rate variability measures how the time between consecutive heartbeats varies. A higher HRV indicates a healthy, adaptable cardiovascular system and a greater ability to respond to stressors. Conversely, a lower HRV is associated with stress, fatigue, and various health issues [59]. As a review, the autonomic nervous system consists of two branches: the sympathetic nervous system and the parasympathetic nervous system. The sympathetic is responsible for the "fight or flight" response, increasing heart rate during stress, whereas the parasympathetic promotes a "rest and digest" state, decreasing heart rate and promoting relaxation. Heart rate variability is a reflection of the balance between these two systems [59]. Research indicates that lower HRV is often associated with higher stress levels and poorer mental health outcomes, which can be particularly relevant in the context of the unique stressors faced by African American communities. These stressors can lead to chronic stress, which negatively impacts HRV [58]. Coping strategies play a crucial role in managing stress and improving heart rate variability; for instance, practices such as mindfulness, deep breathing exercises, and community support can enhance HRV by promoting relaxation and activating the parasympathetic nervous system [58]. Additionally, cultural factors may influence coping mechanisms, as many African Americans may rely on spiritual practices and strong community ties to deal with stressors [60]. Understanding the relationship between HRV, stress, and coping within the African American context is essential for developing culturally sensitive interventions that promote mental well-being and resilience. Focusing on effective coping strategies and fostering supportive environments can improve heart rate variability and overall health outcomes in this community.

12.3 Increased Exposure to Death

One of the more serious life stresses is the death of a family member. African Americans have increased exposure to death and bereavement due to several interrelated factors. Firstly, racial disparities in life expectancy mean that African Americans are more likely to experience the deaths of family members at younger ages compared to other racial and ethnic groups. This includes the death of parents, siblings, children, and spouses from childhood through later life.

Additionally, African Americans face higher rates of premature death due to various causes, including chronic diseases, homicide, and accidents. For example, homicide rates among young African American men are significantly higher, contributing to frequent and early exposure to traumatic loss. Homicide is the number one cause of death in African American males from ages 1–44 [61–63]. This increased exposure to death and bereavement can lead to adverse health outcomes, including higher risks of psychological distress, social isolation, and cardiometabolic conditions. Debra Umberson and colleagues at the University of Texas at Austin outlined the significantly increased exposure to the death of a parent, spouse, or child and its impact on the African American psyche and health [64]:

> This study provides a population-based documentation of earlier and repeated bereavement experiences for (African) Americans, who are more likely to experience the deaths of mothers, fathers, siblings, spouses, and children and to experience multiple family member deaths. Moreover, racial differences in exposure to death of mothers, fathers, and siblings appear early in childhood. By early to mid-adulthood, racial differences in exposure to the death of children and spouses are also significant. Understanding exposure to family deaths from childhood through mid to later life is important because bereavement experiences almost certainly add to cumulative disadvantage in multiple life outcomes. Past research has generally focused on the effects of only one loss on subsequent life outcomes, clearly demonstrating adverse effects of bereavement on socioeconomic status, mental health, health behaviors, physical health, and mortality risk. [64]

The death of only one critical family member has been shown to negatively impact the life course of an individual. African Americans, for medical reasons we have already reviewed, deal with multiple deaths of critical family and friends throughout their lives, burying parents, siblings, spouses, and offspring. The psychiatric burden should be, and is, great, but for "whatever reason" acceptance prevails.

12.4 Sleep Differences

Sleep health disparities among African Americans are a significant health concern, as this population experiences higher rates of sleep disorders. There are sleep differences with African Americans having "shorter sleep duration, greater onset latency, and higher awakening after sleep onset" [65]. There was also a decreased ability to phase shift African Americans' sleep cycles when exposed to jet-lag and shift work situations, and the total duration of the cycle was smaller, a study by Eastman and colleagues at Rush University Medical Center found [66].

These researchers surmised that the differences in sleep architecture grew from thousands of years of genetic modifications resulting from, for Africans, exposure to year-around consistent 12-h light-dark cycles, versus Europeans coming for northern regions with significant variability in the day length, dawn, and dusk times. The shifting circadian periods in non-equatorial regions instilled a genetically modified increased tolerance for variable light-dark productivity hours:

> The magnitude and direction of the phase shift was related to the free-running circadian period, and European-Americans had a longer circadian period than African-Americans. Circadian period was related to the percent Sub-Saharan African and European ancestry from DNA samples. We speculate that a short circadian period was advantageous during our evolution in Africa and lengthened with northern migrations out of Africa. The differences in circadian rhythms remaining today are relevant for understanding and treating the modern circadian-rhythm-based disorders which are due to a misalignment between the internal circadian rhythms and the times for sleep, work, school and meals. [66]

In another study, Eastman exposed African Americans and European Americans to a 9-h delayed light-dark sleep-wake and meal schedule, similar to traveling from Chicago to Japan [67]. Essentially what would take 10 days for full adjustment in European Americans would take 15 days for African Americans to adjust. The need to adjust to time zone changes is only periodic in most people, and there are methods to make this adjustment smoother, but shift work seen in factory workers, police and fire positions, healthcare staff, and other positions place an additional health burden on these workers. Shift working was found to add an additional 40% risk of cardiovascular disease as compared to non-shift work [68].

A study by Halder and colleagues at the University of Pittsburgh found that African genetic ancestry is associated with indices of sleep depth in African Americans, specifically lower percent slow-wave sleep and delta EEG power, suggesting that genetic ancestry influences sleep architecture [69]. Another study identified specific DNA methylation sites associated with daytime sleepiness that were unique to African Americans, indicating potential epigenetic mechanisms [70].

Shift work is more prevalent in the African American community and is associated with worse health outcomes including increased smoking, elevated blood pressures, obesity, increased alcohol use, decreased physical activity, depression, and work stress [71]. Getting a thorough work history and looking for shift work and then counseling and screening for these increased disease propensities can provide a significant benefit for your patient. By incorporating a planned exercise schedule and diet, reaffirming the dangers of smoking (particularly in shift workers), and providing better insight into the social impact of these schedules, many of the detriments of shift work can be tempered. And the few individuals that continually fail to adjust to shift work may find solace in the possible existence of a genetic inability to ever adjust.

12.5 Alcohol and Drug Use

Alcohol consumption among the races, based on the "National Survey on Drug Use and Health" data, range from European Americans at almost 57% using alcohol to a low among Asian Americans at 40%. African American alcohol consumption rests at 44% of the population [72].

In African Americans, the number of underage drinkers is low and there is also low reported heavy on-going alcohol use [73]. A higher number report episodic binge drinking, and this behavior adds to higher social consequences in African Americans. Because of the lower drinking in adolescence, African Americans have fewer earlier age DUIs but catch up later in life and ultimately show higher social consequences of drinking [74]. Particularly, there is a higher male-to-female and female-to-male intimate partner violence reported [75].

One important medical consequence of alcohol in African Americans is liver cirrhosis. African Americans have a greater risk for developing alcohol-related liver disease than European Americans [76]. Additionally, rates of alcohol-related esophageal cancer and pancreatic disease are also higher for African American men than European American men [77].

Drug use among African Americans is a complex issue influenced by various social, economic, and historical factors. Research indicates that African Americans are disproportionately affected by substance use disorders compared to other racial groups, but patterns of drug use can vary significantly [78]. For instance, while crack cocaine use was historically more prevalent in African American communities during the 1980s and 1990s, today, opioid misuse has become a growing concern across all demographics, including African Americans. Cocaine-related treatment admissions and overdose deaths are notably higher among African Americans, particularly men, compared to other racial and ethnic groups [79].

Substance use among African American adolescents is influenced by factors such as racial discrimination and peer pressure, which increase the risk of alcohol and marijuana use. Furthermore, urban stress and environmental factors significantly contribute to substance use among young adult African American men [80]. African Americans often encounter barriers to accessing addiction treatment services due to mistrust of the healthcare system, cultural differences, and a shortage of culturally competent care providers.

Moreover, the criminal justice system has played a significant role in shaping narratives about drug use within African American communities. The "War on Drugs," for instance, has resulted in higher incarceration rates for African Americans,

12.5 Alcohol and Drug Use

affecting not only individuals but also disrupting families and communities. This systemic issue often leads to cycles of addiction and incarceration, further complicating recovery efforts.

Drug overdose death rates among African Americans have been increasing and show significant disparities compared to other racial and ethnic groups. According to recent data, overdose deaths among African Americans rose to 1.4 times the rate seen among European Americans by 2022. This increase is largely driven by the polysubstance use of fentanyl combined with stimulants and other synthetic substances [81].

From 2019 to 2020, drug overdose death rates increased by 44% among African Americans. Specifically, African American males aged ≥65 years had a rate of 52.6 per 100,000, nearly seven times that of European American males of the same age group [82]. Additionally, the opioid epidemic has disproportionately impacted African American communities with cocaine/opioid mortality increasing by 575% from 2007 to 2019 [83].

To address these disparities, it is crucial to implement culturally tailored prevention and treatment programs that resonate with African American communities. Increasing access to healthcare through community-based initiatives and reducing stigma around seeking help can also have a significant impact. Furthermore, reforming policies to emphasize treatment over incarceration for drug-related offenses could help break the cycles of addiction and incarceration.

Stress, Mental Illness, Sleep, and Substance Abuse in African Americans
- Experiences of systemic racism can lead to increased rates of anxiety and depression, while financial insecurity results in chronic stress that exacerbates health conditions like hypertension and cardiovascular disease.
- Stressors can lead to unhealthy coping mechanisms, such as substance abuse or avoidance behaviors, further deteriorating health outcomes.
- Stress-induced inflammation in African Americans is influenced by a complex interplay of genetic predispositions, epigenetic modifications, and social stressors, which collectively heighten the risk of inflammation-related diseases.
- Stress is increasingly recognized as a potential factor related to both cancer risk and recurrence, although it is not a direct cause of cancer.
- Stress is a significant contributing factor to the prevalence of cardiometabolic conditions among African Americans, who experience higher rates of hypertension, diabetes, and cardiovascular disease. It activates the hypothalamic-pituitary-adrenal (HPA) axis and the sympathetic nervous system, leading to elevated levels of cortisol and catecholamines.
- African Americans have fewer mental illnesses with significantly less anxiety, depression, and suicide than other populations.

(continued)

- When African Americans have depression, the symptoms are more severe and persistent and are more resistant to treatment.
- Insomnia, fatigue, overeating, and an array of other complaints may be a manifestation of depression.
- African Americans are much more likely to be diagnosed with a schizophrenia-spectrum diagnosis (psychoses) than an affective diagnosis (depression, bipolar, anxiety) when compared to European Americans.
- Heart rate variability (HRV) is an essential physiological measure that reflects the body's ability to respond to stress. African Americans tend to have a lower HRV, which is associated with higher stress levels and poorer mental health outcomes.
- African Americans have shorter sleep duration, greater onset latency, and higher awakening after sleep onset.
- African Americans have a decreased tolerance for jet lag and shift work.
- Shift work is more prevalent in the African American community and is associated with worse health outcomes including increased smoking, elevated blood pressures, obesity, increased alcohol use, decreased physical activity, depression, and work stress.
- African Americans face a higher risk of developing alcohol-related liver disease, esophageal cancer, and pancreatic disease compared to European Americans.
- Cocaine-related treatment admissions and overdose deaths are notably higher among African Americans, particularly men, compared to other racial and ethnic groups.
- Drug overdose death rates among African Americans have substantially increased over the last 20 years, and it is essential that we address this problem.

References

1. Muscatell KA, Alvarez GM, Bonar AS, Cardenas MN, Galvan MJ, Merritt CC, Starks MD. Brain–body pathways linking racism and health. Am Psychol. 2022;77(9):1049–60. https://doi.org/10.1037/amp0001084.
2. Goosby BJ, Cheadle JE, Colter M. Stress-related biosocial mechanisms of discrimination and African American health inequities. Ann Rev Sociol. 44(1):319–40. https://doi.org/10.1146/annurev-soc-060116-053403.
3. Juliette MC, Chang Katharine J, Michael B, Oltmanns TF, Ryan B. Black-White racial health disparities in inflammation and physical health: cumulative stress social isolation and health behaviors. Psychoneuroendocrinology. 131:105251. https://doi.org/10.1016/j.psyneuen.2021.105251.
4. Simons RL, Man-Kit L, Eric K, Beach Steven RH, Gibbons FX, Philibert RA. The effects of social adversity discrimination and health risk behaviors on the accelerated aging of African Americans: further support for the weathering hypothesis. Soc Sci Med. 282:113169. https://doi.org/10.1016/j.socscimed.2020.113169.

5. Olutosin A, Lavner JA, Carter SE, Beach Steven RH. Stress accumulation depressive symptoms and sleep problems among Black Americans in the rural south. Clin Psychol Sci. 12(3):421–34. https://doi.org/10.1177/21677026231170839.
6. Shervin A, Mohsen B. Unequal associations between educational attainment and occupational stress across racial and ethnic groups. Int J Environ Res Public Health. 2019;16(19):3539. https://doi.org/10.3390/ijerph16193539.
7. Dean R, Luis V, Lamont S, David B. The role of work in gender identity stress and health in low-income middle-aged African-American men. Health Promot Int. 2020;36(5):1231–42. https://doi.org/10.1093/heapro/daaa144.
8. Murkey JA, Beverly-Xaviera W, Dorice V, Bernadette B-A. Disparities in allostatic load telomere length and chronic stress burden among African American adults: a systematic review. Psychoneuroendocrinology. 140:105730. https://doi.org/10.1016/j.psyneuen.2022.105730.
9. Patrick K, Evan R, Christopher W. Systemic discrimination among large U.S. employers. Q J Econ. 2023;137(4):1963–2036.
10. US Bureau of Labor Statistics. https://www.bls.gov/opub/reports/race-and-ethnicity/2022/
11. Center for Economic and Policy Research. https://cepr.net/publications/high-joblessness-for-black-youth-more-than-500000-jobs-are-needed/
12. Guzman G, Kollar M. U.S. Census Bureau, current population reports, P60-282, income in the United States: 2023. Washington, DC: U.S. Government Publishing Office, September 2024.
13. The Annie E. Casey Foundation. Children in single-parent families by race and ethnicity in United States. https://datacenter.aecf.org/data/bar/107-children-in-single-parent-families-by-race-and-ethnicity
14. Katherine LM, Sorensen D'AA, Fatima T, Nafeesa A, Lauren B-R, Carmen G. The physiological toll of arrests: an examination of arrest history on midlife allostatic load. Ann Epidemiol. 96:1–12. https://doi.org/10.1016/j.annepidem.2024.05.007.
15. Boen CE. Criminal justice contacts and psychophysiological functioning in early adulthood: health inequality in the carceral state. J Health Soc Behav. 61(3):290–306. https://doi.org/10.1177/0022146520936208.
16. Pamplin John R, Clancy KN, Keyes Katherine M, Bates Lisa M, Prins Seth J. Race criminalization and urban mental health in the United States. Curr Opin Psychiatry. 36(3):219–36. https://doi.org/10.1097/YCO.0000000000000857.
17. Thames AD, Irwin MR, Breen EC, Cole SW. Experienced discrimination and racial differences in leukocyte gene expression. Psychoneuroendocrinology. 106:277–83. https://doi.org/10.1016/j.psyneuen.2019.04.016.
18. Martz CD, Yijie W, Chung Kara W, Jiakponnah NN, Danila Maria I, Tamika W-D, Allen AM, Chae DH. Incident racial discrimination predicts elevated C-reactive protein in the Black Women's experiences Living with Lupus (BeWELL) study. Brain Behav Immun. 11:277–84. https://doi.org/10.1016/j.bbi.2023.06.004.
19. Aronoff JE, Quinn EB, Forde AT, Glover LM, Alexander R, McDade TW, Mario S. Associations between perceived discrimination and immune cell composition in the Jackson Heart Study. Brain Behav Immun:10328–36. https://doi.org/10.1016/j.bbi.2022.03.017.
20. Irena S, Baker EH, Simoni ZR, Aowen Z, Rutland SB, Mario S, Wilkinson LL. The role of perceived discrimination in obesity among African Americans. Am J Prevent Med. 52(1):S77–85. https://doi.org/10.1016/j.amepre.2016.07.034.
21. Woods-Giscombe CL, Marci L, Catherine Z, Jada B, Karen S-A, Ganga B, Lilian B, Charity L, Raven S, Taleah F, Amnazo M. Use of food to cope with culturally relevant stressful life events is associated with body mass index in African American Women. Nurs Res. 70(5S):S53–62. https://doi.org/10.1097/NNR.0000000000000532.
22. Kronenfeld LW, Lauren R-H, Ann VH, Lynn RM, Bulik CM. Ethnic and racial differences in body size perception and satisfaction. Body Image. 7(2):131–6. https://doi.org/10.1016/j.bodyim.2009.11.002.
23. Esdaille AR, Kevin KN, Ifunanya AV, Ecem K, Omer K. The interplay between structural inequality allostatic load inflammation and cancer in Black Americans: a narrative review. Cancers. 2024;16(17):3023. https://doi.org/10.3390/cancers16173023.

24. Harris AR, Pichardo CM, Jamirra F, Huaitian L, William W, Gatikrushna P, Lawrence WR, Pichardo MS, Jenkins BD, Dorsey TH, Ioffe OB, Yfantis HG, Tanya A-C, Stefan A. Multilevel stressors and systemic and tumor immunity in Black and White women with breast cancer. JAMA Netw Open. 8(2):e2459754. https://doi.org/10.1001/jamanetworkopen.2024.59754.
25. Lord BD, Harris AR, Stefan A. The impact of social and environmental factors on cancer biology in Black Americans. Cancer Causes Control. 34(3):191–203. https://doi.org/10.1007/s10552-022-01664-w.
26. Fuemmeler BF, Jie S, Hua Z, Robert W. Neighborhood deprivation racial segregation and associations with cancer risk and outcomes across the cancer-control continuum. Mol Psychiatry. 28(4):1494–501. https://doi.org/10.1038/s41380-023-02006-1.
27. Davis KM, Katherine K, Lena L, Michael P, Lauren P, Francesca L, Joseph NT, Heather F, Malcolm C, Lance R, Phillip L, Engeland CG, Samuele Z. The heart of Detroit study: a window into urban middle-aged and older African Americans' daily lives to understand psychosocial determinants of cardiovascular disease risk. BMC Psychiatry. 2023;23(1) https://doi.org/10.1186/s12888-023-05148-2.
28. Lockwood KG, Marsland AL, Matthews KA, Gianaros PJ. Perceived discrimination and cardiovascular health disparities: a multisystem review and health neuroscience perspective. Ann N Y Acad Sci. 1428(1):170–207. https://doi.org/10.1111/nyas.13939.
29. Wang N, Xinyi Y, Kellie I, Xu T, Shuang L, Julia G, Wang R, Lee S, Yang L, Chao C. Racial and ethnic disparities in prevalence and correlates of depressive symptoms and suicidal ideation among adults in the United States 2017–2020 pre-pandemic. J Affect Disord. 345:272–83. https://doi.org/10.1016/j.jad.2023.10.138.
30. Boyd DT, Quinn CR, Durkee MI, Williams E-DG, Andrea C, Durrell W, Butler-Barnes ST, Ewing AP. Perceived discrimination mental health help-seeking attitudes and suicide ideation planning and attempts among black young adults. BMC Public Health. 2024;24(1):2019. https://doi.org/10.1186/s12889-024-19519-1.
31. Bommersbach TJ, Rosenheck RA, Greg RT. Racial and ethnic differences in suicidal behavior and mental health service use among US adults 2009–2020. Psychol Med. 53(12):5592–602. https://doi.org/10.1017/S003329172200280X.
32. National Institute of Mental Health. https://www.nimh.nih.gov/health/statistics/major-depression
33. Hankerson SH, Suite D, Bailey RK. Treatment disparities among African American men with depression: implications for clinical practice. J Health Care Poor Underserved. 2015;26(1):21–34.
34. Curtin SC, Brown KA, Jordan ME. Suicide rates for the three leading methods by race and ethnicity: United States, 2000–2020. NCHS Data Brief. 2022;450:1–8.
35. Nguyen AW, Joseph TR, Chatters LM, Owen TH, Lincoln KD, Mitchell UA. Extended family and friendship support and suicidality among African Americans. Soc Psychiatry Psychiatr Epidemiol. 52(3):299–309. https://doi.org/10.1007/s00127-016-1309-1.
36. Lincoln KD, Joseph TR, Chatters LM, Sean J. Suicide negative interaction and emotional support among black Americans. Soc Psychiatry Psychiatr Epidemiol. 47(12):1947–58. https://doi.org/10.1007/s00127-012-0512-y.
37. Frietchen RE, Kinkel-Ram SS, Aziz E, McDermott TJ, Negar F, Abigail P, Lathan EC. Race-related stress dissociation symptoms and suicidal thoughts and behaviors in a community sample of Black Americans. Psychol Trauma. 2025;17:866. https://doi.org/10.1037/tra0001880.
38. Hollingsworth DW, Lillian P-R. Ethnic identity protects against feelings of defeat and entrapment on suicide ideation in African American young adults. Cultur Divers Ethnic Minor Psychol. 2022;28(2):217–26. https://doi.org/10.1037/cdp0000523.
39. Nan W, Xinyi Y, Imm Kellie X, Tianlin LS, Julia G, Ruixuan W, Lee S, Lin Y, Chao C. Racial and ethnic disparities in prevalence and correlates of depressive symptoms and suicidal ideation among adults in the United States 2017–2020 pre-pandemic. J Affect Disord. 345:272–83. https://doi.org/10.1016/j.jad.2023.10.138.

40. Abhery D, Shutong H, Brenda B, Mandana M, Bruckner Tim A, Allison S. Racialized economic segregation and Black youth suicide in the US. Am J Epidemiol. 2025; https://doi.org/10.1093/aje/kwae476.
41. Jester DJ, Kohn JN, Lize T, Thomas ML, Brown LL, Murphy JD, Jeste DV. Differences in social determinants of health underlie racial/ethnic disparities in psychological health and well-being: study of 11143 older adults. Am J Psychiatry. 180(7):483–94. https://doi.org/10.1176/appi.ajp.20220158.
42. Brandon P, Robyn MC, Moyses S. Associations between socioeconomic status markers and depressive symptoms by race and gender: results from the Multi-Ethnic Study of Atherosclerosis (MESA). Ann Epidemiol. 28(8):535–42.e1. https://doi.org/10.1016/j.annepidem.2018.05.005.
43. Whaley AL. Effects of gender-matching and racial self-labeling on paranoia in African American men with severe mental illness. J Natl Med Assoc. 2006;98(4):551–8.
44. Suite DH, La Bril R, Primm A, Harrison-Ross P. Beyond misdiagnosis, misunderstanding and mistrust: relevance of the historical perspective in the medical and mental health treatment of people of color. J Natl Med Assoc. 2007;99(8):879–85.
45. Barnes DM, Bates LM. Do racial patterns in psychological distress shed light on the Black-White depression paradox? A systematic review. Soc Psychiatry Psychiatr Epidemiol. 2017;52(8):913–28.
46. Jackson J, Knight K, Rafferty J. Race and unhealthy behaviors: chronic stress, the HPA Axis, and physical and mental health disparities over the life course. Am J Public Health. 2010;100(5):933–9. https://doi.org/10.2105/ajph.2008.143446.
47. Burgess D, Crowley-Matoka M, Phelan S, et al. Patient race and physician's decisions to prescribe opioids for chronic low back pain. Soc Sci Med. 2008;67(11):1852–60. https://doi.org/10.1016/j.socscimed.2008.09.009.
48. Clark TT. Perceived discrimination depressive symptoms and substance use in young adulthood. Addict Behav. 39(6):1021–5. https://doi.org/10.1016/j.addbeh.2014.01.013.
49. Schuler MS, Schell TL, Wong EC. Racial/ethnic differences in prescription opioid misuse and heroin use among a national sample 1999–2018. Drug Alcohol Depend. 221:108588. https://doi.org/10.1016/j.drugalcdep.2021.108588.
50. Gibbs TA, Mayumi O, Oquendo MA, Lawson WB, Shuai W, Felicity TY, Carlos B. Mental health of African Americans and Caribbean Blacks in the United States: results from the national epidemiological survey on alcohol and related conditions. Am J Public Health. 103(2):330–8. https://doi.org/10.2105/AJPH.2012.300891.
51. Johnson-Lawrence V, Griffith D, Watkins D. The effects of race, ethnicity, and mood/anxiety disorders on the chronic physical health conditions of men from a national sample. Am J Mens Health. 2013;7(4_suppl):58S–67S. https://doi.org/10.1177/1557988313484960.
52. Breslau J, Aguilar-Gaxiola S, Kendler KS, et al. Specifying race-ethnic differences in risk for psychiatric disorder in a USA national sample. Psychol Med. 2006;36(1):57–68.
53. Williams DR, Gonzalez HM, Neighbors H, et al. Prevalence and distribution of major depressive disorder in African Americans, Caribbean blacks, and non-Hispanic whites: results from the National Survey of American Life. Arch Gen Psychiatry. 2007;64(3):305–15.
54. Minsky S, Vega W, Miskimen T, et al. Diagnostic patterns in Latino, African American, and European American psychiatric patients. Arch Gen Psychiatry. 2003;60(6):637–44.
55. Schwartz EK, Docherty NM, Najolia GM, Cohen AS. Exploring the racial diagnostic bias of schizophrenia using behavioral and clinical-based measures. J Abnorm Psychol. 2019;128(3):263–71.
56. Olbert CM, Nagendra A, Buck B. Meta-analysis of Black vs. White racial disparity in schizophrenia diagnosis in the United States: do structured assessments attenuate racial disparities? J Abnormal Psychol. 2018;127(1):104–15.
57. Faber SC, Anjalika KR, Michaels TI, Williams MT. The weaponization of medicine: early psychosis in the Black community and the need for racially informed mental healthcare. Front. Psychiatry. 2023:14. https://doi.org/10.3389/fpsyt.2023.1098292.

58. Brownlow BN, Cheavens JS, Vasey MW, Thayer JF, Hill LBK. Culturally compelled coping and depressive symptoms in Black Americans: examining the role of psychophysiological regulatory capacity. Emotion. 2024;24(4):1003–15. https://doi.org/10.1037/emo0001323.
59. Rajendra AU, Paul JK, Kannathal N, Min LC, Suri JS. Heart rate variability: a review. Med Biol Eng Comput. 44(12):1031–51. https://doi.org/10.1007/s11517-006-0119-0.
60. Cooper DC, Thayer JF, Waldstein SR. Coping with racism: the impact of prayer on cardiovascular reactivity and post-stress recovery in African American women. Ann Behav Med. 47(2):218–30. https://doi.org/10.1007/s12160-013-9540-4.
61. Strassle PD, Parkes K, Baumann MM, Kelly YO, Zhuochen L, Chris S, Sylte DO, Kelly C, Bertolacci GJ, Wichada LM-K, Farah D, Mohsen N, Rodriquez EJ, Mensah GA, Murray Christopher JL, Mokdad Ali H, Laura D-L, Pérez-Stable Eliseo J. Homicide rates across county race ethnicity age and sex in the US. JAMA Netw Open. 8(2):e2462069. https://doi.org/10.1001/jamanetworkopen.2024.62069.
62. Light MT, Karl V, Alberto D-CC. Increased homicide played a key role in driving Black-White disparities in life expectancy among men during the COVID-19 pandemic. PLoS One. 2024;19(8):e0308105. https://doi.org/10.1371/journal.pone.0308105.
63. Kegler SR, Simon TR, Zwald ML, Chen MS, Mercy JA, Jones CM, Mercado-Crespo MC, Blair JM, Stone DM, Ottley PG, Jennifer D. MMWR Morb Mortal Wkly Rep. 2022;71(19):10.15585/mmwr.mm7119e1.
64. Umberson D, Olson J, Crosnoe R, Liu H, Pudrovska T, Donnelly R. Death of family members as an overlooked source of racial disadvantage in the United States. Proc Natl Acad Sci. 2017;114(5):915–20.
65. Fuller-Rowell T, Curtis D, El-Sheikh M, Chae D, Boylan J, Ryff C. Racial disparities in sleep: the role of neighborhood disadvantage. Sleep Med. 2016;27–28:1–8. https://doi.org/10.1016/j.sleep.2016.10.008.
66. Eastman C, Suh C, Tomaka V, Crowley S. Circadian rhythm phase shifts and endogenous free-running circadian period differ between African-Americans and European-Americans. Sci Rep. 2015;5(1):8381. https://doi.org/10.1038/srep08381.
67. Eastman C, Tomaka V, Crowley S. Circadian rhythms of European and African-Americans after a large delay of sleep as in jet lag and night work. Sci Rep. 2016;6(1):36716. https://doi.org/10.1038/srep36716.
68. Knutsson A. Health disorders of shift workers. Occup Med. 2003;53(2):103–8. https://doi.org/10.1093/occmed/kqg048.
69. Indrani H, Matthews KA, Buysse DJ, Strollo PJ, Victoria C, Reis SE, Hall MH. African genetic ancestry is associated with sleep depth in older African Americans. Sleep. 2015;38(8):1185–93. https://doi.org/10.5665/sleep.4888.
70. Richard B, Heming W, Yongmei L, Brody Jennifer A, Brenton S, Ruitong L, Bartz Traci M, Nona S, Chen Yii-der I, Cade Brian E, Han C, Patel Sanjay R, Xiaofeng Z, Gharib Sina A, Craig JW, Rotter Jerome I, Richa S, Shaun P, Xihong L, Susan R, Tamar S. Epigenome-wide association analysis of daytime sleepiness in the multi-ethnic study of atherosclerosis reveals African-American-specific associations. Sleep. 2019;42(8) https://doi.org/10.1093/sleep/zsz101.
71. Books C, Coody LC, Kauffman R, Abraham S. Night shift work and its health effects on nurses. Health Care Manag. 2017;36(4):347–53.
72. Substance Abuse and Mental Health Services Administration. Key substance use and mental health indicators in the United States: results from the 2016 National Survey on Drug Use and Health, HHS publication no. SMA 17-5044, NSDUH series H-52. Rockville: Center for Behavioral Health Statistics and Quality, Substance Abuse and Mental Health Services Administration; 2017. Retrieved from https://www.samhsa.gov/data/
73. Chartier K, Hesselbrock M, Hesselbrock V. Ethnicity and adolescent pathways to alcohol use. J Stud Alcohol Drugs. 2009;70(3):337–45. https://doi.org/10.15288/jsad.2009.70.337.
74. Welty L, Harrison A, Abram K, et al. Health disparities in drug- and alcohol-use disorders: a 12-year longitudinal study of youths after detention. Am J Public Health. 2016;106(5):872–80. https://doi.org/10.2105/ajph.2015.303032.

75. Caetano R, Cunradi C, Schafer J, Clark C. Intimate partner violence and drinking patterns among White, Black, and Hispanic couples in the U.S. J Subst Abus. 2000;11(2):123–38. https://doi.org/10.1016/s0899-3289(00)00015-8.
76. Flores Y, Yee H, Leng M, et al. Risk factors for chronic liver disease in Blacks, Mexican Americans, and Whites in the United States: results from NHANES IV, 1999–2004. Am J Gastroenterol. 2008;103(9):2231–8. https://doi.org/10.1111/j.1572-0241.2008.02022.x.
77. Polednak A. Secular trend in U.S. Black-White disparities in selected alcohol-related cancer incidence rates. Alcohol Alcohol. 2007;42(2):125–30. https://doi.org/10.1093/alcalc/agl121.
78. Xueqin MAG, Steve S. A comparative analysis of perceived risks and substance abuse among ethnic groups. Addict Behav. 25(3):361–71. https://doi.org/10.1016/S0306-4603(99)00070-2.
79. Jones AA, Shearer RD, Segel JE, Santos-Lozada A, Strong-Jones S, Vest N, Teixeira da Silva D, Khatri UG, Winkelman TNA. Opioid and stimulant attributed treatment admissions and fatal overdoses: using national surveillance data to examine the intersection of race sex and polysubstance use 1992–2020. Drug Alcohol Depend. 249:109946. https://doi.org/10.1016/j.drugalcdep.2023.109946.
80. Elizabeth J, Fatima V. African American adolescent substance use: the roles of racial discrimination and peer pressure. Addict Behav. 101:106154. https://doi.org/10.1016/j.addbeh.2019.106154.
81. Friedman JR, Jordan NTM, Helena H. Understanding and addressing widening racial inequalities in drug overdose. Am J Psychiatry. 181(5):381–90. https://doi.org/10.1176/appi.ajp.20230917.
82. Mbabazi K, Davis NL, Sagar K, Puja S, Mattson CL, Farnaz C, Jones CM. MMWR Morb Mortal Wkly Rep. 2022;71(29):940–7. https://doi.org/10.15585/mmwr.mm7129e2.
83. Tarlise T, David K, Ariadne R-A, Bunting Amanda M, Mauro Pia M, Marshall Brandon DL, Martins Silvia S, Magdalena C. Racial/ethnic and geographic trends in combined stimulant/opioid overdoses 2007–2019. Am J Epidemiol. 2022;191(4):599–612. https://doi.org/10.1093/aje/kwab290.

Chapter 13
Pain and Its Management in African Americans: Important Facts, Differences, and Disparities

Staja Q. Booker and Simone Jackson

Contents

13.1	Introduction..	263
	13.1.1 The Deception of Pain Perception..	264
	13.1.2 Public Health-Human-Civil Rights Issue...	266
13.2	Differences in the Experience of Pain...	267
	13.2.1 Perception and Communication of Pain..	267
	13.2.2 Barriers to Care..	268
	13.2.3 Cultural Considerations...	269
13.3	Psychosocial Aspects of Pain..	271
	13.3.1 Patient Advocacy...	272
13.4	Best Practices for African Americans: Interventions and Treatment Approaches........	273
	13.4.1 Pain Affirming Care..	273
	13.4.2 Assessment..	274
	13.4.3 Diagnosis...	274
	13.4.4 Treatment...	274
13.5	Conclusion...	277
13.6	Resources and Tools..	277
	13.6.1 Information Sheet..	277
	13.6.2 Websites (See Box 13.2)	279
References..		279

13.1 Introduction

You have likely heard the term "pain is pain," suggesting that all pain is the same for all people. But this could not be further from the truth. While physical pain is a universal experience, it is individually and subjectively expressed and felt. So, then *what is pain*? According to the International Association for the Study of Pain, "An unpleasant sensory and emotional experience associated with, or resembling that associated with, actual or potential tissue damage" [1]. Pain is categorized as either acute or chronic, with several subclassifications. In terms of acute pain, African Americans are more likely to use the emergency department or urgent care, often waiting until it was severe and unresolving [2, 3]. For instance, African American Veterans had a 58% higher risk of visiting the emergency department for chronic pain-related diagnoses compared to European American Veterans [4]. However, encountering inequities in the acute care setting was inescapable as African Americans have reported feeling like their pain is downplayed, inadequately treated, and assumed to be tolerable [2]. The classification and diagnosis of pain has been archaic to put it nicely. Within the last 5 years, a bold step was taken to better organize and classify diagnostic codes for chronic pain. The ICD-11 diagnostic codes categorize chronic pain as primary or secondary [5]. Primary chronic pain is defined by three criteria: "pain has persisted for more than 3 months, is associated with significant emotional distress and/or functional disability, and the symptoms are not better accounted for by another diagnosis" [6]. These are further delineated into more specific codes: chronic widespread pain, complex regional syndrome, chronic primary headache or orofacial pain, chronic primary visceral pain, and chronic primary musculoskeletal pain. Example health conditions are fibromyalgia, complex regional syndrome types 1 and 2, chronic migraine, irritable bowel syndrome, and chronic primary low back pain. Primary secondary pain is pain that may at least initially be conceived as a symptom or sign secondary to an underlying disease [5]. For example, chronic cancer-related pain, chronic neuropathic pain, chronic secondary visceral pain, chronic posttraumatic and postsurgical pain, chronic secondary headache and orofacial pain, and chronic secondary musculoskeletal pain.

In the USA, up to 50 million Americans have chronic pain, and approximately 20 million have high-impact chronic pain, which is pain that significantly limits life or work activities on most days or every day [7, 8]. In analysis of National Health Interview Survey data from 2016, Black/African Americans (African Americans) had the highest age-adjusted prevalence of high-impact chronic pain (8.1%), followed by Hispanics (7.9%) and Whites (7.1%) [7]. A more recent analysis of 2021 data shows that African Americans had the second highest age-adjusted prevalence of high-impact chronic pain (7.6%), only below American Indian/Alaska Native at 12.6% and above non-Hispanic White (6.5%), Hispanic or Latino (5.7%), and Asian (2.1%) [8].

13.1.1 The Deception of Pain Perception

Historically, Black/African Americans were believed to be insensitive or less sensitive to pain and able to endure pain because they had an inferior biology. This slavery-era myth and perception has unfortunately persisted through stereotypes today, and numerous studies continue to show racial bias in pain attitudes and management toward African Americans [9–11]. Even in Black children racial biases are

13.1 Introduction

observed—a sample of mostly White individuals believed that Black children lived more adverse or harder lives and this did not mediate their perception that 4- to 6-year-old Black children felt less pain than 4- to 6-year-old White children. [12] Several examples include:

- White people were rated as being more sensitive to pain and more willing to report pain than the average Black person [10].
- African Americans nerve endings are less sensitive than whites, have a stronger immune system, and skin is thicker than Whites [9].
- African American women are less sensitive to pain during childbirth [11].
- African Americans are more susceptible to drug addiction, including opioid misuse and addiction.

These beliefs are a result of not only learned racialized differences but a thriving system of social and medical racism that leads to gross racial profiling, underassessment, and undertreatment. Given these stereotypes and fallacious beliefs, it is no surprise that there is also a significant racial disparity in the treatment of pain. Here are the facts about pain in African Americans:

- Central nervous system has less inhibitory control and more facilitatory processes, leading to central sensitization, greater pain sensitivity, lower tolerance, hyperalgesia, and heightened nociception [13–15].
- Pain is felt, perceived, and reported as more severe—often higher in intensity compared to Whites and other racialized groups.
- African American women report higher pain intensities and experience pain at lower experimental temperatures [16].
- Opioid misuse is lower in African Americans, although recent studies show a growing trend in use [17].

In simpler terms, African Americans are more sensitive to pain and noxious stimuli. Despite this knowledge, African Americans are more likely to have their pain discounted or underestimated and less likely to be screened for pain—a form of treatment neglect. Even well-known nursing and medical textbooks perpetuate stereotypic images and nonevidence-based descriptions of pain; such racist statements warranted an apology from the publisher (see Inside Higher Ed [18]). Mitigating this bias requires evidence-based education of health professionals. Knowing and understanding, and effectively demonstrating the pain core competencies for major health disciplines (e.g., medicine, nursing, physical therapy, pharmacy, psychology) can help improve knowledge, attitudes, and behaviors (See Table 13.2 for Interprofessional Core Competencies for Pain Management). Training in cultural sensitivity and implicit bias can facilitate better provider-patient interactions and foster an environment where patients feel heard and respected [19].

13.1.2 Public Health-Human-Civil Rights Issue

Chronic pain itself has been declared a public health problem [20]; however, chronic pain inequities, while readily known, have not been deemed as a public health or national health disparity [21, 22]. For disparity populations like African Americans, mistreatment of pain, whether chronic, acute, or cancer, is not only a public health problem, but also a human rights violation, civil rights issue, and a moral imperative. The unequal treatment of pain in African Americans spans their lifetime and life stage (from pregnancy to end-of-life). Dr. Carmen Green and colleagues' seminal 2003 review paper uncovered the unequal burden of pain and its mistreatment in "racial/ethnic minorities" [23], and in a follow-up article 20 years later, she assigned the "genesis" or origin of the unequal burden with the chief complaint of "structural and institutional racism, and race-based disparities in healthcare, pain, and policing" [24]. Disparities in pain management extend to hospice and nursing homes [25, 26]. The growing concern over poor pain management in the early-mid 1990s prompted the Joint Commission to make pain "visible" and promoted pain as the fifth vital sign. While this campaign was successful at increasing pain assessment and documentation rates, it failed to capture other dimensions of pain's impact, overemphasized treating pain based on a numerical intensity, and still neglected to make African Americans' pain "visible" in the healthcare system. Misdiagnosis and underdiagnosis, under-assessment, mistreatment and undertreatment, low referral rate to pain specialists, and fewer opportunities to participate in pain clinical trials resulted.

Further, quality and fair pain treatment is a basic patient right. Yet, African American adults and children are way less likely to receive adequate amounts of analgesic medications and opioids for acute and chronic pain conditions [27, 28]. When prescribed for cancer pain, African Americans were likely to receive morphine (33% vs. 14%) vs. oxycodone (38% vs. 64%) compared to Whites, respectively, and those with concomitant chronic kidney disease experienced disproportionate adverse effects due to the toxic metabolite in morphine [29, 30]. Indeed, even the treatment of African Americans with opioid misuse disorder (Box 13.1) is laden with racial bias and criminalization while Whites are more likely to be provided opportunities for rehabilitation and treatment [31]; Jones describes these racialized approaches to opioid use disorder and opioid misuse management as barriers to pharmacoequity [32]. The verified decreased use of pain medications in a population with an objectively lower threshold for pain, and a protracted need due to increased comorbidities, is unusually ironic and incredibly cruel. On the contrary, a more recent analysis did not find significant differences in pain medication prescribing between African Americans and Whites presenting to primary care [33]. Ensuring bias-free awareness of this problem and optimal pain care for all, especially those most impacted like African Americans, are critically important for public health and policy making.

13.1 Introduction

Box 13.1: Signs of Opioid Misuse

"At risk" or "high risk" signs of potential opioid abuse	Behavioral signs of opioid misuse
Co-occurring psychiatric disorders (depression, bipolar, etc.) Past cocaine use or abuse Convictions for driving under the influence Past alcohol or drug problems Daily nicotine use Obesity Long-term use of benzodiazepines Long-term use of sleep aids including zolpidem, zaleplon, and eszopiclone	Increasing tolerance Visiting multiple healthcare providers to obtain prescriptions for opioids or other controlled substances Frequent or unexplained prescription refills Secrecy or deception about how much or how often opioids are used or where the medications come from Withdrawal from social or occupational activities or having difficulty meeting daily obligations due to opioid use Engaging in risky behaviors such as driving under the influence Mood swings or personality changes Frequent requests for medication refills Excessive sleepiness, difficulty staying awake, or lethargy, especially when it seems disproportionate to the situation

13.2 Differences in the Experience of Pain

13.2.1 Perception and Communication of Pain

Pain perception and communication are heavily influenced by cultural beliefs and social norms. African American patients may adopt coping strategies rooted in their cultural background, such as prioritizing strength, resilience, and prayer, which may impact their willingness to report pain accurately or seek treatment promptly [34]. This cultural inclination often results in healthcare providers underestimating the severity of the pain or misunderstanding how it is expressed [9]. Social determinants of health, including socioeconomic status, racism and racialized identity, gender identity, education and neighborhood environment all play a profound role in shaping an individual's experience of pain [35, 36]. As noted earlier, any type of pain is likely to be more intense and impactful in African Americans. While pain conditions may not significantly vary in prevalence, African Americans have a greater incidence of conditions associated with chronic pain, neuropathic pain, and pain flares: knee osteoarthritis, sickle cell disease, lupus, sarcoidosis, hypertension, diabetes, and cancer.

Undoubtedly, their perception of pain influences their communication and verbal expression of pain. In one study of osteoarthritis communication, African Americans were more likely to talk about the location, intensity, and timing of pain and few used medical terminology [37]. Puia and McDonald concluded "Practitioners might assist older black adults with persistent osteoarthritis pain to communicate important clinical pain information by helping them to use relevant medical terminology and more explicit pain descriptions when discussing pain management" [37]. To refute this ethnocentric recommendation, providers should instead (1) ensure that African Americans are comfortable to report pain, (2) empower African Americans to report pain using terms consistent with their culture, language, and literacy level, (3) educate African Americans on the nature and treatment of pain, and (4) minimize using medical jargon. In an unpublished pilot study by Booker (first author of this chapter), the author found that African Americans used words like burning, tingling, and numbness, to describe the sensations of knee pain while Whites used terms such as dull ache, pressure, and sharp. It is important that African Americans' descriptions of pain are noted and believed as they provide key information about the type of pain and the subsequent best treatment to treat that type of pain. For example, sensations of burning, numbness, or electric shocks may signify neuropathic pain and a need for antidepressant medications, such as gabapentin; while throbbing or pulsating may indicate muscle-related inflammation and treatment with NSAIDs.

13.2.2 Barriers to Care

Whether it is due to access issues and insurance, bias and discrimination in the healthcare system, or poor-quality communication with their providers, African Americans are more likely to have whatever pain they have go undertreated or untreated. Many barriers to care are cloaked in structural racism and driven by adverse social determinants of health. Indeed, disparities and inequities in the treatment of pain are due to a confluence of patient-, provider- and system-level factors [38]. Early studies documented difficulties in accessing neighborhood pharmacies that carried controlled pain medications [38]. Two recent qualitative studies revealed how forms of racism, discrimination, and microaggressions manifest in the physician-patient relationships with African American patients [39]. Racial discrimination in healthcare has been associated with several unfavorable pain and psychosocial outcomes including lower patient activation, lower communication self-efficacy with physicians, higher pain intensity, and lower pain management self-efficacy [40]. They concluded that "a strong physician-patient relationship did not buffer Black individuals from the consequences of perceiving discrimination" [40]. After completing a tailored, virtual intervention to reduce race-based and socioeconomic disparities in pain treatment decision-making, providers in the tailored intervention group had 85% lower odds of exhibiting a racialized treatment bias against Black patients [41]. These collective studies demonstrate the need for system- and provider-level interventions to address misleading perceptions of racial mistreatment in pain care.

13.2.3 Cultural Considerations

Because pain has historically been undertreated in African Americans, there are important considerations about beliefs, behaviors, and biology that providers should keep in mind. In many Black communities, there may be a cultural and religious expectation of endurance and strength, especially in the face of adversity. Chronic pain might be seen as something to endure, "bear" or live with, sometimes leading individuals to downplay the severity of their pain or to avoid expressing vulnerability [39, 42].

- It may be difficult for African Americans to openly express or communicate pain due to fear of being dismissed, silenced, or not believed. Be aware of potential cultural differences in communication styles (e.g., using more indirect expressions of pain, or having a more reserved manner in the clinical setting). Cultural expressions of pain can vary, and this may be misunderstood by providers who are unfamiliar with these differences.
- They may use different terminology or descriptors to explain the type and amount of pain experienced.
- May underestimate the importance of and fail to prioritize managing pain due to beliefs about "normal aging," God's will (and transcended through faith), or inability to access needed healthcare.
- May fear and avoid or delay surgical or invasive interventions for pain. Many African Americans may prefer or rely on holistic, alternative, or complementary medicine approaches, but they are not opposed to pharmacological treatments and should be offered medications at the same rate as other racial groups. Providers should be open to discussing and integrating different approaches, when possible, while still ensuring evidence-based care (Table 13.1).

Table 13.1 Common questions and answers related to pain in African Americans

Do African Americans feel more pain than other racialized or cultural groups?
Current research suggests that African Americans are more sensitive to pain and painful stimuli. The majority of experimental pain studies in the USA have been conducted in African American and European American samples; thus, it is widely unknown how other racial groups experience pain. African Americans also report higher pain intensities and worse interference on function
Do African Americans use different words or terms to describe pain?
They may use the word pain, but more than likely they will refer to "hurting," "aching," "sore/ness," or "paining"
How do African Americans cope with pain?
African Americans cope with pain using a number of different strategies, including distraction/diverting attention, prayer, calming self-statements, exercise, and expressing gratitude. Because African Americans exhibit great strength and perseverance amid adversity, it is assumed that they are emotionally and physically strong and therefore do not feel pain in the same manner as others. Yet they have poorer physical health and higher pain

(continued)

Table 13.1 (continued)

Can you tell African Americans are in pain by looking at facial expressions?
Nonverbal behaviors may help to identify the presence of pain, but it is not a consistent or reliable form of pain assessment. Furthermore, there are not enough studies to catalog facial expressions as a pain indicator in African Americans. Only a few small studies have examined nonverbal pain expressions in older African Americans with dementia [43]. While African Americans have dynamic facial expressions in general, when in pain, they may display stoicism (particularly older African Americans) whether due to learned behaviors or medical silencing. For instance, a more verbal or animated expression of pain or distress could be misinterpreted as exaggeration or emotional distress (e.g., loud, "angry Black woman," "drama queens," or faking) rather than an authentic sign of physical suffering
How do familial and psychosocial experiences impact pain in African Americans?
A recently published study found that family support and average support were linked to decreased odds of pain incidence while parent-child strain was a risk factor for increased incidence [44]. Family and community support can buffer the negative impacts of pain by providing emotional reassurance, practical assistance, and motivation for adherence to treatment plans. Other research indicates that pain catastrophizing, discrimination, and chronic stress all have variable effects on pain
Are African Americans resistant to taking opioids?
Research shows that African Americans are less likely to take opioids consistently or to use the prescribed amount to reduce possible addiction, dependence, and adverse effects [45, 46]. They may also voice concern about not wanting to take a lot pills, the need to save pills for severe pain, or ration medications due to inability to afford. However, they are not opposed to taking opioids and other pain medications. While attitudes and patterns of use and self-management differ, they should be offered the most effective pain medications.
What disparities or inequities do African Americans experience when it comes to prescription pain meds?
They are more often labeled and viewed as "drug-seeking" and "drug users/addicts," be prescribed less medications or less-effective medications, subjected to random drug screenings, or have greater limitations in access

Table 13.2 Interprofessional core competencies for pain management

Domain 1: multidimensional nature of pain	Domain 2: pain assessment and measurement	Domain 3: management of pain	Domain 4: clinical conditions
Explain the complex, multidimensional, and individual-specific nature of pain	Use valid and reliable tools for measuring pain and associated symptoms to assess and reassess related outcomes as appropriate for the clinical context and population	Demonstrate the inclusion of patient and others, as appropriate, in the education and shared decision-making process for pain care	Describe the unique pain assessment and management needs of special populations
Present theories and science for understanding pain	Describe patient, provider, and system factors that can facilitate or interfere with effective pain assessment and management	Identify pain treatment options that can be accessed in a comprehensive pain management plan	Explain how to assess and manage pain across settings and transitions of care

(continued)

13.3 Psychosocial Aspects of Pain

Table 13.2 (continued)

Domain 1: multidimensional nature of pain	Domain 2: pain assessment and measurement	Domain 3: management of pain	Domain 4: clinical conditions
Define terminology for describing pain and associated conditions	Assess patient preferences and values to determine pain-related goals and priorities	Explain how health promotion and self-management strategies are important to the management of pain	Describe the role, scope of practice, and contribution of the different professions within a pain management care team
Describe the impact of pain on society	Demonstrate empathic and compassionate communication during pain assessment	Develop a pain treatment plan based on benefits and risks of available treatments	Implement an individualized pain management plan that integrates the perspectives of patients, their social support systems, and health care providers in the context of available resources
Explain how cultural, institutional, societal, and regulatory influences affect assessment and management of pain		Monitor effects of pain management approaches to adjust the plan of care as needed	Describe the role of the clinician as an advocate in assisting patients to meet treatment goals
		Differentiate physical dependence, substance use disorder, misuse, tolerance, addiction, and nonadherence	
		Develop a treatment plan that takes into account the differences between acute pain, acute-on-chronic pain, chronic/persistent pain, and pain at the end of life	

13.3 Psychosocial Aspects of Pain

Chronic pain is often intertwined with emotional and psychological suffering. For African Americans, this can include generational trauma related to racism, discrimination, and societal oppression, which can exacerbate both physical pain and emotional distress. Mental health concerns like depression and anxiety are common comorbidities for individuals with chronic pain and have a bidirectional relationship [47]. These conditions are sometimes underdiagnosed in Black populations, partly due to stigma or lack of access to mental health resources. In addition, other psychosocial factors that are shown to impact pain and interact in varying ways include pain catastrophizing, chronic stress, and discrimination. Chronic exposure to these stressors has been linked to heightened pain sensitivity and poorer mental health outcomes [35]. Several studies show a relationship between chronic pain or experimental pain and either perceived or everyday discrimination [48–50]. Having family support and less family strain may mitigate not only the trauma associated with chronic pain but might also reduce the risk of development and persistence of chronic pain particularly in older African Americans. One study found that family support and average support decreased the odds of pain incidence and pain persisting over time, suggesting that family-based and intergenerational interventions might be of benefit [44]. Research tells us that individuals with strong social networks report better pain coping and overall well-being [35]. Clinicians must assess mental health as part of pain management protocols, recognizing that untreated psychological conditions can impair pain treatment outcomes [50, 51].

13.3.1 Patient Advocacy

Advocacy involves ensuring patients' voices are heard, their pain is validated, and they are supported throughout their treatment journey. Patients should be educated about their pain condition and treatment options to take an active role in their care. Health literacy varies among individuals, and patients from marginalized communities, including African Americans, may have limited access to pain management education. Providers should take time to explain pain management options clearly at the level at which patients can understand and apply the knowledge. Providing written resources in plain language or using visual aids can also help. Healthcare providers can play an important role in advocating for better access to pain management resources, such as physical therapy, counseling, and alternative therapies, particularly for patients who may face systemic and structural barriers.

- *Create a space for open dialogue*: Encourage patients to share their pain experiences in their own words and validate their reports. Active listening fosters trust and leads to a more accurate diagnosis.
- *Encourage shared decision-making*: Involve the patient in decisions about pain management. Discuss treatment options openly, and address concerns or fears they may have about specific therapies, such as medications or surgical interventions.
- *Normalize treatment for mental health*: Mental health issues in African Americans communities are sometimes stigmatized, and seeking help for emotional distress or chronic pain can be viewed negatively. Providers should normalize mental health care as part of pain management and offer resources for counseling, therapy, and support groups in a culturally sensitive manner.

13.4 Best Practices for African Americans: Interventions and Treatment Approaches

13.4.1 Pain Affirming Care

It is important to address the whole person: mind, body, spirit. Pain affirming care is an empathy-driven, nonjudgmental approach that goes beyond accepting and believing patients' report of pain, but affirms the person's identity in their fullness, validates their lived experience of pain and culture, and respects their natural or preferred way of presenting with pain [52]. Pain affirming care acknowledges a person's lived experience and the pain-related harms or mistreatment they have experienced and seeks to reconcile those through affirmation of their experience. This also entails incorporating aspects of trauma-informed care into the overall approach to pain management planning and monitoring.

How does this apply to African Americans? Using this care philosophy, providers should:

- *Acknowledge racial disparities in healthcare* and the harm it has caused to generations of African Americans. Affirm that as a healthcare provider or researcher a commitment to improving pain care and removing biases. Offer opportunities for second opinion and respect their decision.
- *Avoid stereotypes by recognition of* unconscious biases or stereotypes about pain tolerance or pain expression in Black patients. Provide a safe space for African American patients to freely discuss their pain and speak up about their care.
- *Consider the effects of medical mistrust* and understand how a patient views medical care—whether they are hesitant to seek it, have past experiences of inadequate care, or are more likely to turn to home remedies—can provide useful context for diagnosing and managing pain. Include their trusted social network of family and friends in their care, who can serve as advocates or caregivers.
- *Engage with cultural humility* and treat each patient as an individual, with respect to their unique experiences, cultural background, and personal perceptions of pain. It is important to listen and take their reports of pain seriously. Respect and affirm African Americans' core values and beliefs, priorities, and goals. Accept that both patient and clinician are "experts" in their own right.
- *Ensure* that Black patients receive the same level of diagnostic workup, pain management options, and referrals to specialists as any other patient. Make the best evidence-informed treatment recommendations considering social determinants of health, abilities, and lifestyle. Identify what they are already doing that is helpful and safe.

The Screen, Intervene, and Reconvene (SIR, Fig. 13.1) cultural model developed by Booker can be used to guide screening/assessment, treatment, and evaluation [53].

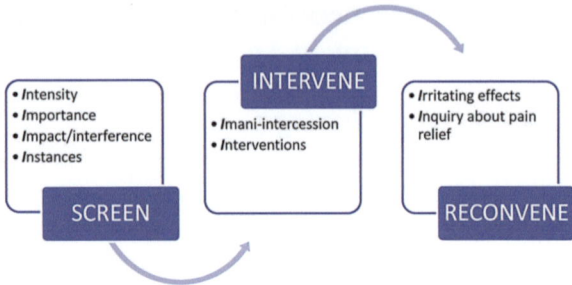

Fig. 13.1 Screen, intervene, and reconvene (SIR) model. (Used with permission from Staja "Star" Booker, ©2014)

13.4.2 Assessment

Clinicians should always take the time to assess pain (Fig. 13.2), then accept and believe their report of pain.

- Use validated and preferred pain assessment tools such as the Defense and Veterans Pain Rating Scale (DVPRS), the Faces Pain Scale-Revised (FPS-R), and the Revised Iowa Pain Thermometer (IPT-R) [54, 55] or the Interventional Pain Assessment (IPA) scale. [56]
- Ask about pain at rest (i.e., spontaneous pain) and during movement to determine the type of pain experience and the appropriate treatment.
- Document characteristics of pain and its impact on mobility, physical function, and quality of life.

13.4.3 Diagnosis

Diagnosing pain in African American patients, like any group, requires a thorough and individualized assessment. However, there are historical, cultural, and social factors that may influence both the way pain is experienced in patients and how it is perceived by healthcare providers. Providers tend to underestimate pain in Black patients, regardless of age, gender, or health condition. It is not uncommon for African Americans to receive substandard workups or diagnostic testing leading to misdiagnosis or delayed diagnosis. The intersection of provider apathy and patients' delayed care seeking can complicate receiving a timely medical diagnosis.

13.4.4 Treatment

The Pain Management Best Practices Inter-Agency Task Force proposed a multimodal approach to pain management using treatments from one or more clinical disciplines incorporated into a comprehensive treatment plan [57]. These approaches

13.4 Best Practices for African Americans: Interventions and Treatment Approaches

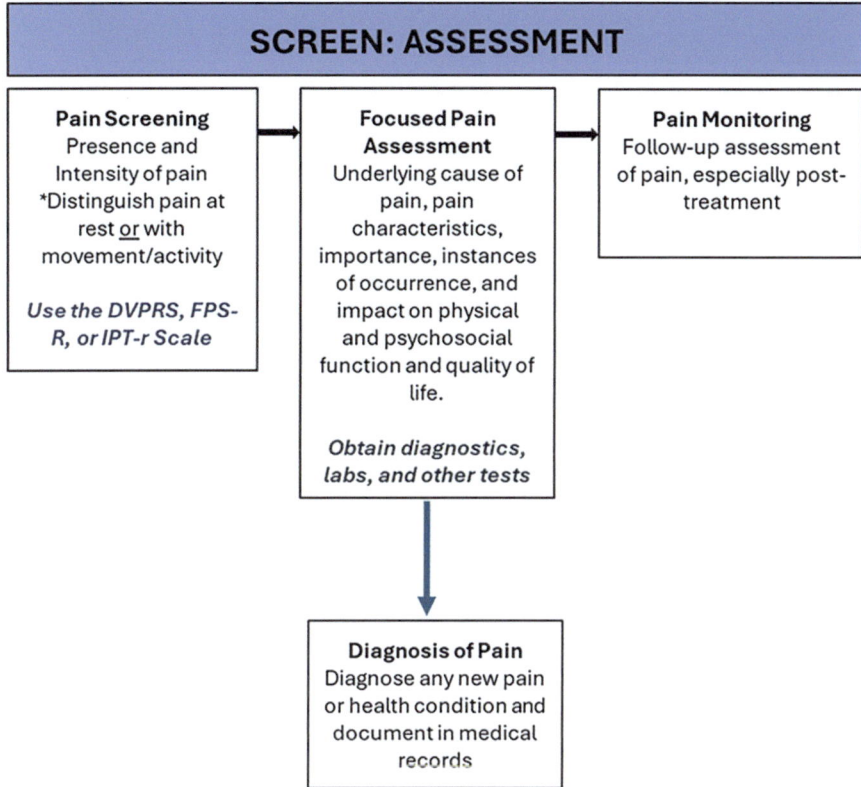

Fig. 13.2 Pain screening

being guided by a risk/benefit assessment, access, and education include medications, restorative therapies, interventional approaches, behavioral health approaches, and complementary and integrative health strategies (Fig. 13.3). Whatever combination of therapies are used, they must be individualized at the patient level but also tailored at the cultural level.

- *Determine acceptable and accessible treatment options* and explain the benefits, risks, and outcomes expected. Common chronic pain strategies that African Americans use include: exercise, over-the-counter pain medications, prayer, heat, topical creams and rubs, and assistive devices [45, 58]. In young Black adults, a considerable number did not use any type of pain reduction strategy [59]. Research is clear on the disproportionate referral rate and subsequent utilization of interventional procedures, such as total joint arthroplasty [60]. Some African Americans may fear being "cut on" or experiencing complications or additional pain [61].
- *Provide timely follow-up evaluations* (within 2–3 weeks vs. 3 months) with patients to determine treatment adherence, effectiveness, and adverse effects and

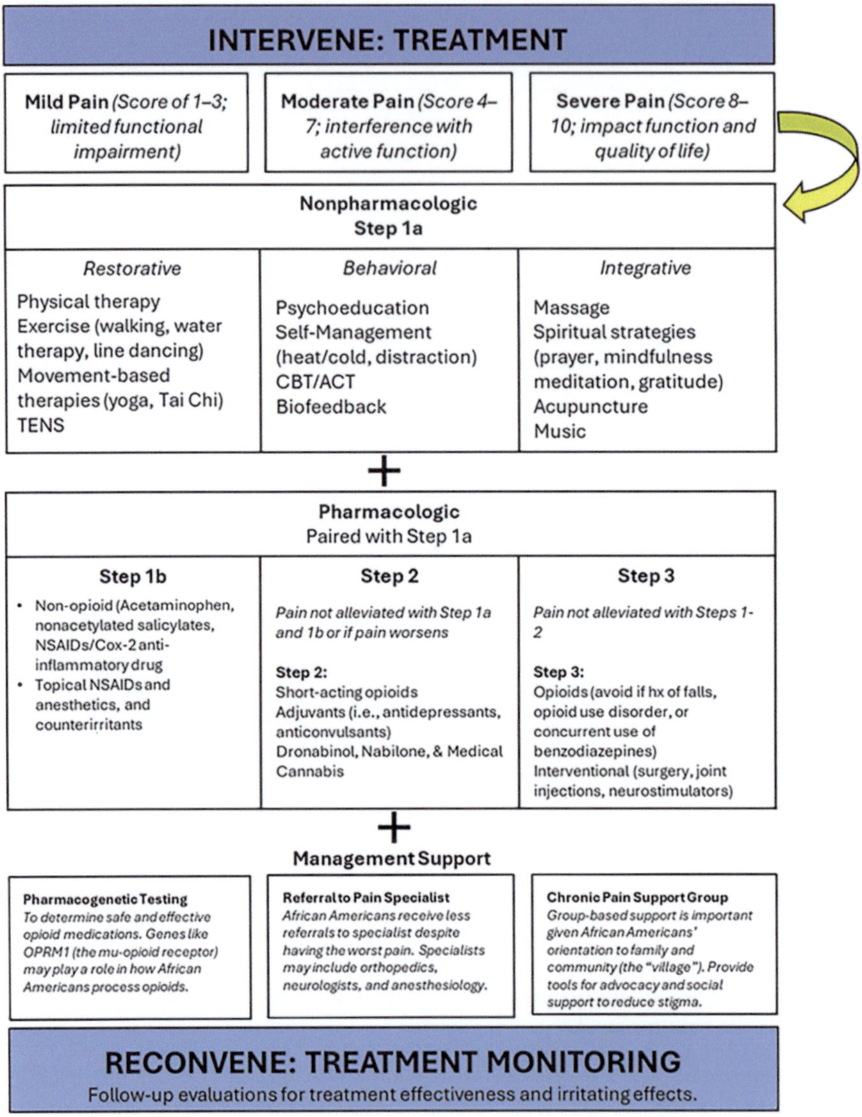

INTERVENE: TREATMENT

Mild Pain *(Score of 1–3; limited functional impairment)*	Moderate Pain *(Score 4–7; interference with active function)*	Severe Pain *(Score 8–10; impact function and quality of life)*

Nonpharmacologic
Step 1a

Restorative	Behavioral	Integrative
Physical therapy Exercise (walking, water therapy, line dancing) Movement-based therapies (yoga, Tai Chi) TENS	Psychoeducation Self-Management (heat/cold, distraction) CBT/ACT Biofeedback	Massage Spiritual strategies (prayer, mindfulness meditation, gratitude) Acupuncture Music

+

Pharmacologic
Paired with Step 1a

Step 1b	Step 2	Step 3
• Non-opioid (Acetaminophen, nonacetylated salicylates, NSAIDs/Cox-2 anti-inflammatory drug • Topical NSAIDs and anesthetics, and counterirritants	Pain not alleviated with Step 1a and 1b or if pain worsens **Step 2:** Short-acting opioids Adjuvants (i.e., antidepressants, anticonvulsants) Dronabinol, Nabilone, & Medical Cannabis	Pain not alleviated with Steps 1-2 **Step 3:** Opioids (avoid if hx of falls, opioid use disorder, or concurrent use of benzodiazepines) Interventional (surgery, joint injections, neurostimulators)

+

Management Support

| **Pharmacogenetic Testing**
To determine safe and effective opioid medications. Genes like OPRM1 (the mu-opioid receptor) may play a role in how African Americans process opioids. | **Referral to Pain Specialist**
African Americans receive less referrals to specialist despite having the worst pain. Specialists may include orthopedics, neurologists, and anesthesiology. | **Chronic Pain Support Group**
Group-based support is important given African Americans' orientation to family and community (the "village"). Provide tools for advocacy and social support to reduce stigma. |

RECONVENE: TREATMENT MONITORING
Follow-up evaluations for treatment effectiveness and irritating effects.

Fig. 13.3 Multimodal treatment pathway

adjust treatment over time. In African American older adults, it is not uncommon to see inappropriate medication prescribing and mismanagement, wherein those who used NSAIDs, 98% experienced potentially inappropriate medication use, 69% had drug duplication, and 65% experienced drug-drug interactions [62].

13.5 Conclusion

The disparities in pain management faced by African Americans are deeply rooted in historical, social, and systemic issues. Addressing these disparities requires an integrated approach that includes culturally competent care, patient advocacy, education, and the consideration of social determinants of health. Caring for African Americans with pain compel providers to view them as human and reliable. Providers should avoid making assumptions based on racial stereotypes, like being more tolerant or are drug-seekers. These biases can lead to undertreatment of pain, poorer outcomes, and further erosion of healthcare trust. Using empathy, standardized pain assessment tools, and active listening to the patient's experiences are crucial. Providers should be patient, open, and respectful when discussing chronic pain. By incorporating evidence-based practices and focusing on equitable treatment, healthcare providers can contribute to closing the gap in pain care for African American patients.

13.6 Resources and Tools

13.6.1 *Information Sheet*

This tip sheet includes a list of pain-related questions and resources developed to improve communication between minoritized family caregivers and healthcare providers.

Information for Family Caregivers

Tips for Communicating with Health Care Providers About Pain
- During health care visits, ask questions about managing or treating your family member's pain. Here are some examples:
  - Pain terminology: "I heard you use the term 'chronic pain.' Can you explain what that means?"
  - Pain communication: "What do I do if a health care provider dismisses my family member's pain complaints?"
  - Medication side effects: "I want to ensure that this medication doesn't negatively interact with other medications or affect memory and thinking. Please tell me its common side effects."
  - Medication alternatives: "What are some safer alternatives to strong pain medications?"
  - Nonprescription treatment: "What are some over-the-counter medications we can use?"
  - Complementary and alternative therapies: "Are there natural remedies for pain that are as effective as medication?"
  - Palliative care: "What is palliative care? Will this help my family member manage pain?"
  - Pain management specialist: "My family member's pain is getting worse and more frequent. When should we consider involving a pain specialist?"
  - Pharmacy: "What should I ask the pharmacist about taking this medication?"
  - Opioids: "What is an opioid? Are opioids safe? When should we consider adding an opioid to the treatment regimen? Are there any opioids among my family member's current medications?"
  - Filling prescriptions: "What if I have difficulty filling a prescription for my family member? Whom should I contact? What pharmacies in my area carry the prescribed medication?"
  - Supportive care: "Are there support groups for people with chronic pain and their caregivers that we can participate in?"
  - Treatment follow-up: "How often should we follow up with you about my family member's pain?"
  - Fair/equitable access to treatment: "What should I do if I feel like my family member is not being treated fairly or receiving the best care possible? Can you provide me with the phone number for patient grievances or complaints?"
- Record the person's pain over time using a pain log (www.theacpa.org/resources/pain-log). The log can be a source of important information for the provider.
- Ask the provider or social worker for community-based resources and programs to assist with pain care.

Resources to Explore
- GeriatricPain.org (https://geriatricpain.org)
- GoodRx: Avoiding 10 Common Prescription Refill Roadblocks: A Doctor's Advice (www.goodrx.com/healthcare-access/pharmacies/problems-filling-prescriptions-what-to-do)
- American Chronic Pain Association (www.theacpa.org)
- National Pain Advocacy Center: Fast Facts About Pain and Opioids (https://nationalpain.org/fast-facts-opioids)
- Pain Connection: National Chronic Pain Support Groups (https://painconnection.org/support-groups/national)

Family caregiver instructional videos about pain can be found on AARP's website:

Caring, for Those in Pain
http://links.lww.com/AJN/A230

What Is Pain?
http://links.lww.com/AJN/A231

For additional information, the AARP Public Policy Institute's Home Alone Alliance website offers publications, training webinars, blog posts, and videos for family caregivers: www.aarp.org/ppi/initiatives/home-alone-alliance.

AJN THE AMERICAN JOURNAL OF NURSING

Reprinted with permission from the authors and the American Journal of Nursing

13.6.2 Websites (See Box 13.2)

> **Box 13.2: Resourceful Websites for Pain Management**
> - BelieveMyPain—a new campaign and website dedicated to increasing awareness of pain injustices and improving pain equity in Black communities. https://www.believemypain.com/.
> - GeriatricPain.org—an educational website with resources for pain assessment, treatment, and in older adults. https://geriatricpain.org/.
> - American Academy of Pain Medicine—list of clinical consensus guidelines. https://painmed.org/clinical-guidelines/.
> - Centers for Disease Control and Prevention (CDC) *Clinical Practice Guidelines for Prescribing Opioids for Pain.* https://www.cdc.gov/overdose-prevention/hcp/clinical-guidance/index.html.

References

1. Raja SN, Carr DB, Cohen M, Finnerup NB, Flor H, Gibson S, Keefe FJ, Mogil JS, Ringkamp M, Sluka KA, Song XJ, Stevens B, Sullivan MD, Tutelman PR, Ushida T, Vader K. The revised International Association for the Study of Pain definition of pain: concepts, challenges, and compromises. Pain. 2020;161(9):1976–82. https://doi.org/10.1097/j.pain.0000000000001939.
2. Agarwal AK, Gonzales RE, Sagan C, Nijim S, Asch DA, Merchant RM, South EC. Perspectives of black patients on racism within emergency care. JAMA Health Forum. 2024;5(3):e240046. https://doi.org/10.1001/jamahealthforum.2024.0046.
3. Mares JG, Lund BC, Adamowicz JL, Burgess DJ, Rothmiller SJ, Hadlandsmyth K. Differences in chronic pain care receipt among veterans from differing racialized groups and the impact of rural versus urban residence. J Rural Health. 2023;39(3):595–603. https://doi.org/10.1111/jrh.12744.
4. Rothmiller SJ, Lund BC, Burgess DJ, Lee S, Hadlandsmyth K. Race differences in Veteran's Affairs emergency department utilization. Mil Med. 2023;188(11–12):3599–605. https://doi.org/10.1093/milmed/usac152.
5. Treede RD, Rief W, Barke A, Aziz Q, Bennett MI, Benoliel R, Cohen M, Evers S, Finnerup NB, First MB, Giamberardino MA, Kaasa S, Korwisi B, Kosek E, Lavand'homme P, Nicholas M, Perrot S, Scholz J, Schug S, Smith BH, Svensson P, Vlaeyen JWS, Wang SJ. Chronic pain as a symptom or a disease: the IASP Classification of Chronic Pain for the international classification of diseases (ICD-11). Pain. 2019;160(1):19–27. https://doi.org/10.1097/j.pain.0000000000001384.
6. Nicholas M, Vlaeyen JWS, Rief W, Barke A, Aziz Q, Benoliel R, Cohen M, Evers S, Giamberardino MA, Goebel A, Korwisi B, Perrot S, Svensson P, Wang SJ, Treede RD, IASP Taskforce for the Classification of Chronic Pain. The IASP classification of chronic pain for ICD-11: chronic primary pain. Pain. 2019;160(1):28–37. https://doi.org/10.1097/j.pain.0000000000001390.
7. Dahlhamer J, Lucas J, Zelaya C, Nahin R, Mackey S, DeBar L, Kerns R, Von Korff M, Porter L, Helmick C. Prevalence of chronic pain and high-impact chronic pain among adults – United States, 2016. MMWR Morb Mortal Wkly Rep. 2018;67(36):1001–6. https://doi.org/10.15585/mmwr.mm6736a2.

8. Rikard SM, Strahan AE, Schmit KM, Guy GP Jr. Chronic pain among adults – United States, 2019–2021. MMWR Morb Mortal Wkly Rep. 2023;72(15):379–85. https://doi.org/10.15585/mmwr.mm7215a1.
9. Hoffman KM, Trawalter S, Axt JR, Oliver MN. Racial bias in pain assessment and treatment recommendations, and false beliefs about biological differences between blacks and whites. Proc Natl Acad Sci USA. 2016;113(16):4296–301.
10. Hollingshead NA, Meints SM, Miller MM, Robinson ME, Hirsh AT. A comparison of race-related pain stereotypes held by White and Black individuals. J Appl Soc Psychol. 2016;46(12):718–23. https://doi.org/10.1111/jasp.12415.
11. Plous S, Williams T. Racial stereotypes from the days of American slavery: a continuing legacy. J App Soc Psychol. 1995;35(9):795–817.
12. Summers KM, Pitts S, Lloyd EP. Racial bias in perceptions of children's pain. J Exp Psychol Appl. 2024;30(1):135–55. https://doi.org/10.1037/xap0000491.
13. Campbell C, Edwards R, Fillingim R. Ethnic differences in responses to multiple experimental pain stimuli. Pain. 2005;113(1):20–6. https://doi.org/10.1016/j.pain.2004.08.013.
14. Meints SM, Wang V, Edwards RR. Sex and race differences in pain sensitization among patients with chronic low back pain. J Pain. 2018;19(12):1461–70. https://doi.org/10.1016/j.jpain.2018.07.001.
15. Bulls HW, Goodin BR, McNew M, Gossett EW, Bradley LA. Minority aging and endogenous pain facilitatory processes. Pain Med. 2016;17(6):1037–48. https://doi.org/10.1093/pm/pnv014.
16. Moss KO, Wright KD, Tan A, Rose KM, Scharre DW, Gure TR, Cowan RL, Failla MD, Monroe TB. Race-related differences between and within sex to experimental thermal pain in middle and older adulthood: an exploratory pilot analysis. Front Pain Res (Lausanne). 2021;2:780338. https://doi.org/10.3389/fpain.2021.780338.
17. Jordan A, Mathis M, Haeny A, Funaro M, Paltin D, Ransome Y. An evaluation of opioid use in Black communities: a rapid review of the literature. Harv Rev Psychiatry. 2021;29(2):108–30. https://doi.org/10.1097/HRP.0000000000000285.
18. Inside Higher Ed (2017) Anger over stereotypes in textbook, October 22. Accessed from https://www.insidehighered.com/news/2017/10/23/nursing-textbook-pulled-over-stereotypes
19. Pham TV, Doorley J, Kenney M, Joo JH, Shallcross AJ, Kincade M, Jackson J, Vranceanu AM. Addressing chronic pain disparities between Black and White people: a narrative review of socio-ecological determinants. Pain Manag. 2023;13(8):473–96. https://doi.org/10.2217/pmt-2023-0032.
20. Institute of Medicine (US) Committee on Advancing Pain Research, Care, and Education. Relieving pain in America: a blueprint for transforming prevention, care, education, and research. Washington, DC: National Academies Press; 2011.
21. Booker SQ, Bartley EJ, Powell-Roach K, Palit S, Morais C, Thompson OJ, Cruz-Almeida Y, Fillingim RB. The imperative for racial equality in pain science: a way forward. J Pain. 2021;22(12):1578–85. https://doi.org/10.1016/j.jpain.2021.06.008.
22. Booker SQ, Merriwether EN, Powell-Roach K, Jackson S. From stepping stones to scaling mountains: overcoming racialized disparities in pain management. Pain Manag. 2024;14(1):5–12. https://doi.org/10.2217/pmt-2023-0098.
23. Green CR, Anderson KO, Baker TA, Campbell LC, Decker S, Fillingim RB, Kalauokalani DA, Lasch KE, Myers C, Tait RC, Todd KH, Vallerand AH. The unequal burden of pain: confronting racial and ethnic disparities in pain. Pain Med. 2003;4(3):277–94. https://doi.org/10.1046/j.1526-4637.2003.03034.x.
24. Green CR. The genesis of the unequal burden of pain: a selective review examining social inequities and unheard voices. Pain. 2023;164(6):1258–63. https://doi.org/10.1097/j.pain.0000000000002869.
25. Dictus C, Cho Y, Baker T, Beeber A. Racial and ethnic disparities in pain management for nursing home residents: a scoping review. Innov Aging. 2021;5(Suppl 1):878.

26. Booker SQ, Herr KA, Wilson Garvan C. Racial differences in pain management for patients receiving hospice care. Oncol Nurs Forum. 2020;47(2):228–40. https://doi.org/10.1188/20.ONF.228-240.
27. Meghani SH, Byun E, Gallagher RM. Time to take stock: a meta-analysis and systematic review of analgesic treatment disparities for pain in the United States. Pain Med. 2012;13(2):150–74. https://doi.org/10.1111/j.1526-4637.2011.01310.x.
28. Goyal MK, Drendel AL, Chamberlain JM, Wheeler J, Olsen C, Grundmeier RW, Cook L, Bajaj L, Babcock L, Zorc JJ, Johnson T, Alpern ER, Pediatric Emergency Care Applied Research Network (PECARN) Registry Study Group. Racial/ethnic differences in ED opioid prescriptions for long bone fractures: trends over time. Pediatrics. 2021;148(5):e2021052481. https://doi.org/10.1542/peds.2021-052481.
29. Meghani SH, Rosa WE, Chittams J, Vallerand AH, Bao T, Mao JJ. Both race and insurance type independently predict the selection of oral opioids prescribed to cancer outpatients. Pain Manag Nurs. 2020;21(1):65–71. https://doi.org/10.1016/j.pmn.2019.07.004.
30. Meghani SH, Kang Y, Chittams J, McMenamin E, Mao JJ, Fudin J. African Americans with cancer pain are more likely to receive an analgesic with toxic metabolite despite clinical risks: a mediation analysis study. J Clin Oncol. 2014;32(25):2773–9. https://doi.org/10.1200/JCO.2013.54.7992.
31. Santoro TN, Santoro JD. Racial bias in the US opioid epidemic: a review of the history of systemic bias and implications for care. Cureus. 2018;10(12):e3733. https://doi.org/10.7759/cureus.3733.
32. Jones KF, Liou KT, Ashare RL, Worster B, Yeager KA, Merlin J, Meghani SH. How racialized approaches to opioid use disorder and opioid misuse management hamper pharmacoequity for cancer pain. J Clin Oncol. 2024;43:JCO2400705. https://doi.org/10.1200/JCO.24.00705.
33. Thompson T, Stathi S, Shin JI, Carvalho A, Solmi M, Liang CS. Racial and ethnic disparities in the prescribing of pain medication in us primary care settings, 1999–2019: where are we now? J Gen Intern Med. 2024;39(9):1597–605. https://doi.org/10.1007/s11606-024-08638-5.
34. Meints SM, Miller MM, Hirsh AT. Differences in pain coping between Black and White Americans: a meta-analysis. J Pain. 2016;17(6):642–53. https://doi.org/10.1016/j.jpain.2015.12.017.
35. Maly A, Vallerand AH. Neighborhood, socioeconomic, and racial influence on chronic pain. Pain Manage Nurs. 2018;19(1):14–22. https://doi.org/10.1016/j.pmn.2017.11.004.
36. Baker TA, Booker SQ, Janevic MR. A progressive agenda toward equity in pain care. Health Psychol Behav Med. 2023;11(1):2266221. https://doi.org/10.1080/21642850.2023.2266221.
37. Puia D, McDonald DD. Older black adult osteoarthritis pain communication. Pain Manag Nurs. 2014;15(1):229–35. https://doi.org/10.1016/j.pmn.2012.09.001.
38. Meints SM, Cortes A, Morais CA, Edwards RR. Racial and ethnic differences in the experience and treatment of noncancer pain. Pain Manag. 2019;9(3):317–34. https://doi.org/10.2217/pmt-2018-0030.
39. Braxton C, Begian-Lewis KM, Marback R, Fritz H. Pain, no gain?: a narrative analysis exploring the accounts of older African American patients and their discussion of pain management related to chronic illness. Rhetor Health Med. 2023;6(2):217–40.
40. Derricks V, Hirsh AT, Perkins AJ, Daggy JK, Matthias MS. Health care discrimination affects patient activation, communication self-efficacy, and pain for African Americans. J Pain. 2024;25:104663. https://doi.org/10.1016/j.jpain.2024.104663.
41. Hirsh AT, Miller MM, Hollingshead NA, Anastas T, Carnell ST, Lok BC, Chu C, Zhang Y, Robinson ME, Kroenke K, Ashburn-Nardo L. A randomized controlled trial testing a virtual perspective-taking intervention to reduce race and socioeconomic status disparities in pain care. Pain. 2019;160(10):2229–40. https://doi.org/10.1097/j.pain.0000000000001634.
42. Booker SQ, Tripp-Reimer T, Herr KA. "Bearing the pain": the experience of aging African Americans with osteoarthritis pain. Glob Qual Nurs Res. 2020;7:2333393620925793. https://doi.org/10.1177/2333393620925793.

43. Booker SQ, Robinson-Lane S, Moss K, Epps F, Taylor J. Missing at random or not?: evidence on pain in Black older adults with dementia and their caregivers. Res Gerontol Nurs. 2024;17(4):162–4. https://doi.org/10.3928/19404921-20240628-01.
44. Woods SB, Roberson PNE, Booker Q, Wood BL, Booker SQ. Longitudinal associations of family relationship quality with chronic pain incidence and persistence among aging African Americans. J Gerontol B Psychol Sci Soc Sci. 2024;79(7):gbae064. https://doi.org/10.1093/geronb/gbae064.
45. Booker S, Herr K, Tripp-Reimer T. Patterns and perceptions of self-management for osteoarthritis pain in African American older adults. Pain Med. 2019;20(8):1489–99. https://doi.org/10.1093/pm/pny260.
46. Meghani SH, Wool J, Davis J, Yeager KA, Mao JJ, Barg FK. When patients take charge of opioids: self-management concerns and practices among cancer outpatients in the context of opioid crisis. J Pain Symptom Manag. 2020;59(3):618–25. https://doi.org/10.1016/j.jpainsymman.2019.10.029.
47. Drazich BF, Jenkins E, Nkimbeng M, Abshire Saylor M, Szanton SL, Wright R, Beach MC, Taylor JL. Exploring the experiences of co-morbid pain and depression in older African American women and their preferred management strategies. Front Pain Res (Lausanne). 2022;3:845513. https://doi.org/10.3389/fpain.2022.845513.
48. Losin EAR, Woo CW, Medina NA, Andrews-Hanna JR, Eisenbarth H, Wager TD. Neural and sociocultural mediators of ethnic differences in pain. Nat Hum Behav. 2020;4(5):517–30. https://doi.org/10.1038/s41562-020-0819-8.
49. Spector AL, Quinn KG, Cruz-Almeida Y, Fillingim RB. Chronic pain among middle-aged and older adults in the United States: the role of everyday discrimination and racial/ethnic identity. J Pain. 2024;25(5):104439. https://doi.org/10.1016/j.jpain.2023.11.022.
50. Hammett PJ, Eliacin J, Saenger M, Allen KD, Meis LA, Krein SL, Taylor BC, Branson M, Fu SS, Burgess DJ. The association between racialized discrimination in health care and pain among black patients with mental health diagnoses. J Pain. 2024;25(1):217–27. https://doi.org/10.1016/j.jpain.2023.08.004.
51. Hood AM, Morais CA, Fields LN, Merriwether EN, Brooks AK, Clark JF, McGill LS, Janevic MR, Letzen JE, Campbell LC. Racism exposure and trauma accumulation perpetuate pain inequities-advocating for change (RESTORATIVE): a conceptual model. Am Psychol. 2023;78(2):143–59. https://doi.org/10.1037/amp0001042.
52. Booker SQ, Okolie T. Pain-affirming care at the intersection of race, aging, and pain management nursing. Pain Manag Nurs. 2024;25(4):323–6. https://doi.org/10.1016/j.pmn.2024.05.012.
53. Booker SS, Herr KA. Pain management for older African Americans in the perianesthesia setting: the "Eight I's". J Perianesth Nurs. 2015;30(3):181–8. https://doi.org/10.1016/j.jopan.2015.01.011.
54. Booker SQ, Herr KA, Horgas AL. A paradigm shift for movement-based pain assessment in older adults: practice, policy and regulatory drivers. Pain Manag Nurs. 2021;22(1):21–7. https://doi.org/10.1016/j.pmn.2020.08.003.
55. Ware LJ, Herr KA, Booker SS, Dotson K, Key J, Poindexter N, Pyles G, Siler B, Packard A. Psychometric evaluation of the revised Iowa pain thermometer (IPT-R) in a sample of diverse cognitively intact and impaired older adults: a pilot study. Pain Manag Nurs. 2015;16(4):475–82. https://doi.org/10.1016/j.pmn.2014.09.004.
56. Boggs L, Fleming J, Geamanu A, Vaidya R. Improving pain assessment after inpatient orthopedic surgery: a comparison of two scales. Am J Nurs. 2024;124:18. https://doi.org/10.1097/01.NAJ.0001094532.56392.71.
57. U.S. Department of Health and Human Services (2019) Pain management best practices inter-agency task force report: updates, gaps, inconsistencies, and recommendations, May 23. Accessed from https://www.hhs.gov/sites/default/files/pmtf-final-report-2019-05-23.pdf
58. Janevic MR, Robinson-Lane S, Murphy S, Piette J. Chronic pain self-management practices and preferences among urban African American older adults. Innov Aging. 2019;3(Suppl 1):S70.

59. Eze B, McDonald DD. African American young adults' pain and pain reduction strategies. Pain Manag Nurs. 2020;21(5):423–7. https://doi.org/10.1016/j.pmn.2020.05.004.
60. Hu DA, Hu JB, Lee A, Rubenstein WJ, Hwang KM, Ibrahim SA, Kuo AC. What factors lead to racial disparities in outcomes after total knee arthroplasty? J Racial Ethn Health Disparities. 2022;9(6):2317–22. https://doi.org/10.1007/s40615-021-01168-4.
61. Figaro MK, Russo PW, Allegrante JP. Preferences for arthritis care among urban African Americans: "I don't want to be cut". Health Psychol. 2004;23:324–9.
62. Yazdanshenas H, Bazargan M, Smith J, Martins D, Motahari H, Orum G. Pain treatment of underserved older African Americans. J Am Geriatr Soc. 2016;64(10):2116–21. https://doi.org/10.1111/jgs.14302.

Chapter 14
Dietary and Nutritional Need Differences in African Americans and Ways to Impact Choices

Contents

14.1	Historical Perspectives	285
14.2	Dietary Components	286
14.3	Fried Foods	288
14.4	Importance of Breakfast	290
	14.4.1 Lactose Intolerance	292
14.5	Beverage Differences	292
14.6	Vitamins, Minerals, and Supplements	295
	14.6.1 Vitamin D Deficiency	295
	14.6.2 Other Vitamin Issues	298
	14.6.3 Mineral Deficiencies	299
References		302

14.1 Historical Perspectives

Dietary differences exist due to cultural differences that can be impacted by region, community, and socioeconomic status. African Americans, by and large, came to America by way of slave ships and originally represented the poorest of the poor. The American poor had limited dietary choices; African American slaves had even less. A significant degree of creativity went into making a meal out of the "leftovers" and discards from plantation owners and their families. Because the plantation was farmland, African Americans had access to a number of fruits and vegetables, but meats were monopolized by the landowners, and only the discarded cuts of meat were reserved for slaves.

Some of the foundations of African Americans' diet stem from these slavery days, but there are also more recent adaptations that have slowly weaved into the fabric of the African American diet. Some of the changes were economic and others more convenient and culture related. To sum up the African American diet by only referring to slave circumstances is to ignore centuries of added influences that made the African American diet what it is today. Food availability, storage, financial independence, health literacy, and a sense of history and heritage all contribute to the ever-changing components of the African American diet.

Being able to positively impact an African American patient's diet will first require a fundamental knowledge of the existing components. The basics of the African American diet mirror an American diet. The "average" meal will have meat, starch, and vegetables in varying proportions [1].

Because of the scarcity of meat as a main course in slavery days, seasoning these cooked vegetable dishes with fatty cuts of low preference meat (whether smoked or not) quickly became a mainstay in the African American diet. Having the lean cuts reserved exclusively for the more affluent, African Americans became accustomed to other cuts of meat. Ham hocks (tibia fibula joint in pigs), neck bones (pork neck vertebrae), ox tails (beef tail), and others became a standard way to "season" and fortify boiled vegetable dishes and beans of various types including navy beans, lima beans, and black eyed peas [2].

Now that the scarcity of meat is much less of a logistical problem, the "habit" or custom of adding meats to vegetables is now merely a standard way to cook them. String beans and collard/mustard/turnip greens almost always have a smoked (and salted) cut of meat in the pot.

Processed meat, which originally represented easily stored meat (and the preserving medium frequently included salt) also found its way to African American dinner tables. For African Americans, having a gene that drives up blood pressure and kidney disease in the presence of salt is an unfortunate reality given the increased presence of salted preserved meats [3].

14.2 Dietary Components

The breakdown in terms of specific meats preferred by African Americans shows a predominance of chicken and turkey, as well as relatively more fish and pork, but less beef than European and Hispanic American diets [2] (Fig. 14.1).

Overall, African Americans eat less grains, fewer eggs, less vegetables, and much less milk, but they consume significantly more meat and fruits [2]. By increasing the amount of vegetables, particularly fresh uncooked in the form of salads, more nutritional balance can be brought to the African American diet fairly easily. The increased consumption of fish and poultry (both chicken and turkey) already represents a beneficial existing tradition [1].

Although African Americans eat relatively fewer vegetables, there are also distinct differences within this category with an increased consumption of fresh green beans, fresh cabbage, and fresh greens when compared with other vegetables [4] (Fig. 14.2).

African Americans prepare more meals "from scratch" when compared to majority of the populations. This increased home cooking leads to comparatively more

14.2 Dietary Components

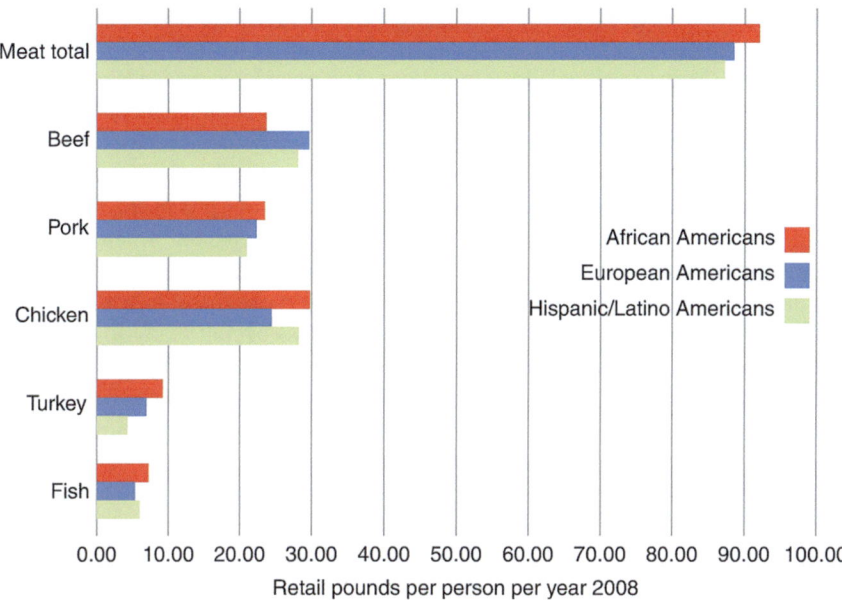

Fig. 14.1 Meat consumption at home by race/ethnicity. (United States Department of Agriculture Economic Research Service. Commodity Consumption by Population Characteristics (by author from raw data). https://www.ers.usda.gov/data-products/commodity-consumption-by-population-characteristics.aspx)

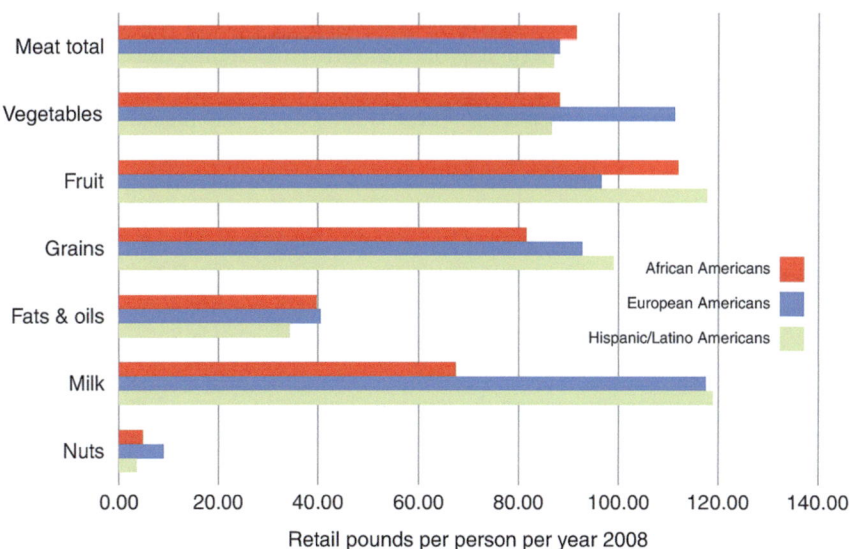

Fig. 14.2 Food consumption at home by race/ethnicity. (United States Department of Agriculture Economic Research Service. Commodity Consumption by Population Characteristics (by author from raw data). https://www.ers.usda.gov/data-products/commodity-consumption-by-population-characteristics.aspx)

purchases of cooking items including spices, seasonings, and oils and preparation items including baking powder, flour, extracts, and sugars in multiple forms [4].

The more "home cooking" done in African American kitchens leads to less consumption of preprocessed or ready-to-eat foods, which is considerably beneficial. Conventionally, when people think of processed and ready-to-eat foods, they generally equate them with poor nutritional quality and lower socioeconomic status. Poti, Mendez, and colleagues looked at the nutritional value of "processed foods" and found they have "higher saturated fat, sugar, and sodium content" when compared to lesser processed foods [5]. Because of the higher proportion of African Americans that are poor, many assumed that they too consume more ready-to-eat foods, but studies reveal that, in fact, African Americans buy less overall ready-to-eat and/or highly processed foods when compared to European Americans [5].

One glaring exception in the purchasing of preprocessed foods was African Americans' tendency to purchase a much higher proportion of preprocessed sugary beverages when compared to European Americans and a much lower volume of milk and dairy purchases [2]. Other exceptions include a significantly higher consumption of bacon and sausages. Finally, there was also an increased purchasing of processed sweeteners including sugar, syrups, jams, and jellies in African American consumers [1].

14.3 Fried Foods

Looking at home preparation patterns, African Americans have an increased propensity to fry meats, potatoes, and other vegetables [6]. From a practical standpoint, frying foods is a fast and flavorful approach to fortifying (adding calories and substance) to almost any food. If you want to increase or stretch the caloric value of a food, flour or batter it, and then fry it. There is little doubt that the scarcity of food for the poor leads to practical approaches to stretching and making more palatable whatever food was present. African Americans have not just fried potatoes, but introduced fried okra, fried mushrooms, fried onions, fried green tomatoes, southern fried steak or pork chops, and a host of other dishes that started merely out of necessity. Now that there is more variety of food and it is presumably more plentiful, the "need" to fry food has diminished, but the habit and culturalization of fried foods are as strong as ever in both the African American and American-at-large communities [6].

Now that we better understand the logic behind fried foods and its place in the African American diet, decreasing the consumption due to its detrimental effects needs to be a higher priority. Sun, Lui, and colleagues at the University of Iowa looked at the impact of fried food consumption on cardiovascular mortality [6]:

> We found a significantly positive association of fried food consumption, especially fried chicken and fried fish/shellfish, with risk of all cause and cardiovascular mortality. These associations were slightly attenuated, but remained significant, after additional adjustment for a variety of factors that were related to mortality, including age, race/ethnicity, socioeconomic status, hormone use, lifestyle factors, health status, and body mass index. [6]

With obesity as a prominent public health risk and African Americans leading the way in obesity prevalence, placing fried foods as a major offender is key. Eating fried foods is dangerous from a number of perspectives. The frying process greatly increases the calorie content, increases the fat content, and significantly increases cardiovascular risk.

A lesser-known problem with frying foods is it facilitates the formation of chemical reaction by-products called advanced glycation end products (AGEs), which seem to be linked to a number of serious health issues [7]. Advanced glycation end products are the subject of ongoing research investigations into its detrimental impact on health including its promotion of cancer cell proliferation in the presence of colorectal, liver, pancreatic, and breast cancer [7]. As cooking oil is heated and used, AGEs form and become more plentiful in the oil. They are then consumed and are highly bioavailable while circulating in the body. These circulating dietary AGEs have been suspected to increase diabetes occurrence, cause premature aging, facilitate further weight gain, advance carotid stenosis and peripheral artery occlusive disease, worsen kidney disease, and promote the development and progression of heart failure [8]. All of these problems, in addition to the poor cancer outcomes, occur disproportionately in African Americans. While the research on AGEs is ongoing, and our understanding rudimentary at this point, it is fairly clear that AGEs are not at all beneficial, and while some AGEs form naturally as part of our aging process, consuming more only advances whatever pathology is present. African Americans can greatly impact the nutritional value of any meal by merely avoiding frying their foods.

Most African American patients acknowledge that fried food is bad for their health, but few know the specifics of why [9, 10]. Beyond the obvious increase in obesity (due to increased caloric content and AGE impact), increased consumption of fried foods directly leads to lower HDL cholesterol levels and higher LDL levels [11]. Increased consumption of fried foods has also been linked to the later development of type 2 diabetes and coronary heart disease [12].

Advanced Glycation End Products (AGEs)
- AGEs are generated through nonenzymatic glycation and oxidation of proteins, lipids, and nucleic acids.
- They alter tissue function and mechanical properties through cross-linking matrix proteins and through binding to their cell surface receptors.
- Enhanced formation and accumulation of AGEs have been reported to occur in conditions such as diabetes mellitus as well as in natural aging, renal failure, and chronic inflammation [8].

It should also be noted that reusing cooking oils is common in African American homes and is associated with added health risks. Heat causes oxidation and degradation of many oils with the formation of increased trans-fatty acids, which have definitively been associated with increased heart disease and stroke [13]. The degradation seen with reusing oils varies based on the oil and the type of food being cooked with olive oil showing great resistance to degradation and soybean (vegetable) oils showing linear degradation with temperature and heating time [14]. Some have suggested that much of the detriment associated with increased restaurant or fast-food consumption is the prolonged and repeated use of oils and comparatively more trans-fat formation [14]. An oil with no trans-fat content can acquire significant trans-fat with heat, time, and reuse. Younger African Americans, like all Americans, find themselves eating fast food with increased frequency; advice to avoid fried fast food and giving a rationale behind the advice should improve compliance. As far as home frying is concerned, discarding oils after a "few" uses is a practical advice that is easily understood and could have a big impact.

The increased preparation of meals in the African American household also offers a big opportunity to make gradual adjustments in cooking techniques and ingredient substitutions that can have a positive impact on health over time. Making different suggestions on each patient visit can improve the adoption of healthier habits. Suggesting to not add meat to cooked vegetables, or at least substituting a lower fat content meat (e.g., switching from fatty pork meat to turkey meat), can impact health and health education. As you would discuss smoking cessation at every visit from a smoking patient, discussing small diet modifications at each visit can more reliably improve compliance and change habits.

Explaining Why Eating Fried Foods Is Bad
- Increases calorie content
- Increases obesity
- Lowers HDL cholesterol and raises LDL cholesterol
- Increases risk for type 2 diabetes
- Increases risk for heart disease
- Adds dietary AGEs
- Increases trans-fatty acids with repeated oil use

14.4 Importance of Breakfast

African Americans more frequently skip breakfast [15, 16]. The reasons range from busy schedules, the added preparation time for an "old-style breakfast" (that could include bacon, sausage, potatoes, pancakes, etc.), or the lack of an appetite. The absence of breakfast has been associated with decreased calcium, dairy, fiber, and fruit consumption [17].

Generally, the percentage of young African American children that eat breakfast starts relatively high, but that number decreases in the teen years [17]. Studies have verified that routinely eating breakfast frequently leads to more regular eating habits later in the day, improved exercise patterns, better cognition, and more healthful food choices [18, 19]. Those changes could result in less weight gain and contribute to a reduced BMI.

Making a positive impact on breakfast in African Americans first requires a starting definition. An agreement reported by the Journal of the Academy of Nutrition and Dietetics defined breakfast [18]:

14.4 Importance of Breakfast

Breakfast is the first meal of the day that breaks the fast after the longest period of sleep and is consumed within 2–3 hours of waking; it is comprised of food or beverage from at least one food group, and may be consumed at any location. [18]

Having one consensus definition of breakfast allows for clinicians and researchers to move forward with recommendations from the same starting point. Before 2014, there were widely variable definitions of breakfast that lead to confusion when proposals for changes were made.

The same report (The Role of Breakfast in Health: Definition and Criteria for a Quality Breakfast) proposed criteria for a quality breakfast but also allowed for much more variability based on "age, sex, activity level, and individual tastes and preferences" [18]. By not specifically listing "what you should eat," the report allows for the realistic cultural differences in meals that already exist. The components of a quality breakfast take into account energy needs, nutrient requirements, food composition and food groups, portion sizes, and the presence of nutrient-dense foods and beverages [18].

Many older African Americans have the time (and inclination) to have a breakfast that includes bacon or sausage, eggs, and toast or pancakes. While from a cholesterol standpoint, this is not an ideal meal, eating a protein-rich breakfast has been shown to help satiety and promote sensible eating throughout the rest of the day [18].

Many Americans believe that skipping meals is a reasonable approach to weight loss and the meal most skipped is breakfast [20]. It is important to stress during weight counseling that there is controversy regarding the benefit or detriment of meal skipping. Krista Casazza and colleagues at the University of Alabama weighed the evidence behind this common belief:

> Beyond observational and single meal studies, very little evidence directly supports or refutes the belief that breakfast eating affects weight. Shorter, single-meal, controlled studies have investigated the links between breakfast consumption and factors related to weight. Some evidence indicates that skipping breakfast results in partial compensation during subsequent meals. [20]

The significantly decreased consumption of milk and dairy products in the African American diet presents a potential increased health risk as "moderate evidence shows that the intake of milk and milk products is associated with a reduced risk of cardiovascular disease, type 2 diabetes, and lower blood pressure in adults" [21]. An assessment of nutrient intake related to dairy consumption showed that African Americans' intake of the required nutrients calcium, vitamin D, and potassium was all lower than that of European Americans and Hispanic/Latino Americans. Be aware that for prostate cancer, high calcium intake has been linked to an increased risk of aggressive prostate cancer in African American men. Batai et al. found that high calcium intake was significantly associated with higher odds of aggressive prostate cancer (OR = 4.28, 95% CI: 1.70–10.80) in African Americans, while high vitamin D intake was inversely associated with aggressive prostate cancer [22]. Similarly, Rowland et al. reported that high dietary calcium intake was associated with an increased risk of both localized and advanced prostate cancer, with a significant dose-response relationship [23].

14.4.1 Lactose Intolerance

The choice for African Americans to avoid milk and related products is not entirely voluntary. Research has consistently shown that 75% or more of African Americans are lactose intolerant [24, 25]. Poor digestion of lactose occurs when insufficient amounts of lactase are available in the small intestine to hydrolyze lactose into its two constituents, galactose and glucose. New evidence is discovering that the proportion of people that are lactose intolerant could be tied to their region of genetic origin [26]. Put simply, regions where dairy herds could be raised safely and efficiently produced people that could digest lactose better. Harsher climates in African and Asia restricted the availability of dairy herds that produced milk and thus produced people with much more lactose intolerance, a study at Cornell University found [26]. Researchers found a wide range of lactose intolerances with as low as 2% of the population of Denmark descendants to as high as 100% of the people with Zambian origin. Their survey "found that lactose intolerance decreases with increasing latitude and increases with rising temperature" [26].

The process of replacing the missing nutrients resulting from low dairy consumption has become fairly easy due to lactase-fortified milks, as well as multiple milk equivalents including soy, almond, coconut, and others that can be used as part of a healthy breakfast. Oatmeal and/or whole grain cereals with milk equivalents can make a fast and nutritionally efficient meal.

14.5 Beverage Differences

As reviewed earlier, there is a substantial difference in the drinking practices of both teen and adult African Americans. Milk and water consumption is particularly low, while sugar-sweetened beverages (SSBs) are all significantly higher [2]. The consumption of fruit juice, soda, sport drinks, and all other sweetened beverages is significantly higher in African Americans [27–29].

An African American woman consumes almost double the sugar-sweetened beverage amounts than European American woman of the same age [28]. A historical review showed decreased consumption of sugar-sweetened beverages in the 1980s with a gradual increase to today's significant surplus [27]. Several studies link the trend directly to targeted and financially disproportional marketing of sugar-sweetened beverages to African Americans [27, 30, 31].

The overconsumption of sugar-sweetened beverages does not start in childhood, in fact European American male children and teens consume more sweetened beverages when compared to African American males of similar ages, but somewhere in their twenties, European Americans decrease their consumption and African Americans increase consumption [28] (Fig. 14.3).

Looking at African American women in particular, there is an across-the-board increased average daily consumption from sugar-sweetened beverages. The Black Women's Health Study found that women who transitioned from drinking "one or

14.5 Beverage Differences

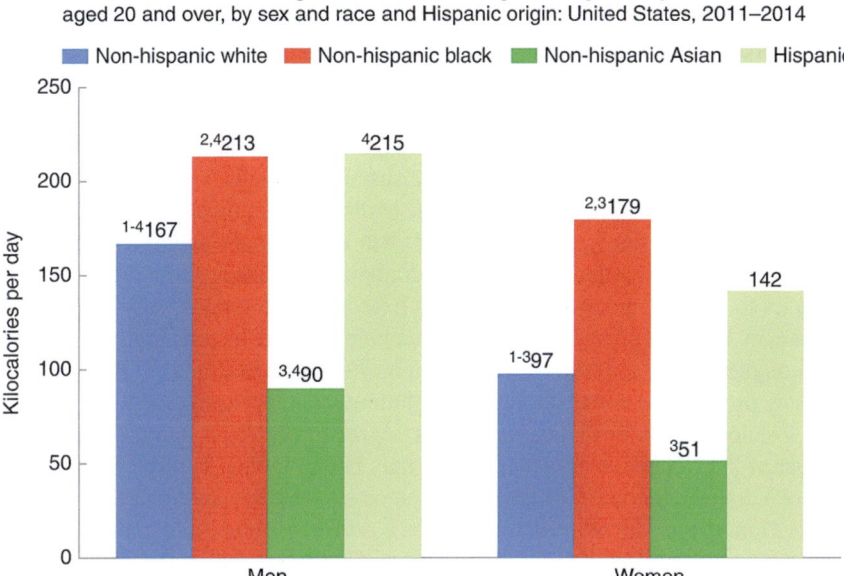

Fig. 14.3 Daily calories from sugar-sweetened beverages by race/ethnicity and sex (https://www.cdc.gov/nchs/data/databriefs/db270.pdf)

fewer soft drinks per week to drinking one or more soft drinks per day" saw the greatest weight gain (15 pounds) [27]. Those who were able to keep their consumption at one soft drink or less per week, or were able to decrease to that level, saw a 9–11 pound weight loss [27].

Making a point of emphasizing the detriment of too many sugar-sweetened beverages in any diet is essential, and passing on data-based information to patients on how they can practically impact their diet is extremely useful [32]. Basic messaging like drinking water when they are thirsty, and having a sugar-sweetened beverage for pleasure (rather than thirst), is a sound advice worth repeating at every visit.

> Sugar-sweetened beverages (SSBs) can lead to weight gain through their high added-sugar content, low satiety, and an incomplete compensatory reduction in energy intake at subsequent meals after intake of liquid calories. On average, SSBs contain 140–150 calories and 35.0–37.5 g sugar per 12-oz serving. In addition, fructose from any sugar or high fructose-content sugar (HFCS) has been shown to promote the development of visceral adiposity and ectopic fat deposition. [32]

Obesity impacts African Americans in a number of ways including increased coronary heart disease, heart failure, hypertension, stroke, and venous thrombosis. The increased obesity rate drives up type 2 diabetes incidence in both adults and children while also increasing the incidence of fatty liver, obstructive sleep apnea, and degenerative joint disease. As research into the specific ways a patient's eating habits impact them continues, applying the knowledge that already exists to patient-centered diet modification suggestions can add up to a significant impact.

While self-perception in African Americans does blunt some degree of trepidation resulting from obesity, there is still a disproportionate amount of helplessness as it relates to getting practical advice for a sustained benefit.

As primary clinical providers, being able to discuss poor dietary habits and physical inactivity with our patients is critical. But any changes suggested should be incremental. Simply telling a patient to dramatically change their diet and daily lifestyles to something completely foreign to them is a complete waste of time for the patient and the provider. Mapping out planned and incremental suggestions based on the patient's preferences and current lifestyle is essential.

Many providers confuse obesity with gluttony and appear to blame patients for their size and health. In reality, a patient's degree of obesity is a combination of a number of interrelated factors that may or may not be in their control. Success will require a delicate mix of interventions based on treating the patient as the center of the solution. Is the patient's risk for diabetes based on genetics, diet, family cooking patterns, or other factors? Only the patient can tell you, and as the provider, you have a unique opportunity to be granted permission by the patient to make a difference.

Sports Drinks May Be Harmful Sports drinks are frequently marketed as a way to replenish the electrolytes and fluids lost during intense physical activity. However, concerns about their sodium content, especially in relation to African Americans, warrant a closer examination. These drinks usually contain sodium, which aids in fluid retention and helps prevent dehydration, but excessive sodium intake can lead to hypertension, a condition that already disproportionately affects African Americans. The American College of Cardiology and the American Heart Association emphasize that salt sensitivity is especially prevalent among African Americans, older adults, and individuals with comorbidities such as chronic kidney disease, diabetes mellitus, or metabolic syndrome [33]. This heightened sensitivity to sodium can contribute to increased blood pressure and a higher risk of cardiovascular disease and stroke. Studies have shown that African Americans exhibit stronger blood pressure responses to sodium intake compared to Americans of European descent [34, 35]. This is supported by findings indicating that African Americans have altered renal sodium handling and vascular responses, which contribute to their increased risk of hypertension and related complications [34–36]. The average sports drink contains about 110–160 mg of sodium per 8-ounce serving. While this amount is designed to aid athletes in recovery and hydration, it can contribute to overall sodium intake if consumed frequently without sufficient physical activity to justify it. For example, if an individual regularly consumes sports drinks during moderate exercise or daily activities, the added sodium may lead to intake exceeding the recommended daily limit, thereby increasing the risk of developing hypertension. It is essential for individuals, particularly African Americans, to consider their overall dietary sodium consumption. While sports drinks can benefit athletes engaged in prolonged, intense exercise, moderation is essential. African Americans, particularly those with existing health concerns, should be mindful of their sodium intake from all sources, including sports drinks, and consider alternatives like water or homemade electrolyte solutions that can replenish fluids without excessive salt.

14.6 Vitamins, Minerals, and Supplements

14.6.1 Vitamin D Deficiency

Vitamin D deficiency has a significant impact on the health of African Americans, contributing to various health disparities. African Americans have a higher prevalence of severe vitamin D deficiency compared to European Americans, primarily due to increased melanin in the skin, which reduces the synthesis of vitamin D from sunlight [37]. Vitamin D is acquired through diet and skin exposure to ultraviolet B light. The skin's production of vitamin D is determined by length of exposure, latitude, season, and degree of skin pigmentation [37]. African Americans produce less vitamin D3 than do European Americans in response to matched levels of sun exposure and have dramatically lower 25-hydroxyvitamin D [25(OH)D] concentrations, with some studies indicating up to 82% of the African American population as deficient [38].

Some hypothesize that vitamin D deficiency is simply a matter of location and skin color. Human skin contains melanin, which provides pigmentation and protects against UV radiation. However, higher levels of melanin can impede the skin's ability to produce vitamin D in response to sunlight exposure. In regions with lower latitudes, where UV radiation is more intense, individuals with lighter skin are typically able to synthesize vitamin D more efficiently. Conversely, as one moves toward higher latitudes, where UV exposure diminishes, individuals with darker skin, including African Americans, struggle to produce adequate vitamin D [37].

Vitamin D Deficiency and Health Disparities
Bruce Ames from the University of California at Berkeley concluded that African Americans should be deliberate about vitamin D replacement as an approach to address multiple health disparities:

> Moderate-to-strong evidence exists that high 25-hydroxyvitamin D levels and/or vitamin D supplementation reduces risk for many adverse health outcomes including all-cause mortality rate, adverse pregnancy and birth outcomes, cancer, diabetes mellitus, Alzheimer's disease and dementia, multiple sclerosis, acute respiratory tract infections, COVID-19, asthma exacerbations, rickets, and osteomalacia. We suggest that people with low vitamin D status, which would include most people with dark skin living at high latitudes, along with their health care provider, consider taking vitamin D3 supplements to raise serum 25-hydroxyvitamin D levels to 30 ng/mL (75 nmol/L) or possibly higher. [37]

While African Americans tend to have lower vitamin D3 levels and are very frequently labeled vitamin D deficient, they also have confirmed stronger bones and fewer fractures. Powe and colleagues at the Brigham and Woman's Hospital in

Cambridge, Massachusetts, looked specifically at this paradox as it related to vitamin D3- and vitamin D-binding proteins and suggested that some of the vitamin D deficiency was exaggerated [39].

Overall, vitamin D deficiency is significantly associated with increased risks of cardiovascular disease, type 2 diabetes, and hypertension in African Americans [40, 41]. Lower serum 25-hydroxyvitamin D [25(OH)D] levels are linked to higher mean arterial pressure, fasting plasma glucose, waist circumference, and lower HDL cholesterol levels. Additionally, vitamin D deficiency is associated with a higher incidence of anemia, particularly anemia with inflammation, among African Americans [42–44].

Freishtat and colleagues found that urban African American youth with asthma had significantly higher rates of vitamin D insufficiency and deficiency compared to controls without asthma, suggesting a strong link between low vitamin D levels and asthma [45]. Additionally, Pillai et al. identified associations between genetic variants in vitamin D metabolism genes and asthma characteristics in young African Americans, further supporting the role of vitamin D in asthma pathogenesis [46].

Vitamin D Deficiency, Calcium, and Prostate Cancer
Ken Batai and colleagues at the University of Arizona, through studying over 2000 patients, found a direct benefit to vitamin D supplementation to preventing prostate cancer in African American men and a *pro-carcinogenic* effect of calcium supplementation on the prostate [22]. These findings were strongest in African Americans:

> Calcium and vitamin D are important nutrients, and they may have preventive effects against many health conditions. Although toxicity from high vitamin D supplementation may be low, high calcium intake is associated with increased prostate cancer risk as well as risk of cardiovascular disease and kidney stones. High calcium consumption might be harmful, and for prostate cancer prevention, high-dose calcium supplementation and fortification should be avoided, especially among (African American) men. [22]

If your African American patient is concerned about prostate cancer, vitamin D supplementation will certainly help, and if your patient is a health nut on multiple supplements or has heartburn and takes a lot of antacids, check to ensure the calcium supplementation is not overly aggressive. High calcium intake in African American men may actually increase the risk for prostate cancer [22, 23].

The genetic basis for this increased risk is linked to polymorphisms in the vitamin D receptor (VDR) gene, specifically the VDR Cdx2 genotype. This genotype influences calcium absorption in the intestine. Studies have shown that African American men with the VDR Cdx2 GG genotype, which is associated with lower calcium absorption, have a significantly lower risk of advanced prostate cancer compared to those with higher calcium absorption genotypes [23, 47]. Additionally, polymorphisms in the calcium-sensing receptor (CaSR) gene have been investigated. Although the CaSR genotypes were not associated with prostate cancer overall, specific polymorphisms like Q1011E were found to be associated with a less aggressive form of prostate cancer among African American men [48]. Furthermore, the TRPV6 calcium channel gene, which has a higher frequency of the ancestral allele in people of African ancestry, may also contribute to the increased risk. This

14.6 Vitamins, Minerals, and Supplements

allele is associated with higher cellular calcium levels, which have been implicated in cancer development [49].

Vitamin D Deficiency and Renal Insufficiency

Vitamin D measurement and appropriate supplementation in African American patients with renal insufficiency have been suggested by the National Kidney Foundation due to its beneficial effects. With the increased kidney disease in African Americans and the concomitant lower vitamin D levels across the African American population, the benefits of vitamin D replacement in these patients are high. Lunyera and colleagues at Duke University looked at vitamin D and chronic kidney disease in the Jackson Heart Study.

> Our data also support a role of low 25(OH)D as an independent risk for faster decline in kidney function in (African) Americans with diabetes. This finding corroborates, in an exclusively (African American) cohort, a growing body of evidence that suggests low 25(OH)D confers greater risk factor for adverse CKD outcomes among individuals with diabetic kidney disease.

Vitamin D Deficiency and Cancer

Another study linked vitamin D level to the patient's risk for ovarian cancer:

> The role of Vitamin D in human cancers, including ovarian cancer, has been widely investigated, where it was proposed to play a protective and antitumorigenic role by regulating cellular proliferation and metabolism. In this review, we have shown that vitamin D status may be an independent predictor of prognosis in ovarian cancer patients. Vitamin D combination therapy improves antitumor effects allowing for potential clinical application. Supplement of vitamin D and calcium combination may be an efficient method for cancer prevention.

Yao and Ambrosone looked at the association between vitamin D deficiency and aggressive breast cancer in African American women and found:

> The relationship of vitamin D with breast cancer risk may be subtype-specific, with emerging evidence of stronger effects of vitamin D for more aggressive breast cancer, particularly in women of African ancestry.

A link between vitamin D and colon cancer exists as well:

> our work provides evidence of differences in transcriptional responses to a fixed dose of (vitamin D) 1α,25(OH)2D3 between African Americans and European Americans ... These inter-ethnic response differences are irrespective of serum 25(OH)D levels suggesting that even if equivalent serum levels are achieved between populations, there could still be differences in response at the tissue level. We provide evidence supporting a genetic mechanism underlying inter-ethnic differences in vitamin D ...

Genetic factors further exacerbate the risk associated with vitamin D deficiency. Bhasin and colleagues at the University of Chicago found that a polymorphism in the UPP1 gene, which is more common among African Americans, reduces the expression of UPP1 in response to vitamin D. This reduction leads to increased uridine-induced DNA damage and a higher risk of colorectal cancer [50]. Similarly, Pibiri et al. identified that genetic variants in vitamin D-related genes, such as CYP2R1, are linked to colorectal cancer risk in African Americans [51].

In breast cancer, Yao et al. demonstrated that specific SNPs in the vitamin D pathway, particularly those in the CYP24A1 gene, are associated with a higher risk of estrogen receptor-negative breast cancer among African American women. This subtype of breast cancer is more aggressive and has fewer treatment options [52]. In prostate cancer, Nelson et al. found that vitamin D deficiency significantly increases the risk of aggressive prostate cancer in African American men, and this risk is further influenced by genetic variants in the vitamin D receptor [53]. These findings underscore the importance of addressing vitamin D deficiency in African Americans, considering both environmental and genetic factors, to potentially reduce the risk of these aggressive cancers.

14.6.2 Other Vitamin Issues

In addition to vitamin D, which is often highlighted due to its crucial role in bone health and immune function, African Americans are also at risk for several other vitamin deficiencies. One significant deficiency is vitamin B12. This vitamin is essential for nerve function, red blood cell production, and DNA synthesis. While the deficiency is less common, it can lead to anemia and neurological issues. African Americans may be at a higher risk due to dietary habits and lower absorption rates, particularly if they consume fewer animal products, which are primary sources of B12 [54, 55]. Another important vitamin deficiency to consider is folate (vitamin B9). Folate is vital for DNA synthesis and repair, as well as for the production of healthy red blood cells. A deficiency in folate can lead to anemia and complications during pregnancy, such as neural tube defects. African Americans, particularly women of childbearing age, may benefit from increased folate intake, especially through fortified foods or supplements [56]. Vitamin A is also a concern, as it plays a crucial role in vision, immune function, and skin health. Deficiencies can lead to night blindness and increased susceptibility to infections. Diets low in fruits and vegetables, especially those rich in beta-carotene (a precursor to vitamin A), can contribute to this deficiency [56]. Lastly, vitamin C deficiency, though not as common, can still pose health risks. Vitamin C is important for collagen synthesis, antioxidant protection, and immune support. Individuals with limited access to fresh fruits and vegetables may not receive sufficient amounts of this vitamin [57]. While vitamin D is a prominent concern, African Americans should also be aware of the potential deficiencies in vitamin B12, folate, vitamin A, and vitamin C.

Vitamin E and an Increased Risk for Prostate Cancer
It is important to note that the Selenium and Vitamin E Cancer Prevention Trial (SELECT) found that vitamin E supplementation significantly increased the risk of prostate cancer among healthy men [58, 59]. Since African American men face a markedly higher risk for prostate cancer, caution is warranted when considering vitamin E supplementation due to these potential risks.

A study on oxidative DNA damage found that African Americans had lower plasma concentrations of vitamin E compared to European Americans, and a positive association between vitamin E and oxidative DNA damage was observed in African American men [60]. This suggests that high levels of vitamin E might be linked to increased oxidative stress in African Americans, potentially leading to adverse health outcomes. Therefore, it is crucial for individuals, particularly African American men, to consult with healthcare professionals before starting vitamin E supplementation. A balanced approach to diet and supplementation can help minimize risks while promoting health and preventing potential adverse effects.

14.6.3 Mineral Deficiencies

Various socioeconomic, dietary, and lifestyle factors influence mineral deficiencies in African Americans. Iron deficiency is especially prevalent among African American women and children, often resulting from inadequate nutritional intake, higher rates of menorrhagia, or elevated physiological needs during pregnancy and growth periods. This deficiency can lead to prolonged anemia, fatigue, and impaired immune function [61]. Several studies have shown that African American women are more likely to experience heavy menstrual bleeding compared to their European American counterparts. Uterine fibroids, which are more common and severe among African American women, play a significant role in this increased incidence of menorrhagia [62]. For example, a study published in the Journal of Women's Health found that African American women with uterine fibroids were significantly more likely to report heavy or prolonged menstruation [63]. Furthermore, the New England Journal of Medicine has noted that fibroids are more frequently encountered and symptomatic in African American women, resulting in higher rates of heavy menstrual bleeding and associated anemia [64]. Studies indicate that African American women have lower average hemoglobin levels and higher rates of iron deficiency. The prevalence of iron deficiency anemia is nearly 20% among African American women, compared to 9–12% among European American women [65]. Additionally, African American women tend to have higher serum ferritin levels despite a greater prevalence of iron deficiency, suggesting differences in iron metabolism [66, 67]. Serum ferritin levels serve as markers of the body's iron stores. High serum ferritin levels in the presence of iron deficiency may indicate inflammation or other underlying conditions that affect iron metabolism.

Another important mineral deficiency is magnesium, which plays a crucial role in various bodily functions, including muscle and nerve function, blood glucose regulation, and bone health. Many African Americans may not meet the recommended dietary intake for magnesium due to diets that are low in whole grains, nuts, seeds, and green leafy vegetables. This deficiency can lead to various health issues, including muscle cramps, fatigue, and an increased risk of heart disease and type 2 diabetes [68, 69]. Additionally, magnesium deficiency can also contribute to imbalances in calcium and potassium levels, further exacerbating health problems.

Several studies have demonstrated this racial difference in serum potassium levels. For instance, a study published in the American Journal of Kidney Diseases found that African Americans had on average 0.162 mmol/L lower serum potassium levels compared to non-African Americans, even after adjusting for demographics, comorbid conditions, and potassium-altering medication use [70]. Another study from the Atherosclerosis Risk in Communities (ARIC) Study reported that African Americans had lower mean serum potassium concentrations (4.2 mEq/L) compared to whites (4.5 mEq/L) [71]. Chronic mild hypokalemia can exacerbate cardiac arrhythmias. The American Heart Association notes that hypokalemia can cause electrocardiographic changes, such as broadening of T waves, ST-segment depression, and prominent U waves, which predispose patients to arrhythmias like ventricular tachycardia and fibrillation [72, 73]. Additionally, arrhythmias induced by hypokalemia are linked to reduced Na/K-ATPase activity, resulting in calcium overload in ventricular myocytes [73]. Hypokalemia can also cause neuromuscular symptoms, including muscle weakness and cramps. Chronically low potassium levels may accelerate the progression of chronic kidney disease and worsen hypertension control. Persistent hypokalemia can lead to hypokalemic nephropathy, characterized by renal cysts, chronic interstitial nephritis, and progressive loss of renal function [74, 75]. Finally, hypokalemia can impair insulin release, leading to glucose intolerance, which is particularly prevalent among African Americans. This effect complicates the management of diabetes and contributes to poor glycemic control [76].

Zinc deficiency can also be problematic, impacting immune function and wound healing; it is often associated with dietary patterns that lack sufficient protein sources. Zinc is essential for various enzymatic functions and plays a critical role in DNA synthesis and cell division. Deficiency can result in stunted growth in children, weakened immunity, and delayed wound healing. Several studies have shown a higher prevalence of zinc deficiency among African Americans compared to other racial groups. For instance, a study by Cole and colleagues found that low-income African American children had a significantly increased risk of zinc deficiency compared to their Hispanic counterparts, with an odds ratio of 3.47 [77]. Furthermore, research by Neggers et al. indicated that low-income African American pregnant women had lower plasma zinc levels compared to European American women [78]. Finally, the Third National Health and Nutrition Examination Survey (NHANES III) reported that African Americans had a lower mean total zinc intake than European Americans [79].

Dietary and Nutritional Need Differences in African Americans
- African Americans eat relatively more chicken and turkey, as well as fish and pork, but less beef than European and Hispanic/Latino American diets.
- African Americans eat relatively more fruit, but fewer vegetables.
- Explain the true impact of frying foods.
- Advise against reusing cooking oil more than twice.
- Dietary AGEs have been suspected to increase diabetes occurrence, cause premature aging, facilitate weight gain, advance carotid stenosis and peripheral artery occlusive disease, worsen kidney disease, and promote the development and progression of heart failure.
- Patient encounters focusing and discussing current dietary habits and physical inactivity is crucial.
- Any change suggestions related to diet and activity levels should be gradual and incremental.
- Dramatic changes from a baseline diet will frequently fail.
- Whenever possible, be specific about the dietary changes you expect.
- Advise a healthy (yet easy) low-fat breakfast daily with a high-fiber food (oatmeal, grits, or fresh fruit).
- African Americans can greatly impact the nutritional value of their meals by simply avoiding frying their foods.
- Quantify your patient's current use of sugar-sweetened beverages, and advise a gradual (yet reasonable) decrease in use.
- An African American woman consumes almost double the sugar-sweetened beverage amounts than European American woman of the same age.
- An African American woman who was able to keep their consumption at one soft drink or less per week, or was able to decrease to that level, saw a sustained 9–11 pound weight loss.
- African Americans exhibit stronger blood pressure responses to sodium intake and should avoid "Sports Drinks" unless they are truly electrolyte deficient.
- Be aware that African Americans frequently will be more content at a larger size and may not be aware of the true impact of their size on their future health.
- African Americans have a higher prevalence of severe vitamin D deficiency compared to European Americans, primarily due to increased melanin in the skin, which reduces the synthesis of vitamin D from sunlight.
- While African Americans tend to have lower vitamin D3 levels and are very frequently labeled vitamin D deficient, they also have confirmed stronger bones and fewer fractures.
- Vitamin D deficiency is significantly associated with increased risks of cardiovascular disease, type 2 diabetes, advancing kidney disease, and hypertension in African Americans.

(continued)

- The Selenium and Vitamin E Cancer Prevention Trial (SELECT) found that vitamin E supplementation significantly increased the risk of prostate cancer among healthy men.
- Studies indicate that African American women have lower average hemoglobin levels and higher rates of iron deficiency.
- Look for magnesium, potassium, and zinc deficiency and suggest replacement, as African Americans have an increased occurrence.

References

1. Standard American Diet. NutritionFacts.org. https://nutritionfacts.org/topics/standard-american-diet/. Accessed 28 May 2019.
2. Commodity consumption by population characteristics. United States Department of Agriculture. Economic Research Service. https://www.ers.usda.gov/data-products/commodity-consumption-by-population-characteristics/. Accessed 28 May 2019.
3. Richardson S, Freedman B, Ellison D, et al. Salt sensitivity: a review with a focus on non-Hispanic blacks and hispanics. J Am Soc Hypertens. 2013;7(2):170–9.
4. African-americans combine tradition with a multimedia approach to shopping. 2016. Retrieved 22 Nov 2018, from https://www.nielsen.com/us/en/insights/news/2016/african-americans-combine-tradition-with-a-multimedia-approach-to-shopping.html
5. Poti J, Mendez M, Ng S, Popkin B. Is the degree of food processing and convenience linked with the nutritional quality of foods purchased by US households? Am J Clin Nutr. 2015;101(6):1251–62.
6. Sun Y, Liu B, Snetselaar LG, et al. Association of fried food consumption with all cause cardiovascular and cancer mortality: prospective cohort study. BMJ. 2019;364:k5420.
7. Chen H, Wu L, Li Y, Meng J, Lin N, Yang D, et al. Advanced glycation end products increase carbohydrate responsive element binding protein expression and promote cancer cell proliferation. Mol Cell Endocrinol. 2014;395(1–2):69–78.
8. Hegab Z, Gibbons S, Neyses L, Mamas M. Role of advanced glycation end products in cardiovascular disease. World J Cardiol. 2012;4(4):90–102.
9. Park A, Eckert TL, Zaso MJ, et al. Associations between health literacy and health behaviors among urban high school students. J Sch Health. 2017;87(12):885–93.
10. Berkman ND, Sheridan SL, Donahue KE, et al. Low health literacy and health outcomes: an updated systematic review. Ann Intern Med. 2011;155(2):97–107.
11. HDL cholesterol: how to boost your 'good' cholesterol. Mayo Clinic 2018. https://www.mayoclinic.org/diseases-conditions/high-blood-cholesterol/in-depth/hdl-cholesterol/art-20046388. Accessed 9 June 2019.
12. Cahill L, Pan A, Chiuve S, et al. Fried-food consumption and risk of type 2 diabetes and coronary artery disease: a prospective study in 2 cohorts of US women and men. Am J Clin Nutr. 2014;100(2):667–75.
13. de Souza RJ, Mente A, Maroleanu A, et al. Intake of saturated and trans unsaturated fatty acids and risk of all-cause mortality, cardiovascular disease, and type 2 diabetes: systematic review and meta-analysis of observational studies. BMJ. 2015;351:h3978.
14. Li A, Ha Y, Wang F, Li W, Li Q. Determination of thermally induced trans-fatty acids in soybean oil by attenuated total reflectance Fourier transform infrared spectroscopy and gas chromatography analysis. J Agric Food Chem. 2012;60(42):10709–13.

15. Affenito SG, Thompson DR, Barton BA, et al. Breakfast consumption by African American and white adolescent girls correlates positively with calcium and fiber intake and negatively with body mass index. J Am Diet Assoc. 2005;105(6):938–45.
16. Rampersaud GC, Pereira MA, Girard BL, et al. Breakfast habits, nutritional status, body weight, and academic performance in children and adolescents. J Am Diet Assoc. 2005;105(5):743–60. https://doi.org/10.1016/j.jada.2005.02.007.
17. Hopkins LC, Sattler M, Anderson Steeves E, et al. Breakfast consumption frequency and its relationships to overall diet quality, using healthy eating index 2010, and body mass index among adolescents in a low-income urban setting. Ecol Food Nutr. 2017;56(4):297–311.
18. O'Neil C, Byrd-Bredbenner C, Hayes D, et al. The role of breakfast in health: definition and criteria for a quality breakfast. J Acad Nutr Diet. 2014;114(12 Suppl):S8–26.
19. Adolphus K, Lawton CL, Champ CL, Dye L. The effects of breakfast and breakfast composition on cognition in children and adolescents: a systematic review. Adv Nutr. 2016;7:590S–612S.
20. Casazza K, Brown A, Astrup A, et al. Weighing the evidence of common beliefs in obesity research. Crit Rev Food Sci Nutr. 2015;55(14):2014–53.
21. Brown-Riggs C. Nutrition and health disparities: the role of dairy in improving minority health outcomes. Int J Environ Res Public Health. 2015;13(1):28. https://doi.org/10.3390/ijerph13010028.
22. Ken B, Murphy AB, Maria R, Jennifer N, Ebony S, Dixon MA, Jacobs ET, Hollowell Courtney MP, Chiledum A, Kittles Rick A. Race and BMI modify associations of calcium and vitamin D intake with prostate cancer. BMC Cancer. 17(1) https://doi.org/10.1186/s12885-017-3060-8.
23. Rowland Glovioell W, Schwartz Gary G, John Esther M, Ann IS. Calcium intake and prostate cancer among African Americans: effect modification by vitamin D receptor calcium absorption genotype. J Bone Miner Res. 2011;27(1):187–94. https://doi.org/10.1002/jbmr.505.
24. Lactose intolerance by ethnicity and region. ProCon.org. 2018. https://milk.procon.org/view.resource.php?resourceID=000661. Accessed 9 June 2019.
25. Baily RK, Fileti CP, Keith J, et al. Lactose intolerance and health disparities among African Americans and Hispanic Americans: an updated consensus statement. J Natl Med Assoc. 2013;105(2):112–27.
26. Lang SS. Lactose intolerance seems linked to ancestral struggles with harsh climate and cattle diseases, Cornell study finds. 2005. http://news.cornell.edu/stories/2005/06/lactose-intolerance-linked-ancestral-struggles-climate-diseases. Accessed 9 June 2019.
27. Kumanyika SK, Grier SA, Lancaster K, Lassiter V. Impact of sugar-sweetened beverage consumption on black American's health. Robert Wood Johnson Foundation; 2011. https://www.rwjf.org/en/library/research/2011/01/impact-of-sugar-sweetened-beverage-consumption-on-black-american.html. Accessed 9 June 2019.
28. Rosinger A, Herrick K, Gahche J, Park S. Sugar-sweetened beverage consumption among US adults, 2011–2014. NCHS Data Brief. 2017;270:1–8.
29. Hartman TJ, Haardörfer R, Greene BM, et al. Beverage consumption patterns among overweight and obese African American women. Nutrients. 2017;9(12):E1344.
30. Harris JL, Bargh JA, Brownell KD. Priming effects of television food advertising on eating behavior. Health Psychol. 2009;28:404–13.
31. Grier SA, Kumanyika SK. The context for choice: health implications of targeted food and beverage marketing to African Americans. Am J Public Health. 2008;98:1616–29.
32. Malik VS, Pan A, Willett WC, Hu FB. Sugar-sweetened beverages and weight gain in children and adults: a systematic review and meta-analysis. Am J Clin Nutr. 2013;98(4):1084–102.
33. Whelton PK, Carey RM, Aronow WS, Casey DE, Collins KJ, Cheryl DH, DePalma Sondra M, Samuel G, Jamerson KA, Jones DW, MacLaughlin EJ, Paul M, Bruce O, Smith SC, Spencer CC, Stafford RS, Taler SJ, Thomas RJ, Williams KA, Williamson JD, Wright JT. ACC/AHA/AAPA/ABC/ACPM/AGS/APhA/ASH/ASPC/NMA/PCNA guideline for the prevention detection evaluation and management of high blood pressure in adults: a report of the American College of Cardiology/American Heart Association Task Force on Clinical Practice guidelines. Circulation. 2017;138(17) https://doi.org/10.1161/CIR.0000000000000596.

34. Wenner MM, Paul EP, Robinson AT, Rose WC, Farquhar WB. Acute NaCl loading reveals a higher blood pressure for a given serum sodium level in African American compared to Caucasian adults. Front Physiol. 2018;9 https://doi.org/10.3389/fphys.2018.01354.
35. Soolim J, Hunter SD, Cook MD, Grosicki GJ, Robinson AT. Salty subjects: unpacking racial differences in salt-sensitive hypertension. Curr Hypertens Rep. 26(1):43–58. https://doi.org/10.1007/s11906-023-01275-z.
36. Cristina P, Karin W, Martin BR, Lisa J, Howard PJ, Munro P, George MC, Weaver CM. Sodium retention in Black and White female adolescents in response to salt intake. J Clin Endocrinol Metab. 89(4):1858–63. https://doi.org/10.1210/jc.2003-031446.
37. Ames BN, Grant WB, Willett WC. Does the high prevalence of vitamin D deficiency in African Americans contribute to health disparities? Nutrients. 2021;13(2):499. https://doi.org/10.3390/nu13020499.
38. Parva Naveen R, Satish T, Pratiksha S, Andrew Q, Rajat J, Hyndavi K, Nookala Vinod K, Pramil C. Prevalence of vitamin D deficiency and associated risk factors in the US population (2011-2012). Cureus. 10:e2741. https://doi.org/10.7759/cureus.2741.
39. Powe CE, Evans MK, Julia W, Zonderman AB, Berg AH, Michael N, Hector T, Dongsheng Z, Ishir B, Ananth KS, Powe NR, Ravi T. Vitamin D–binding protein and vitamin D status of Black Americans and White Americans. New Engl J Med. 369(21):1991–2000. https://doi.org/10.1056/NEJMoa1306357.
40. Scragg R, Sowers M, Bell C. Serum 25-hydroxyvitamin D ethnicity and blood pressure in the third national health and nutrition examination survey. Am J Hypertens. 20(7):713–9. https://doi.org/10.1016/j.amjhyper.2007.01.017.
41. Kimmie N, Scott Jamil B, Drake Bettina F, Chan Andrew T, Hollis Bruce W, Chandler Paulette D, Bennett Gary G, Giovannucci Edward L, Elizabeth G-S, Meyerhardt Jeffrey A, Emmons Karen M, Fuchs Charles S. Dose response to vitamin D supplementation in African Americans: results of a 4-arm randomized placebo-controlled trial. Am J Clin Nutr. 99(3):587–98. https://doi.org/10.3945/ajcn.113.067777.
42. Khan Rumana J, Gebreab Samson Y, Pia R, Mario S, Amadou G, Ruihua X, Davis Sharon K. Associations between vitamin D and cardiovascular disease risk factors in African Americans are partly explained by circulating adipokines and C-reactive protein: the Jackson heart study. J Nutr. 146(12):2537–43. https://doi.org/10.3945/jn.116.239509.
43. Harris Susan S. Does vitamin D deficiency contribute to increased rates of cardiovascular disease and type 2 diabetes in African Americans? Am J Clin Nutr. 93(5):1175S–8S. https://doi.org/10.3945/ajcn.110.003491.
44. Smith EM, Alvarez JA, Martin GS, Zughaier SM, Ziegler TR, Tangpricha V. Vitamin D deficiency is associated with anaemia among African Americans in a US cohort. Br J Nutr. 2015;113(11):1732–40. https://doi.org/10.1017/S0007114515000999. Epub 2015 Apr 16. PMID: 25876674; PMCID: PMC4465993.
45. Freishtat RJ, Iqbal SF, Pillai DK, Klein CJ, Ryan LM, Benton AS, Teach SJ. High prevalence of vitamin D deficiency among inner-city African American youth with asthma in Washington DC. J Pediatr. 156(6):948–52. https://doi.org/10.1016/j.jpeds.2009.12.033.
46. Pillai DK, Iqbal SF, Benton AS, Jennifer L, Andrew W, Matthew F, Tugba O, Holbrook HP, Payne PW, Heather G-D, Teach SJ, Freishtat RJ. Associations between genetic variants in vitamin D metabolism and asthma characteristics in young African Americans: a pilot study. J Investig Med. 59(6):938–46. https://doi.org/10.2310/JIM.0b013e318220df41.
47. Rowland GW, Schwartz GG, John EM, Ann IS. Protective effects of low calcium intake and low calcium absorption vitamin D receptor genotype in the California collaborative prostate cancer study. Cancer Epidemiol Biomarkers Prev. 2013;22(1):16–24. https://doi.org/10.1158/1055-9965.EPI-12-0922-T.
48. Schwartz GG, John EM, Glovioell R, Ingles SA. Prostate cancer in African-American men and polymorphism in the calcium-sensing receptor. Cancer Biol Ther. 2014;9(12):994–9. https://doi.org/10.4161/cbt.9.12.11689.
49. Francis-Lyon PA, Fahreen M, Xiaoyun C, Alireza G, Feihan X, Rafiki C. TRPV6 as a putative genomic susceptibility locus influencing racial disparities in cancer. Cancer Prev Res. 2020;13(5):423–8. https://doi.org/10.1158/1940-6207.CAPR-19-0351.

50. Nobel B, Dereck A, Gray OA, Kupfer SS. Vitamin D regulation of the uridine phosphorylase 1 gene and uridine-induced DNA damage in colon in African Americans and European Americans. Gastroenterology. 155(4):1192–204.e9. https://doi.org/10.1053/j.gastro.2018.06.049.
51. Fabio P, Kittles RA, Sandler RS, Keku TO, Kupfer SS, Xicola RM, Xavier L, Ellis NA. Genetic variation in vitamin D-related genes and risk of colorectal cancer in African Americans. Cancer Causes Control. 25(5):561–70. https://doi.org/10.1007/s10552-014-0361-y.
52. Song Y, Gary Z, Bovbjerg Dana H, Lina J, Chen HC, Hua Z, Sucheston Lara E, Li T, Michelle R, Gregory C, Warren D, Helena H, Johnson Candace S, Trump Donald L, McCann Susan E, Foluso A, Pawlish Karen S, Bandera Elisa V, Ambrosone Christine B. Variants in the vitamin D pathway serum levels of vitamin D and estrogen receptor negative breast cancer among African-American women: a case-control study. Breast Cancer Res. 2012;14(2) https://doi.org/10.1186/bcr3162.
53. Shakira N, Ken B, Chiledum A, Tanya A-C, Rick K. Association between serum 25-Hydroxyvitamin D and aggressive prostate cancer in African American men. Nutrients. 2017;9(1):12. https://doi.org/10.3390/nu9010012.
54. Stabler Sally P, Allen Robert H, Fried Linda P, Marco P, Kittner Steven J, WJH PB, Guralnik Jack M. Racial differences in prevalence of cobalamin and folate deficiencies in disabled elderly women. Am J Clin Nutr. 70(5):911–9. https://doi.org/10.1093/ajcn/70.5.911.
55. Ann JM, Hausman DB, Davey A, Poon LW, Allen RH, Stabler SP. Vitamin B12 deficiency in African American and white octogenarians and centenarians in Georgia. J Nutri Health Aging. 14(5):339–45. https://doi.org/10.1007/s12603-010-0077-y.
56. Yanni P, James B, Carroll R, Fulgoni VL. Comparison of inadequate nutrient intakes in non-Hispanic Blacks vs. non-Hispanic Whites: an analysis of NHANES 2007–2010 in U.S. children and adults. J Health Care Poor Underserved. 26(3):726–36. https://doi.org/10.1353/hpu.2015.0098.
57. Rock CL, Jahnke MG, Gorenflo DW, Swartz RD, Messana JM. Racial group differences in plasma concentrations of antioxidant vitamins and carotenoids in hemodialysis patients. Am J Clin Nutr. 65(3):844–50. https://doi.org/10.1093/ajcn/65.3.844.
58. Klein EA, Thompson IM, Tangen CM, Crowley JJ, Scott LM, Goodman PJ, Minasian LM, Ford LG, Parnes HL, Michael GJ, Karp DD, Lieber MM, Walther PJ, Laurence K, Kellogg PJ, Chin JL, Darke AK, Lippman SM, Goodman GE, Meyskens FL, Baker LH. Vitamin E and the risk of prostate cancer. JAMA. 306(14):1549. https://doi.org/10.1001/jama.2011.1437.
59. Lippman Scott M, Klein Eric A, Goodman Phyllis J, Scott LM, Thompson Ian M, Ford Leslie G, Parnes Howard L, Minasian Lori M, Michael GJ, Ann HJ, Kellogg PJ, Bearden James D, David CE, Goodman Gary E, Jaime C, Eric W, Cook Elise D, Karp Daniel D, Philip W, Lieber Michael M, Kristal Alan R, Darke Amy K, Arnold Kathryn B, Ganz Patricia A, Santella Regina M, Demetrius A, Taylor Philip R, Probstfield Jeffrey L, Jagpal TJ, Crowley John J, Meyskens Frank L, Baker Laurence H, Coltman Charles A. Effect of selenium and vitamin E on risk of prostate cancer and other cancers. JAMA. 301(1):39. https://doi.org/10.1001/jama.2008.864.
60. Antwi SO, Steck SE, Joseph SL, Hébert JR, Hongmei Z, Fontham Elizabeth TH, Smith GJ, Bensen JT, Mohler JL, Lenore A. Dietary supplement and adipose tissue tocopherol levels in relation to prostate cancer aggressiveness among African and European Americans: the North Carolina-Louisiana Prostate Cancer Project (PCaP). Prostate. 75(13):1419–35. https://doi.org/10.1002/pros.23025.
61. Michael A, DeLoughery Thomas G, Tirnauer JS. Iron deficiency in adults. JAMA. https://doi.org/10.1001/jama.2025.0452.
62. Peng Anqi H, Peipei SC, Angela V, Guodong D, Yongjun Z. Socio-demographic determinant factors for serum iron copper zinc and selenium concentrations among U.S. women of childbearing age. Nutrients. 2024;16(23):4243. https://doi.org/10.3390/nu16234243.
63. Stewart EA, Nicholson WK, Linda B, Borah BJ. The burden of uterine fibroids for African-American women: results of a national survey. J Women's Health. 22(10):807–16. https://doi.org/10.1089/jwh.2013.4334.
64. O'Malley PG, Stewart EA, Laughlin-Tommaso SK. Uterine fibroids. New Engl J Med. 391(18):1721–33. https://doi.org/10.1056/NEJMcp2309623.

65. Killip S, Bennett JM, Chambers MD. Iron deficiency anemia. Am Fam Phys. 2007;75(5):671–8. Erratum in: Am Fam Physician. 2008 Oct 15;78(8):914
66. Gordeuk Victor R, Brannon Patsy M. Ethnic and genetic factors of iron status in women of reproductive age. Am J Clin Nutr. 106:1594S–9S. https://doi.org/10.3945/ajcn.117.155853.
67. Barton JC, Wiener HH, Acton RT, Adams PC, Eckfeldt JH, Gordeuk VR, Harris EL, McLaren CE, Helen H, McLaren GD, Reboussin DM, Connor JR. Prevalence of iron deficiency in 62685 women of seven race/ethnicity groups: the HEIRS study. PLoS One. 2020;15(4):e0232125. https://doi.org/10.1371/journal.pone.0232125.
68. Jackson SE, Lee S, Igor G, Sandra H, Jacopo D, López-Sánchez GF, Pinar S, Sarah R, Turan IA, Lin Y. Ethnic differences in magnesium intake in U.S. older adults: findings from NHANES 2005–2016. Nutrients. 2018;10(12):1901. https://doi.org/10.3390/nu10121901.
69. Song AY, Crews DC, Ephraim PL, Dingfen H, Greer RC, Lewis BLP, Jessica A, Gayles DJ, Valerie S, Carson KA, Michael A, Yang L, Cooper LA, Ebony BL. Sociodemographic and kidney disease correlates of nutrient intakes among urban African Americans with uncontrolled hypertension. J Renal Nutr. 29(5):399–406. https://doi.org/10.1053/j.jrn.2018.12.004.
70. Yan C, Yingying S, Ballew SH, Adrienne T, Chang AR, Kunihiro M, Josef C, Kamyar K-Z, Molnar MZ, Grams ME. Race serum potassium and associations with ESRD and mortality. Am J Kidney Dis. 70(2):244–51. https://doi.org/10.1053/j.ajkd.2017.01.044.
71. Ranee C, Hsin-Chieh Y, Tariq S, Cheryl A, Pankow James S, Miller Edgar R, David L, Elizabeth S, Brancati Frederick L. Serum potassium and the racial disparity in diabetes risk: the Atherosclerosis Risk in Communities (ARIC) Study. Am J Clin Nutr. 93(5):1087–91. https://doi.org/10.3945/ajcn.110.007286.
72. Sandau KE, Marjorie F, Andrew A, Barsness GW, Kay B, Maria C, Rachel L, May JL, McDaniel GM, Perez MV, Sue S, Sommargren CE, Wang PJ. Update to practice standards for electrocardiographic monitoring in hospital settings: a scientific statement from the American Heart Association. Circulation. 136(19) https://doi.org/10.1161/CIR.0000000000000527.
73. Aronsen JM, Skogestad J, Lewalle A, Louch WE, Hougen K, Stokke MK, Swift F, Niederer S, Smith NP, Sejersted OM, Sjaastad I. J Physiol. 593(6):1509–21. https://doi.org/10.1113/jphysiol.2014.279893.
74. Abdo A, Rajesh M, Wingo CS. A physiologic-based approach to the treatment of a patient with hypokalemia. Am J Kidney Dis. 60(3):492–7. https://doi.org/10.1053/j.ajkd.2012.01.031.
75. Fervenza FC, Ralph R. The role of growth factors and ammonia in the genesis of hypokalemic nephropathy. J Renal Nutr. 12(3):151–9. https://doi.org/10.1053/jren.2002.33511.
76. Palmer BF. A physiologic-based approach to the evaluation of a patient with hypokalemia. Am J Kidney Dis. 56(6):1184–90. https://doi.org/10.1053/j.ajkd.2010.07.010.
77. Cole Conrad R, Grant Frederick K, Dawn S-EE, Smith Joy L, Anne J, Northrop-Clewes Christine A, Caldwell Kathleen L, Pfeiffer Christine M, Ziegler Thomas R. Zinc and iron deficiency and their interrelations in low-income African American and Hispanic children in Atlanta. Am J Clin Nutr. 91(4):1027–34. https://doi.org/10.3945/ajcn.2009.28089.
78. Neggers YH, Dubard MB, Goldenberg RL, Tsunenobu T, Johnston Kelley E, Copper Rachel L, Hauth John C. Factors influencing plasma zinc levels in low-income pregnant women. Biol Trace Elem Res. 55(1–2):127–35. https://doi.org/10.1007/BF02784174.
79. Briefel RR, Karil B, Jocelyn K-S, McDowell MA, Bethene ER, Wright JD. Zinc Intake of the U.S. population: findings from the third national health and nutrition examination survey 1988–1994. J Nutr. 130(5):1367S–73S. https://doi.org/10.1093/jn/130.5.1367S.

Chapter 15
Connecting with African American Patients Using Emotional Intelligence and Stories: Improving Adherence and Compliance

Contents

15.1	Emotional and Cultural Intelligence	307
15.2	Storytelling	310
	15.2.1 Storytelling Influences Start Early	311
15.3	Marketing for Good Health	311
	15.3.1 The Patient's Perspective	314
	15.3.2 Hypertension and Diabetes Examples	315
	15.3.3 Worldview = Culture = Cultural Intelligence	317
References		319

15.1 Emotional and Cultural Intelligence

Effective communication with African American patients greatly benefits from emotional intelligence (EI) and cultural sensitivity. Emotional intelligence involves recognizing and managing one's own emotions while also understanding the emotions of others. In a healthcare context, this entails being self-aware, practicing self-regulation, developing social awareness, and refining relationship management skills [5]. For example, when interacting with an African American patient, healthcare clinicians should invest time in building trust and rapport by clearly introducing themselves and maintaining open body language. See Fig. 15.1.

Cultural sensitivity entails understanding and respecting the diverse cultural backgrounds and experiences of patients. This is crucial in healthcare as it enables clinicians to deliver personalized care that acknowledges and honors patients' values and beliefs. Establishing trust with patients is essential since it creates a safe and supportive environment where they feel comfortable sharing personal information. This trust allows us to gather accurate and comprehensive health histories, resulting in more effective diagnoses and treatment plans. Furthermore, when patients trust us, they are more likely to adhere to prescribed treatments and follow-up

© The Author(s), under exclusive license to Springer Nature
Switzerland AG 2025
G. L. Hall, *Precision Medicine for African Americans*,
https://doi.org/10.1007/978-3-031-95774-1_15

Fig. 15.1 Emotional intelligence components

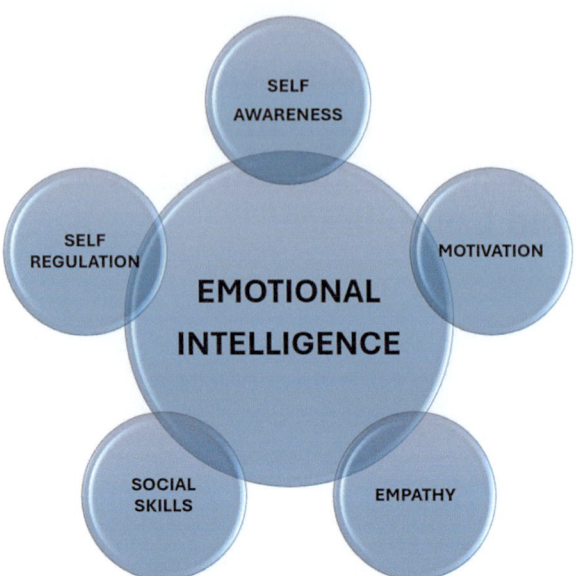

recommendations, ultimately enhancing health outcomes. Studies have shown that higher levels of emotional intelligence in clinicians are associated with better interactions [6–8]. For instance, Al-Aamri and colleagues found that emotional intelligence was positively correlated with the quality of patient-provider interactions among African American patients with hypertension, which in turn influenced self-management behaviors and medication adherence [6]. This suggests that clinicians with higher emotional intelligence are better equipped to engage in meaningful, empathetic communication, which is essential for building trust and improving health outcomes.

The Presence 5 for Racial Justice framework emphasizes the importance of emotional intelligence in anti-racist communication practices. This framework includes practices such as preparing intentionally, listening attentively, and exploring emotional cues, all of which require a high level of emotional intelligence to effectively address the unique challenges faced by African American patients and to build trusting relationships [8]. Research by Johnson et al. highlights that African American patients often experience less patient-centered communication and lower levels of positive affect during medical visits compared to patients of European descent [7]. Additionally, research by Asare et al. found that the patient-provider relationship, which includes elements of emotional support and communication, significantly influenced health outcomes and perceived quality of care among African American cancer survivors. The study indicated that the quality of care mediated the relationship between the patient-provider relationship and health outcomes, suggesting that emotional intelligence in providers can enhance the perceived quality of care and subsequently improve health outcomes [9].

By improving their emotional and cultural intelligence, healthcare professionals can enhance communication, minimize misunderstandings, and ultimately improve patient satisfaction and outcomes. This approach also aids in fostering long-term relationships between patients and providers, cultivating a sense of mutual respect and understanding. Ultimately, this approach contributes to better health outcomes by addressing the unique needs of African Americans.

Acknowledge Historical Misdoings as a Way to Build Trust
A vital component of emotional intelligence is the capacity to empathize with the patient. Empathy encompasses both cognitive understanding and emotional resonance [10]. The widespread mistrust of medicine and healthcare professionals stems from a history of intentional abuse, as discussed in Chap. 2. It is crucial to acknowledge historical mistrust in healthcare. This can resonate deeply with African Americans due to past unethical medical experiments and systemic discrimination. Recognizing these misdoings can help rebuild trust, demonstrate respect, and encourage patients to engage more openly with healthcare professionals, ultimately improving health outcomes and reducing disparities. This can be achieved by openly discussing past injustices, offering sincere apologies, and committing to equitable and inclusive care.

Active Listening
Active listening also plays a vital role in fostering effective communication [5]. We should be intentional about paraphrasing patient concerns to confirm understanding, such as saying, "So, you're feeling anxious about your upcoming procedure. Is that right?" This not only validates the patient's feelings but also encourages open dialogue. Additionally, healthcare professionals can use active listening techniques to build rapport and trust with patients. This involves maintaining eye contact, nodding in acknowledgment, and avoiding interruptions. By doing so, patients feel heard and valued, which can lead to better communication and ultimately improve health outcomes.

Using Understandable Language
Using simple, jargon-free language is essential [11]. Instead of saying, "You have hypertension," a provider might say, "Your blood pressure is higher than normal, which we need to manage." This clarity ensures that patients fully understand their health conditions and treatment options. Data has shown that over 50% of African Americans have basic or lower health literacy, so do not assume that terms like hypertension, renal insufficiency, or heart failure are understood with their true implications [12]. Additionally, incorporating visual aids or written materials can further enhance comprehension, especially for patients with low health literacy or those who better process information through visual or written formats. Emotional support is critical, especially when discussing chronic conditions [5]. Clinicians can say, "It's understandable to feel overwhelmed. We can take this one step at a time together," reinforcing that the patient is not alone.

Continuous engagement, such as scheduling follow-up appointments and checking in with patients about their feelings and progress, further enhances the patient experience. Utilizing technology, like text reminders or patient portals, can maintain communication and support adherence to treatment plans. In summary, by integrating emotional intelligence and cultural sensitivity into their practice, healthcare providers can create a more equitable and supportive environment for African American patients, ultimately improving health outcomes and fostering trust.

15.2 Storytelling

The African American tradition extends deeply into African tribal customs. The telling of stories to convey knowledge and experience is as old as time [13, 14]. For the African people, the oral tradition defined their cultural heritage. The spoken word was how traditions, folktales, histories, and religious convictions were passed from one generation to the next [14]. Family histories and stories were learned, memorized, and recounted as a way to remember the past, and in many parts of Africa, that tradition continues to this day. If the story did not evoke an emotion, be it laughter, agreement, concern, or some other feeling, the story was lost to the listener. So the storyteller and their proper preparation were critical to the success of the story.

In general, stories are easier to remember than facts. Stories come with a context and details meant to include the listener. Because stories are told with more than just words, the listener remembers the details and the emotions. This is in sharp contrast to histories, which are merely an account of events. Clinicians deal in histories all the time.

> The patient was cutting his grass when he began to have chest pain, sat down, and then called 911.

We've been trained to listen to the history, pull out key elements, ask relevant questions, and then come up with helpful recommendations. Stories, or narratives, require forethought, are usually better organized, and have a moral and an intended outcome in the listener. Many patients with viral upper respiratory infections come to clinicians with "stories" designed to prompt a desired outcome: prescribed antibiotics. They know that certain elements of their story will trigger the antibiotic button in us and the absence of those triggers will not. By embellishing their history into a story, patients will frequently get what they want.

If a story can be told to manipulate trained clinicians into action, surely we can build our arsenal of accurate, motivational narratives to tell and inspire our patients.

JoAnne Banks-Wallace believed stories and storytelling were also a cornerstone of qualitative research [14]:

> Story creation and storytelling enable us to give unique expression to our experiences, the wisdom gleaned through living, and truths passed on from generation to generation. Storytelling steeped in oral traditions provides unique opportunities to contribute to the development and testing of theories or interventions while promoting the health of study participants [14]

In African history, the storytellers played a significant role as the human voice, and presentation style was critical to the successful communication of the details and sentiment of a story. Stories were organized, rehearsed, and presented as a way to perpetuate tribal histories, herbal medicine ingredients, and healing techniques through a conduit story that, if misremembered, would impact not just one, but all subsequent generations.

15.2.1 Storytelling Influences Start Early

This predilection for stories starts early in the African American culture, and educators have found reliable and persistent differences in the learning and advancement of African American children and their ability to tell and interpret a story [15, 16]. African American children tell stories that are "vivid, elaborate, and rich in imagery" says Nicole Gardner-Neblett from the University of North Carolina's Frank Porter Graham Child Development Institute. She found distinct differences in how early storytelling skills in African American children impacted later literacy. Dr. Gardner-Neblett states:

> The strong storytelling skills of African-American children may stem from the cultural and historic influences that have fostered a preference for orality among African Americans [15]

By considering African American's "preference for orality" and the imagery and mastery of stories as a way to connect and learn, we clinicians will merely be taking a path of least resistance when it comes to connecting with the many patients that appreciate stories.

Abject data, like most of the information we give our patients, is decontextualized from the standpoint of our listeners. We have spent years learning basic sciences and have progressed to superspecialized clinicians. When explaining the impact of any particular medical intervention, we speak from a very learned context, one that is dramatically distant from most of our patients. Taking the time and energy to translate that information into actionable stories will be an impactful and efficient use of our time. Once well-crafted contextualized stories are developed, they can be individually refined and used repeatedly on countless patients.

15.3 Marketing for Good Health

Salesmen and marketers have touted the importance of using stories to improve a brand, sell a product, inspire interest, and advance long-term product loyalty. In medicine, the goals for our patients are strikingly similar. We want to inspire them to understand their disorder and make the appropriate changes in their lifestyle. We need to motivate them to take their medications regularly, modify their diet, and increase their exercise in a way that is stimulating and memorable.

By using a storytelling approach, we can help our patients better internalize their medical problem, see where they are impacting it negatively, and then inspire them to make the appropriate changes that will have a lasting positive impression.

Interviews of successful physicians across racial populations find that storytelling is a valuable and integral part of educating patients about the merit of a clinical intervention [17]. Successful physicians tell stories all the time. These physicians, with high patient satisfaction scores, frequently tell relatable stories and personal disclosures about their family and friends as a way to connect with their patients.

Many successful physicians report that they "stumbled" onto stories as a tactic to help them convince a skeptical patient and, after seeing early and consistent success, incorporated the telling of stories into their daily routine. Encouraging physicians to tell stories is not new. John Steiner wrote about the use of stories in clinical settings and proposed many of the same components emphasized in marketing: getting the customer's point of view through a clinical interrogation and then telling a good story based on a narrative competence [18].

Kenneth Calman compared stories to viruses:

> It is suggested that behavior can change because of ideas transmitted, often in the form of stories from one person to another. Such a mechanism may involve transmids (transmitted ideas). The analogy can be developed further, in that such contagion depends on virulence, and on the resistance of the listener. Like micro-organisms, some ideas are dangerous [17]

Patients will frequently be told a story by a neighbor or friend that is completely counterproductive. A patient hobbling on a knee that needs replacement will reject the suggestion because of a horrific story of a bad outcome. Much of the success of herbs and home remedies rely on stories of healing.

Physicians have a long history of submitting interesting "case reports" to journals and colleagues as a way to stimulate discussion, gather input, and generally form the foundation for future research. These accounts of unusual clinical outcomes are merely well-crafted stories. Steiner wrote:

> Clinical stories are used in many ways: to inform, to share, to inspire, to educate, and to persuade. Physicians constantly use the stories they hear to inform decisions and actions that directly affect the patient subject. [18]

Professional marketers are specifically instructed to tell stories as an early approach to establish trust and allegiance [19]. There are countless articles and books on marketing stories as a way to sell almost anything. In marketing, the telling of stories as a way to "connect" to the customer is fully accepted as the only true path to success. A good story contains these five components:

1. A subject or hero
2. A goal
3. A conflict or obstacle
4. A mentor
5. A moral

When applying these marketing elements to a clinical approach to storytelling, we see a natural fit. The *hero* is *always* the patient or, more often, a surrogate for the

15.3 Marketing for Good Health

patient, someone "just like the patient" who had similar challenges and overcame them.

The *goal* is the "transformation" that the hero is seeking: good health, more energy, longer life, better endurance, etc. It is critical that clinicians fully elucidate and understand our hero/patient's goal. In hypertension, it usually is *not* controlled blood pressure (that is the clinician's goal). Their goal is more likely to "feel healthier," as evidenced by more energy, stamina, fewer discomforts, and/or the absence of life-threatening events (heart attacks and strokes).

The *obstacles* in our story may be internal or external in origin. With most of our stories dealing with internal motivational obstacles that must be overcome to reach a healthy steady state, it is the obstacles that make the story motivational.

The clinician is the *mentor*, and rightfully so. We have the knowledge, training, and expertise to help the subject overcome health obstacles. If the patient is Luke Skywalker, then the physician is Obi-Wan Kenobi. We are the wise mentors who can provide essential information and tools that allow the hero subject to attain their goal.

And finally, marketers stress that the *moral* of any story should be clear and concise. In the beginning, the patient was *less* than what they should have been, and while their goal was to have a transformation, there were obstacles in the form of motivation, understanding, and trust. Ultimately these barriers were overcome and a remarkable and honest *truth* evolved.

Adapting this generally accepted model for motivational clinical stories has wide-ranging potential for better communication, understanding, compliance, and improved outcomes. Researchers are currently investigating the impact of storytelling on a host of problems including smoking cessation [20] at a VA hospital in Massachusetts, hypertension [21] control by using successful personal narratives in a theater setting, a compilation of patient-reported storytelling of their success with smoking cessation, and much more. As the power of storytelling and its relation to African American influence improves, the ways to apply stories in pursuit of better health will grow.

While these components of a story are popularly linked to marketing approaches, Jerome Bruner, noted psychologist, author, and law professor from Harvard, wrote that "it is no surprise that story is the coin and currency of culture." In his book, *Making Stories: Law, Literature, Life*, Bruner examines the usefulness of stories as they relate to business strategies, legal success with judges and juries, and their application in effective writing [22].

Bruner emphasized that the key component of a story is the obstacle… "For there to be a story something unforeseen must happen. There is an unexpected turn of events, a peripeteia as Aristotle said" [22]. In our clinical world, the peripeteia is the medical intervention, because without its presence, the patient's life course was headed in a dire direction. The uncontrolled hypertension was spiraling toward a fatal stroke or heart attack. The unbridled smoking was feeding cancerous cells in their infancy. And then we, the clinicians, arrive with life-saving advice.

Bruner also stressed that the cultural perspective of the narrator and the subject must be considered as culture explains both the origin of the problem as well as the key to the solution. Trying to convince a person that comes from a family where everyone smokes is a greater challenge due to their cultural affirmation that smoking is "okay." Getting a thorough family history that shows premature death from smoking-related illnesses and approaching the patient with the long-livers in their family who did not smoke uses a logical "you-gave-me-the-history" evidence-based argument that few could refute.

Finally, Bruner stressed that the story is bound by its verisimilitude (and yes I had to look that word up too). Culture's "myths and its folktales, its dramas and its pageants memorialize both its norms and notable violations of them" [22]. Verisimilitude means the story must "ring true" to the listener, or the impact will be lost. Therefore, the culture and history of the listener must be artfully embedded into the story respectfully and with regard for the cultural perspectives assigned to the narrator by the listener. This explains why reformed alcoholics are the best mentors and teachers for current alcoholics. They both have a common historical perspective and a number of stories to tell to motivate action. Someone who never drank alcohol comes with little perspective to convince others … unless they have a really good story.

15.3.1 The Patient's Perspective

I don't want medicine … is there a vitamin I can take?

I have frequently told my patients to not discriminate against the medications I prescribe "just because they've been proven to work." After the FDA has approved a medication for use and demonstrated that it works across a population, it has to be monitored and regulated, whether prescription or over-the-counter. It seems that as soon as a medication requires a prescription, many of my patients want to avoid it. Somehow the medication has become tainted, and rather than be energetic about the proven prospects for a longer life and good health, they become depressed and bemoan the fact that they have to take a medication for "the rest of their life." This reaction, however dysfunctional, is based on a learned and trained response that we clinicians taught them.

When presented with elevated blood pressure in African Americans, our response is casual and typical. After all, the vast majority of African Americans we see in the medical environment have hypertension, as do almost half of all African Americans. Hypertension is so commonplace in African Americans that we do not take the time to frame the problem properly, explain the far-reaching implications, or fully praise the miraculous potential of antihypertensive medications.

Studies have repeatedly shown that controlled blood pressure increases energy and stamina, reduces fatigue, and bolsters well-being [23, 24]. In addition, hypertensive therapy saves a resounding number of lives and dramatically decreases cardiovascular events including heart attack, stroke, and congestive heart failure [23, 24]. What this data confirms across racial populations is even more impactful in

African Americans who have a disproportionate percentage with these deadly diseases.

The reality of hypertension is it does progressive damage to the circulatory system, and the proper functioning of the circulatory system is essential to the basic functions of both major and minor organs. The medical establishment frequently says that hypertension is asymptomatic ... the silent killer, but studies have confirmed that it actually negatively impacts a patient's quality of life [25]. Put simply, there are symptoms in untreated hypertension that improve after therapy.

In striking contrast, the stories patients typically have heard about blood pressure medications are all sad. "They make you have to go to the bathroom all the time." "They kill an erection." "They make you tired." These narratives drain all of the excitement and motivation from patients. Rather than thinking of the prospect of living a longer, healthier life, they are now burdened with feeling that they will be taking a pill for the rest of their life.

In medicine, our usual approach is one of lecturing. Since we know the truth about what ails our patients, we simply present our solution ... take it or leave it. Unfortunately, many African Americans will "leave it." Because of the fundamental lack of trust for the medical establishment that many African Americans feel, just giving out "the facts" of our ailment is far from adequate. We need to take the time to formulate an inspirational story that is patient centered and diagnostically appropriate.

Interviewing the patient to elicit their perception of their exercise tolerance, baseline energy levels, and activities of daily living, and then offering an opportunity to improve their function, can shed an entirely new light on antihypertensive therapy. By going one step further and determining the patient's emotional wants (feeling better) versus their simple needs (lowering blood pressure), and then aiming therapeutic goals and future discussions at their wants rather than the needs, clinicians can positively impact overall compliance and satisfaction.

15.3.2 Hypertension and Diabetes Examples

When telling the story about hypertension,
... talk about thestress that high blood pressure places on arteries and veins throughout their body ...day in and day out ... the wearing down of the basic foundations of their systems. The unrelenting strain that their vessels see as they try to stay intact and properly deliver organ-saving oxygen and nutrients to their muscles, brain, heart, liver, bone marrow, and much more. The literal abuse of their bodies running on overdrive all the time, yet yearning for relief. It is no wonder there is fatigue, irritation, anxiety, inefficiency, and sporadic malfunctions in patients with hypertension.

By starting clinically proven medications for blood pressure, we restore normal blood and vessel function, boost endurance, and fortify the bodies' normal performance. In addition to safely and effectively improving everyday function, these medications will extend life through dramatically decreased stroke, heart attack, and kidney failure.

After starting antihypertensionmedications, some patients feel a little fatigued. If they do, it is because their body has been strained for an extended period of time and is finally able (and needs) to rest. Calling the initial physiological response to finally feeling a normal blood pressure, a medication side effect, is wholly inaccurate and misleading. The body is finally, after years of progressive unrelenting strain, seeing normality … give it a chance to recover and rest. Be thankful that no permanent damage was done in overdrive. Let the body recover.

Needless to say, every story does not fit every person. The interview that elicits the details of our patient's emotional wants will drive the content of each story. It is also important to use what author Richard Bayan calls "Words that Sell" [26]. These are time-tested words that paint a positive picture. Marketers know and agree that certain words have more energy, are more inspiring, and can move more people into action. Purposely adding these words to your stories for health will improve communication and help compliance.

When telling the story about diabetes,

… talk about how African Americans are disproportionately impacted with diabetes being 80% more likely to be diagnosed initially, four times more likely to be diagnosed with kidney disease leading to dialysis, and 3.5 times more likely to have a leg amputation. African Americans are twice as likely to die from diabetes than European Americans [27].

Patients with uncontrolled diabetes lead topoor quality lives for a number of reasons. In addition to the inefficient processing of sugars in the blood, the elevated sugars have a devastating impact on health in a number of ways. Based on the list below,determine which are affected in your patient.

- *The increased sugar impairs kidney function, which causes increased water loss through excessive urination … both day and night … leading to dehydration.*
- *Kidney function: The elevated glucose impacts the body's ability to filter water.*
- *Poor digestion: Because of dehydrationand nerve damage, diabetes impacts the enjoyment and digestion of food.*
- *High blood glucose levels contribute tothe formation of fatty deposits in blood vessel walls that can restrict blood flow and increase the risk of hardening of the blood vessels.*
- *The lack of blood flow causes decreased exercise tolerance, walking distances, and wound healing.*
- *Diabetes causes changes in the skin withdrying and cracking, increased boils, ulcers, and calluses.*
- *Diabetes causes damage to the nerves, which can affect the perception of heat, cold, and pain and makes you more susceptible to accidental injury.*
- *Swollen, leaky blood vessels in the eye (diabetic retinopathy) can damage your vision and even lead to blindness.*
- *People with diabetes tend to developcataracts at an earlier age.*

15.3 Marketing for Good Health

Your goal will be to fix whichever problems (obvious and subtle) you find are most negatively impacting the patient. But also try to quantify how negatively impacted is their overall quality of life, emphasizing the background damage occurring that is not among their complaints, but present nonetheless.

How often are tasks you want to complete interrupted by the need to urinate? How has your perception of heat or cold changed? You can clearly see that your quality of life is a mere fraction of what it was?

Metformin takes the most natural approach to lowering your elevated blood sugars by having your body naturally absorb the excess sugar. It hasthe added benefit that if you take in food that worsens the diabetes, your body will quickly flush it out of your system. All of the medicines for diabetes have been clinically tested and proven to be safe and effective. In no time, you will feel invigorated and energized, while your metabolism and immune system are enhanced.

15.3.3 Worldview = Culture = Cultural Intelligence

Marketers talk about approaching potential customers by using their "worldview." Market and branding author Jeff Korhan defines a worldview as "a philosophy or set of values through which people interpret and interact with the world" [28].

The approach to convincing anyone of anything involves discerning their worldview and then framing the approach appropriately, a marketer would say. A person's cultural history is just another term for worldview ... how the person, or patient, sees things. If we are to be successful in convincing our patients of anything, we need to understand their life's perspective, their worldview ... their culture. We do this by developing our own cultural intelligence.

African American cultural intelligence signifies the ability to navigate and comprehend the diverse cultural nuances, histories, and experiences of African American communities [29]. This form of cultural intelligence comprises several key components. Firstly, cognitive cultural intelligence entails understanding historical contexts, such as the impact of slavery, segregation, and the civil rights movement, which shape the collective identity and cultural expressions of African Americans [30]. For example, recognizing how these historical events influence contemporary social dynamics and issues like systemic racism is essential for effective engagement. Emotional cultural intelligence is also significant, as it involves empathizing with the unique challenges faced by African Americans, such as discrimination and cultural misrepresentation [30]. This may manifest in healthcare settings where clinicians demonstrate sensitivity to the stressors faced by African American patients living in dangerous neighborhoods. Such sensitivity fosters a supportive and inclusive environment. Behavioral cultural intelligence emphasizes the importance of adapting communication and interaction styles to align with African American cultural norms and values, including the significance of storytelling and oral tradition in conveying messages [30]. For example, a clinician who integrates storytelling into patient care can foster a more relatable and engaging atmosphere. Lastly, motivational cultural intelligence signifies an individual's commitment to comprehending and valuing African American culture, which can be shown through active participation in community events or educational initiatives focused on African American history and contributions [30].

By looking at clinicians' perspective for why African Americans do or do not do anything, the reason is embedded in their culture. When clinicians look at their own clinical behavior and outcomes, the explanations for their successes and failures are embedded in their culture as well. The "value" that clinicians place on a distinguished gentleman with chest pain versus a homeless alcoholic smoker with chest pain is dramatically different, and clinical outcome data confirm it consistently [31, 32]. The decreased value, whether conscious or subconscious, drives the speed, number, and quality of the subsequent interventions.

Objective protocols for serious presentations, like angina, have dramatically decreased disparities in outcomes for chest pain in the emergency department [33]. The subjective "clinical calls" that used to be made when an individual presented with chest pain resulted in differences in myocardial infarction outcomes based on race and sex. By removing the clinicians' personal cultural perspective from the equation, health disparities shrunk.

But removing the clinician's cultural perspective from the encounter essentially removes the clinician, which needless to say, also results in poor clinical outcomes. The obvious answer is to open the clinicians' perception to other worldviews, or cultural perspectives, so that they can consider how their culture colors the clinical picture at hand. Overall, cultivating African American cultural intelligence is crucial for fostering social cohesion, respect, and constructive clinical relationships within a diverse society, ultimately improving health outcomes.

Cultural competence and patient-centered care are really pseudonyms for knowing a patient's worldview before advancing or framing an approach to their care. We currently are telling patients what they should do and in many ways are trying to sell a person something they do not want. Instead, we need to understand their cultural view and then tailor our approach to be complementary. Connect with your patients by understanding their personal culture, and then adapt your educational approach accordingly.

> **Connecting with African American Patients Using Emotional Intelligence and Stories**
> - Emotional intelligence is the ability to perceive and manage one's emotions and comprises five key elements: self-awareness, self-regulation, motivation, empathy, and social skills.
> - Cultural sensitivity entails understanding and respecting the diverse cultural backgrounds and experiences of patients.
> - By using a storytelling approach, we can help our patients better internalize their medical problems and help them make the appropriate changes.

(continued)

- A good story has these five components:
  1. A subject or hero
  2. A goal
  3. A conflict or obstacle
  4. A mentor
  5. A moral
- To be successful in convincing our patients, we need to understand their life's perspective (their culture).

References

1. Kaczynski MA, Benitez G, Shehadeh F, Mylonakis E, Fiala MA. Perceived discrimination in the healthcare setting and medical mistrust: findings from the health information National Trends Survey, 2022. J Gen Intern Med. 2025;21:1–8.
2. Mundy LM, Judd SE, Clay OJ, Howard VJ, Durant RW, Ballard EE, Crowe M. Correlates of patient trust in doctors: demographic factors and experiences of medical care discrimination. J Gen Intern Med. 2025;31:1–7.
3. Brown Jordyn A, Taffe Brianna D, Richmond Jennifer A, Roberson Mya L. Racial discrimination and health-care system trust among American adults with and without cancer. JNCI J Natl Cancer Inst. 2024;116(11):1845–55. https://doi.org/10.1093/jnci/djae154.
4. Hall GL, Heath M. Poor medication adherence in African Americans is a matter of trust. J Racial Ethn Health Disparities. 2021;8(4):927–42.
5. Dott C, Mamarelis G, Karam E, Bhan K, Akhtar K. Emotional intelligence and good medical practice: is there a relationship? Cureus. 2022;14(3)
6. Alaamri M, Martin RJ, Burant C, Dolansky MA, Hickman RL Jr. Emotional intelligence: a novel factor influencing hypertension self-management. West J Nurs Res. 2023;45(7):618–25.
7. Johnson RL, Roter D, Powe NR, Cooper LA. Patient race/ethnicity and quality of patient–physician communication during medical visits. Am J Public Health. 2004;94(12):2084–90.
8. Brown-Johnson C, Cox J, Shankar M, Baratta J, De Leon G, Garcia R, Hollis T, Verano M, Henderson K, Upchurch M, Safaeinili N. The presence 5 for racial justice framework for anti-racist communication with black patients. Health Serv Res. 2022;57:263–78.
9. Asare M, Fakhoury C, Thompson N, Culakova E, Kleckner AS, Adunlin G, Reifenstein K, Benavidez GA, Kamen CS. The patient–provider relationship: predictors of black/African American cancer patients' perceived quality of care and health outcomes. Health Commun. 2020;35(10):1289–94.
10. Roberts BW, Puri NK, Trzeciak CJ, Mazzarelli AJ, Trzeciak S. Socioeconomic, racial and ethnic differences in patient experience of clinician empathy: results of a systematic review and meta-analysis. PLoS One. 2021;16(3):e0247259.
11. Gilligan T, Coyle N, Frankel RM, Berry DL, Bohlke K, Epstein RM, Finlay E, Jackson VA, Lathan CS, Loprinzi CL, Nguyen LH. Patient-clinician communication: American Society of Clinical Oncology consensus guideline. J Clin Oncol. 2017;35(31):3618–32.
12. Muvuka B, Combs RM, Ayangeakaa SD, Ali NM, Wendel ML, Jackson T. Health literacy in African-American communities: barriers and strategies. HLRP. 2020;4(3):e138–43.
13. Alvarez. African story telling. 2014. https://prezi.com/uq3pxvnigfoq/african-story-telling/. Accessed 9 June 2019.

14. Banks-Wallace J. Talk that talk: storytelling and analysis rooted in African American oral tradition. Qual Health Res. 2002;12(3):410–26.
15. Gardner-Neblett N. Why storytelling skills matter for African-American kids. 2018. Retrieved November 22, 2018, from https://theconversation.com/why-storytelling-skills-matter-for-african-american-kids-46844 .
16. Champion T. Understanding storytelling among African American children. n.d. Retrieved November 22, 2018, from https://books.google.com/books?hl=en&lr=&id=5XuRAgAAQBAJ&oi=fnd&pg=PP1&dq=tempiichampionbook&ots=u6FexFy8Kh&sig=nUUvxu4HI6vjdjbcxSVkJTA9OqM#v=onepage&q=tempii champion book&f=false
17. Calman K. A study of storytelling, humour and learning in medicine. Clin Med (Lond). 2001;1(3):227–9.
18. Steiner JF. The use of stories in clinical research and health policy. JAMA. 2005;294(22):2901. https://doi.org/10.1001/jama.294.22.2901.
19. Godin S. All marketers are liars (tell stories). The underground classic that explains how marketing really works – and why authenticity is the best marketing of all. New York: Portfolio; 2012.
20. Cherrington A, Williams J, Foster P. Narratives to enhance smoking cessation interventions among African-American smokers, the ACCE project. BMC Res Notes. 2015;8(1):567. https://doi.org/10.1186/s13104-015-1513-1.
21. Fix G, Houston T, Barker A, et al. A novel process for integrating patient stories into patient education interventions: incorporating lessons from theater arts. Patient Educ Couns. 2012;88(3):455–9.
22. Bruner JS. Making stories: law, literature, life. Cambridge: Harvard University Press; 2003.
23. Fryar CD, Ostchega Y, Hales CM, et al. Hypertension prevalence and control among adults: United States, 2015–2016. NCHS Data Brief. 2017;289:1–8.
24. Zhang Y, Moran AE. Trends in the prevalence, awareness, treatment, and control of hypertension among young adults in the United States, 1999–2014. Hypertension. 2017;70(4):736–42.
25. Hypertension (normal Vs. high blood pressure). n.d. Retrieved November 22, 2018, from https://my.clevelandclinic.org/health/diseases/4314-hypertension-high-blood-pressure
26. Bayan R. Words that sell. 2nd ed. New York: McGraw-Hill Education; 2006.
27. Office of Minority Health. n.d. Retrieved November 22, 2018, from https://minorityhealth.hhs.gov/omh/browse.aspx?lvl=4&lvlid=18
28. Korhan J. Marketing to the worldview of your customers – Jeff Korhan. 2014. Retrieved November 22, 2018, from http://www.jeffkorhan.com/2014/06/marketing-to-worldview-your-customers.html
29. Sternberg RJ, Siriner I, Oh J, Wong CH. Cultural intelligence: what is it and how can it effectively be measured? J Intelligence. 2022;10(3):54.
30. Ang S, Van Dyne L, Koh C. Personality correlates of the four-factor model of cultural intelligence. Group Org Manag. 2006;31(1):100–23.
31. Ghail JK, Cooper RS, Kowatly I, Liao Y. Delay between onset of chest pain and arrival to the coronary care unit among minority and disadvantaged patients. J Natl Med Assoc. 1993;85(3):180–4.
32. Pawlik TM, Olver IN, Storm CD, Rodriguez MA. Can physicians refuse treatment to patients who smoke? J Oncol Pract. 2009;5(5):250–1.
33. 2015 National Healthcare Quality and Disparities Report Chartbook on Health Care for Blacks. Rockville: Agency for Healthcare Research and Quality; 2016. AHRQ Pub. No 16-0015-1-EF.

Chapter 16
An "Oath" and a Responsibility to All Patients

Contents

16.1	Foundations of Medical Ethics	323
16.2	Misunderstandings	324
16.3	Recognizing and Correcting Barriers to Good Care	325
16.4	Small Improvements Within a Population Can Yield Impressive Gains	326
References		329

I swear to fulfill, to the best of my ability and judgment, this covenant:

I will respect the hard-won scientific gains of those physicians in whose steps I walk, and gladly share such knowledge as is mine with those who are to follow.

I will apply, for the benefit of the sick, all measures which are required, avoiding those twin traps of overtreatment and therapeutic nihilism.

I will remember that there is art to medicine as well as science, and that warmth, sympathy, and understanding may outweigh the surgeon's knife or the chemist's drug.

I will not be ashamed to say "I know not," nor will I fail to call in my colleagues when the skills of another are needed for a patient's recovery.

I will respect the privacy of my patients, for their problems are not disclosed to me that the world may know. Most especially must I tread with care in matters of life and death. Above all, I must not play at God.

I will remember that I do not treat a fever chart, a cancerous growth, but a sick human being, whose illness may affect the person's family and economic stability. My responsibility includes these related problems, if I am to care adequately for the sick.

I will prevent disease whenever I can but I will always look for a path to a cure for all diseases.

I will remember that I remain a member of society, with special obligations to all my fellow human beings, those sound of mind and body as well as the infirm.

If I do not violate this oath, may I enjoy life and art, respected while I live and remembered with affection thereafter. May I always act so as to preserve the finest traditions of my calling and may I long experience the joy of healing those who seek my help.

(This "modern version" of the Hippocratic Oath was written in 1964 by Louis Lasagna, Dean of the School of Medicine at Tufts University.)

The honor and responsibilities of being a clinical provider are best characterized by the centuries-old Hippocratic Oath. Written as a welcoming to new physicians to medical practice, updated versions of this Greek medical text are mainstays at medical graduations across the world [1–4].

While recited at the end of a long and grueling educational process, many repeat the oath without much thought or reflection. But the content of the oath sets the stage for a very rewarding and successful clinical practice, a common thread of decency, humility, respect, and responsibility course through the passages. The fact that this "oath" in its various translations has lasted over 2000 years is a testament to the foundational truths it dictates.

Not adhering to these tenets has resulted in many of the deficiencies and disparities we see in modern medicine. Avoiding "therapeutic nihilism" in its many forms including defensive medicine and therapies for profit all represents the downsides of clinical care. The lack of respect for privacy in the Tuskegee Syphilis Study resounds as one of the many incredible injustices that were overseen by physicians. And the "special obligations" providers have to fellow human beings must transgress political parties, sexual orientations, and other differences that make humans human. Re-centering our care to best treat a specific population by "all measures which are required" is an obligation by oath, as well as a recipe for a successful clinical practice.

The oath also describes our added responsibilities that include "the person's family and economic stability." While some providers consider these as "outside" of their control, the presumption is to merely "consider" these modifiers of health and include them in your treatment discussion and plan. Consider a patient's spouses' ability to influence their diet and include them in discussions related to nutrition. Consider the patient's ability to travel to consultants or for studies, and discuss what needs to take place in order for there to be a successful follow-through.

> The major attributes of Hippocratic morality can be summarized as follows: the first characteristic is that Hippocratic medicine is individualistic, that is, the physician acts always in the best interest of the patient, which implies the moral obligation of beneficent and consequently nonmaleficent. The aim of any medical procedure is the good of the patient independently of other factors, such as the ability to pay or the background of the patient [4]

None of these doctrines are new, and they essentially amount to basic common sense. We have sacred responsibilities that are almost as old as time itself, and while perspectives vary, with all of the advancements and technologies at our disposal, the basic ethics of the Hippocratic Oath have not changed.

The "Florence Nightingale Pledge" developed in 1893 for nurses has the same ethical tone and central themes [5]:

I solemnly pledge myself before God and in the presence of this assembly, to pass my life in purity and to practice my profession faithfully. I will abstain from whatever is deleterious and mischievous, and will not take or knowingly administer any harmful drug. I will do all in my power to maintain and elevate the standard of my profession, and will hold in confidence all personal matters committed to my keeping and all family affairs coming to my knowledge in the practice of my calling. With loyalty will I endeavor to aid the physician, in his work, and devote myself to the welfare of those committed to my care [5].

16.1 Foundations of Medical Ethics

From an ethics standpoint, the four basic principles of medical ethics developed by Beauchamp and Childress also nicely describe the foundations of good clinical care [6]:

- *Beneficence* describes the concept of acting for the patient's good.
- *Nonmaleficence* describes the concept of doing no harm.
- *Autonomy* conveys the idea that each patient has a right to voice his or her own values and choices about care.
- *Justice* expresses the idea that healthcare resources should be equitably distributed among patients and that patients should be treated fairly.

These four foundations of medical ethics are also in line with health equity teachings. By following prescriptions and recommendations tailored for African American outcomes, we act for the "patient's good," and by appropriately changing our care to align with published research that shows inferior outcomes, we do less harm. Building trust with our patients involves, among other things, identifying with their values and priorities. And finally, true justice in medicine is personified by every patient having access to medical care and a choice when decisions are made about their life.

It is certainly not unusual for providers to be unaware of nuances that apply to isolated special populations. Primary care providers are occasionally presented with patients with Down's syndrome or HIV and may not be the best authority on their care due to a very low volume presenting to their practice. When presented with a patient with a unique clinical demographic, providers will usually brush up quickly on the topic and then refer to a specialist for more definitive interventions. When we repeatedly see the same presentations or unique populations, we slowly become authorities in the nuances of care in that population.

There is no question that many providers "anecdotally" saw that ACE inhibitors were inferior to calcium channel blockers when trying to reach blood pressure goals in African Americans. Oncologists saw more aggressive presentations of breast and prostate cancer in African Americans as well. Many of these clinical observations led to the research that verified their suspicions. Clinicians then incorporate those differences into their clinical practice for the betterment of their patient population. Somehow incorporating this nuanced care for African Americans' benefit has eluded some clinicians' threshold of notice, and numerous research outcomes continue to confirm this. By recognizing these important differences and applying them appropriately, everyone wins.

16.2 Misunderstandings

It is also important to note that some of the poor outcomes seen in African Americans result from misguided assumptions and misunderstandings that ultimately undermine a clinicians' best intentions when trying to provide quality care. Health literacy may be a stronger predictor of personal health than age, employment status, education level, race, or income. While a student's literacy is frequently tied to their teacher's ability to teach, a patient's health literacy is frequently proportional to their clinician's ability to communicate the nuances of medical care in ways that their patients can understand. For example, patient education and health literacy were shown to greatly improve the nutrient quality of many patients' diet, a study by Kuczmarski and colleagues at the University of Delaware determined [7]. Health literacy leads to improved patient self-management support in chronic diseases like diabetes, heart failure, and hypertension and is critical to improving long-term quality outcomes [8–13].

Some degree of poor compliance with medications in African Americans can be attributed to cultural misunderstandings of the known causes of many conditions. A clinician's knowledge of these common misperceptions can greatly facilitate provider-patient conversations and allow for much more efficient visits and productive outcomes. Beliefs that are generationally embedded in a culture will take repetition and trust-building during clinical visits to dispel.

Causes of hypertension according to African American focus groups [9]:

1. Stress (100% of groups interviewed)
2. Heredity (83%)
3. Consumption of pork (67%)
4. Salt intake (67%)
5. Excessive use of alcohol (67%)
6. Overweight (67%)
7. Evil spirits (42%)

The most commonly perceived treatments for hypertension according to African American focus groups included [9]:

1. Garlic (92% of groups)
2. Herbs/vitamins (92%)
3. Physician-prescribed medications (83%)
4. Vinegar (75%)
5. Diet or weight loss (67%)

Gbenga Ogedegbe and colleagues at Columbia University looked at prevalent African American beliefs of the causes and treatments for common conditions [14].

For example, a great number confirm that African Americans attribute "stress" to many ailments including hypertension, stroke, myocardial infarctions, and more [15–17]. While some research has suggested that "stress" leads to increased cortisol, which worsens obesity, hypertension, kidney failure, and others, patients pin their cure for the stress-induced condition on becoming "stress-free." Achieving the nirvana of becoming stress-free has eluded African Americans, and everyone else, since the beginning of time. When looking at the perceived best treatment for hypertension, the knowledge/literacy disconnect persists. A full 92% of respondents reported that hypertension was "best" treated with garlic, herbs, and vitamins, while physician-prescribed medicines ranked third. The disconnect driving health literacy issues greatly impact compliance and acceptance of advice [18].

16.3 Recognizing and Correcting Barriers to Good Care

Researchers at the Cleveland Clinic developed a framework for looking at compliance in patients and categorized four types of barriers [18]:

1. Patient-specific barriers
2. Medication-specific barriers
3. Disease-specific barriers
4. Logistical barriers

Patient-Specific Barriers
This included (1) forgetfulness; (2) beliefs that medications were associated with impotence or drug dependence/addiction or are not needed when one feels well; and (3) attitudes such as denial or feelings that medications are not needed if there is no family history of hypertension and that medications are associated with other poor outcomes such as development of kidney disease or diabetes mellitus, as well as being required to take medications for the rest of one's life.

Medication-Specific Barriers
This included side effects such as allergies, dizziness, headaches, and loss of sexual drive or desire.

Disease-Specific Barriers
This included the absence of symptoms, which was interpreted as implying the lack of need for treatment.

Logistical Barriers
This included the burden of filling prescriptions, making office visits, having to use the restroom while away from home, and having to carry extra medications to avoid missing a dose [18].

When discussing poor compliance with medications, try to categorize the patient's barriers to taking the medication. If it is forgetfulness, examine their routine and try to develop a better approach. Ashish Atreja and colleagues wrote about ways to improve compliance and grouped the interventions into categories that could be remembered by the mnemonic "SIMPLE" [18]:

- Simplify the regimen
- Impart knowledge
- Modify beliefs
- Provider communication is ineffective
- Leave the bias
- Evaluate adherence

Many patients believe that their hypertension medications need to be taken with food and will carry their pills around with them "until they eat." Amlodipine and hydrochlorothiazide are usually well tolerated on an empty stomach. If the patient brushes their teeth daily, have them associate the taking of medication with teeth brushing instead of food. Suggest buying a weekly pill dispenser so that patients can more accurately track missed doses and improve overall compliance [19]. A large percentage of African Americans never eat breakfast [20], so discuss their perception of when to take their morning medications if they don't eat until later in the day. Suggest and agree on an acceptable solution. Have the patient make that modification and reevaluate their adherence at their next visit.

Emmanuel Fai and colleagues looked at attitudes of patients and their intention to stay on diabetes medications [21]:

> The findings suggest that attitudes, intentions and perceived behavioral control predict adherence to the use of oral antihyperglycemic regimens in African Americans. In addition, the findings suggest that individuals who perceive taking their type 2 diabetes medications as easy and those with a positive perception about taking their type 2 diabetes medications have high adherence to the use of oral antihyperglycemic regimens [21]

The attitude and intention of African American patients were shown to be directly correlated with improved compliance. Seeing the task as "easy" greatly improved outcomes. Explaining the rationale and simple mechanism of action for a particular medicine will greatly improve outcomes both individually and across a population [22].

16.4 Small Improvements Within a Population Can Yield Impressive Gains

The effects of a positive impact in the health of African Americans can have wide-ranging and highly sustainable benefits. For example, Hardy and colleagues in the *Journal of the American Heart Association* used multivariate linear regression to estimate benefit from a 1 mm Hg lowering of blood pressure and a 10% proportional reduction in the hypertensive awareness, untreated and uncontrolled [23]. They found that very modest decreases in blood pressure can have dramatic improvements in outcomes particularly in African Americans, likely because there is much more disease to prevent. If all patients did just a little bit better, dramatic

16.4 Small Improvements Within a Population Can Yield Impressive Gains

improvements in outcomes can be expected. For example, taking the reported 33% of African Americans currently on ACE inhibitors for monotherapy of hypertension and shifting them to a more efficacious medication will undoubtedly save lives.

Lowering the HbA1c has been proven to improve outcomes across populations including decreased heart failure [24], lower extremity amputations [25], and other benefits. With African Americans having a higher incidence of diabetes, achieving better glycemic control will substantially decrease disease burden.

Steven Woolf and colleagues wrote about "the health impact of resolving racial disparities" by analyzing mortality data [26]:

> The US health system spends far more on the "technology" of care (e.g., drugs, devices) than on achieving equity in its delivery. For 1991 to 2000, we contrasted the number of lives saved by medical advances with the number of deaths attributable to excess mortality among African Americans. Medical advances averted 176,633 deaths, but equalizing the mortality rates of Whites and African Americans would have averted 886,202 deaths. Achieving equity may do more for health than perfecting the technology of care [26]

By determining that five deaths could be avoided for every life saved by medical advances, Woolf put the country's healthcare priorities into perspective. By saving lives with what we know already, we can advance as a society.

Looking at life expectancy, African Americans have made great improvements over the last 50 years in large part due to improved medical care. In short, our efforts thus far have produced significant benefits. In 1960, the average life expectancy of African Americans was 63.6 years, while European Americans' lifespan was 70.6 years [27]. Most recent data shows a gain of 8 years (71.2) for African Americans versus just under 7 years for European Americans (76.7 years). These improvements came at the hand of clinicians across the country who cared enough to improve access to hospitals, nursing facilities, physician practices, and other healthcare entities. While access is still an issue in some places in the USA, our next step is to identify clinical differences and through research and reviewed quality outcomes apply nuanced care to this special population. Figure 16.1 shows a significantly decreased death rate for African Americans over a 16-year span [28].

Despite the numerous differences described in the preceding chapters, there are far more clinical treatment similarities between African Americans and the other racial groups. Infections, orthopedics, muscle disorders, head and neck pathologies, and much more generally have very similar clinical prevalence, approaches to therapy, and outcomes, when compared with a racial or ethnic eye.

But African Americans still carry the unique and unenviable distinction of being the population in America that has the worst clinical outcomes. Finding ways to reverse this heavy burden should be a priority of every clinician that sees African American patients.

As individual providers, attempting to change society's approach to race and ethnicity is a daunting task, but adjusting our care for patients sitting in front of us and asking for our help is completely within our capacity and responsibility. While no clinician intentionally provides poor medical care, giving good care to all patients in a practice requires thoughtful alacrity. Parents frequently find that raising multiple children in one household successfully requires an array of approaches

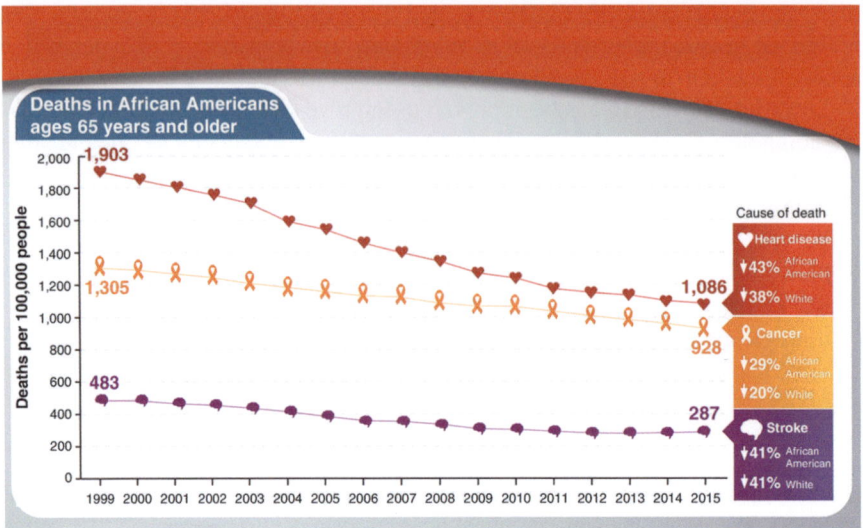

Fig. 16.1 The leading causes of death for African Americans have decreased from 1999 to 2015 [29]

depending on the child—what worked for one may completely fail another. Using the same approach with all patients will also show variable outcomes.

Quality providers also recognize the "differences" in patients and adjust their approach and care accordingly. Recognizing these differences and applying validated nuanced approaches in care is the pure and simple purpose of this text.

The age-old Hippocratic Oath ends with:

> If I do not violate this oath, may I enjoy life and art, respected while I live and remembered with affection thereafter. May I always act so as to preserve the finest traditions of my calling and may I long experience the joy of healing those who seek my help.

An "Oath" and a Responsibility to All Patients
- Recognizing the important differences that exist among populations and applying them appropriately ensures quality patient care for everyone.
- The disconnect driving health literacy issues greatly impact compliance and acceptance of advice.
- African Americans have the worst overall clinical outcomes. Reducing this disparity should be the priority of every clinician that sees African American patients.
- Four basic principles of medical ethics:
  - *Beneficence* describes the concept of acting for the patient's good.
  - *Nonmaleficence* describes the concept of doing no harm.

(continued)

- *Autonomy* conveys the idea that each patient has a right to voice his or her own values and choices about care.
- *Justice* expresses the idea that healthcare resources should be equitably distributed among patients and that patients should be treated fairly.

- Some poor outcomes seen in African Americans result from misguided assumptions and misunderstandings on the patient's part. Gaining insight into some of the more common misconceptions can be beneficial.
- African Americans attribute "stress" to many ailments including hypertension, stroke, myocardial infarctions, and more.
- Improve patient compliance by using the mnemonic "SIMPLE":

  - *S*implify the regimen
  - *I*mpart knowledge
  - *M*odify beliefs
  - *P*rovider communication is ineffective
  - *L*eave the bias
  - *E*valuate adherence

- Modest decreases in blood pressure can have dramatic improvements in outcomes particularly in African Americans.
- African Americans have made great improvements over the last 50 years with an 11-year increase in life expectancy.

References

1. Clark S. The impact of the Hippocratic Oath in 2018: the conflict of the ideal of the physician, the knowledgeable humanitarian, versus the corporate medical allegiance to financial models contributes to burnout. Cureus. 2018;10(7):e3076.
2. Miles SH. Hippocrates and informed consent. Lancet. 2009;374:1322–3.
3. Antoniou SA, Antoniou GA, Granderath FA, et al. Reflections of the Hippocratic oath in modern medicine. World J Surg. 2010;34(12):3075–9.
4. Jotterand F. The Hippocratic Oath and contemporary medicine: dialectic between past ideals and present reality? J Med Philos. 2005;30(1):107–28.
5. Sessanna L. Incorporating Florence Nightingale's theory of nursing into teaching a group of preadolescent children about the negative peer pressure. J Pediatr Nurs. 2004;19(3):225–31.
6. Beauchamp T, Childress J. Principles of biomedical ethics. 6th ed. New York: Oxford University Press; 2008.
7. Kuczmarski M, Adams E, Cotugna N, et al. Health literacy and education predict nutrient quality of diet of socioeconomically diverse, urban adults. J Epidemiol Prev Med. 2016;2(1):13000115.
8. Hoover DS, Vidrine JI, Shete S, et al. Health literacy, smoking, and health indicators in African American adults. J Health Commun. 2015;20(Suppl 2):24–33.
9. Baker DW, Parker RM, Williams MV, et al. The relationship of patient reading ability to self-reported health and use of health services. Am J Public Health. 1997;87(6):1027–30.

10. Bennett IM, Chen J, Soroui JS, White S. The contribution of health literacy to disparities in self-rated health status and preventive health behaviors in older adults. Ann Fam Med. 2009;7(3):204–11.
11. Berkman ND, Sheridan SL, Donahue KE, et al. Low health literacy and health outcomes: an updated systematic review. Ann Intern Med. 2011;155(2):97–107.
12. Berkman ND, Sheridan SL, Donahue KE, et al. Health literacy interventions and outcomes: an updated systematic review, vol. 155. Rockville: Agency for Healthcare Research and Quality; 2011. p. 97.
13. Stewart DW, Vidrine JI, Shete S, et al. Health literacy, smoking, and health indicators in African American adults. J Health Commun. 2015;20(02):24–33.
14. Ogedegbe G, Harrison M, Robbins L, et al. Barriers and facilitators of medication adherence in hypertensive African Americans: a qualitative study. Ethn Dis. 2004;14(1):3–12.
15. Wilson RP, Freeman A, Kazda MJ, et al. Lay beliefs about high blood pressure in a low- to middle-income urban African-American community: an opportunity for improving hypertension control. Am J Med. 2002;112(1):26–30.
16. Dutta M, Sastry S, Dillard S, et al. Narratives of stress in health meanings of African Americans in Lake County, Indiana. Health Commun. 2017;32(10):1241–51.
17. Dubbin L, McLemore M, Shim JK. Illness narratives of African Americans living with coronary heart disease: a critical interactionist analysis. Qual Health Res. 2017;27(4):497–508.
18. Atreja A, Bellam N, Levy SR. Strategies to enhance patient adherence: making it simple. MedGenMed. 2005;7(1):4.
19. Conn VS, Ruppar TM, Chan KC, Dunbar-Jacob J, Pepper GA, De Geest S. Packaging interventions to increase medication adherence: systematic review and meta-analysis. Curr Med Res Opin. 2015;31(1):145–60.
20. Rampersaud GC, Pereira MA, Girard BL, et al. Breakfast habits, nutritional status, body weight, and academic performance in children and adolescents. J Am Diet Assoc. 2005;105(5):743–60.
21. Fai EK, Anderson C, Ferreros V. Role of attitudes and intentions in predicting adherence to oral diabetes medications. Endocr Connect. 2017;6(2):63–70.
22. Rimando PM. Perceived barriers to and facilitators of hypertension management among underserved African American older adults. Ethn Dis. 2015;25(3):329.
23. Hardy ST, Loehr LR, Butler KR, et al. Reducing the blood pressure–related burden of cardiovascular disease: impact of achievable improvements in blood pressure prevention and control. J Am Heart Assoc. 2015;4(10):e002276.
24. Zhao W, Katzmarzyk PT, Horswell R, et al. HbA1c and coronary heart disease risk among diabetic patients. Diabetes Care. 2013;37(2):428–35.
25. Zhao W, Katzmarzyk PT, Horswell R, et al. HbA1c and lower-extremity amputation risk in low-income patients with diabetes. Diabetes Care. 2013;36(11):3591–8.
26. Woolf SH, Johnson RE, Fryer GE, et al. The health impact of resolving racial disparities: an analysis of US mortality data. Am J Public Health. 2004;94:2078–81.
27. Arias E, Xu J, Kochanek K. United States Life Tables, 2021. Natl Vital Stat Rep. 2023 Nov;72(12):1–64. PMID: 38048433.
28. African American Health. Centers for Disease Control and Prevention. 2017. https://www.cdc.gov/vitalsigns/aahealth/index.html. Accessed 25 May 2019.
29. Cunningham TJ, Croft JB, Liu Y, Lu H, Eke PI, Giles WH. Vital Signs: Racial Disparities in Age-Specific Mortality Among Blacks or African Americans - United States, 1999-2015. MMWR Morb Mortal Wkly Rep. 2017 May 5;66(17):444–456. https://doi.org/10.15585/mmwr.mm6617e1. Erratum in: MMWR Morb Mortal Wkly Rep. 2017 May 12;66(18):490. PMID: 28472021; PMCID: PMC5687082. https://doi.org/10.15585/mmwr.mm6618a11.

Index

A
ABCG2 gene, 155
Abdominal aortic aneurysms (AAAs), 65, 66
Abuse, 17, 18
Active listening, 309
Acute chest syndrome, 198
Advanced glycation end products (AGEs), 289, 290
African American Study of Kidney Disease and Hypertension (AASK), 136, 137
African Americans
    decreased death rate, 328
    dietary differences (*see* Dietary differences)
    folate deficiency, 298
    fried food health risks, 288–289
    lactose intolerance, 292
    life expectancy, 327
    mineral deficiencies, 299–300
    positive health impact, 326
    sports drinks, 294
    vitamin A deficiency, 298
    vitamin B12 deficiency, 298
    Vitamin C deficiency, 298
    vitamin D deficiency, 295–298
Agency for Healthcare Research and Quality (AHRQ), 7
Alcohol consumption, 254
Alpha-fetoprotein (AFP), 189
Alpha thalassemia, 202, 203
American Association for the Study of Liver Diseases (AASLD), 226
American Diabetes Association (ADA), 91
American Urological Association, 116
Amlodipine, 326
Ancestral genomics, 3, 4
Angiotensin-converting enzyme (ACE) inhibitors, 52, 53
Ankylosing spondylitis (AS), 152
Antimalarial drugs, 152
Antinuclear antibodies (ANA), 151
Aplastic crisis, 197–198
Apolipoprotein 1 (APOL1) gene, 134–137, 139, 150, 193
Arthritis, 150
Asthma, 169–171
Atrial fibrillation, 59, 60

B
Barrett's esophagus, 230
Barriers
    to care, 268
    to medical care, 325–326
Benign ethnic neutropenia, 184–185
Beta blockers, 53
Beta thalassemia, 202, 203
Bias, 265, 277
    against Black patients, 268
    racial, 264, 266
    unconscious, 273
Black Women's Health Study, 292
Blood pressure, categories, 52
Body mass indices (BMIs), 173
Breakfast, 290–292
Breast cancer, 109–112
B-type natriuretic peptide (BNP), 56

C

Calcinosis cutis, Raynaud's phenomenon, esophageal dysmotility, sclerodactyly, and telangiectasia (CREST) syndrome, 153
Calcium channel blockers (CCBs), 137
Calcium supplementation, 296
Cancer
    breast, 109, 111, 112
    chemotherapy, 123
    colon, 112–114
    lung
        African American smoking paradox, 120, 121
        incidence, 117
        industrial exposure, 119
        low-dose computed tomography, 119
        small cell carcinoma, 119
        smoking, 118, 119
        tobacco cessation, 119
    multiple myeloma, 121–123
    prostate, 116, 117
    stress and, 244
Cancer antigen 125 (CA-125), 188
Carbohydrate antigen 19-9 (CA 19-9), 189
Cardiometabolic disease, stress and, 245
Cardiovascular care, 47, 48, 51
    ACE medications, 52, 53
    ARB medications, 52
    atrial fibrillation, 59, 60
    blood pressure
        categories, 52
        control, 52
    DVT and pulmonary embolism, 68
    lipids, 57, 58
    peripheral vascular disease, 65
    stroke, 61–63
Chemotherapy, 123
Chronic bronchitis, 166, 168
Chronic inflammatory bowel disease, 227
Chronic kidney disease (CKD), 183
Chronic Kidney Disease Epidemiology Collaboration (CKD-EPI), 182
Chronic obstructive pulmonary disease (COPD), 166–169
Chronic pain, 266, 271
    inequities, 266
    primary, 264
Chronic stress, 244, 245
Chronic stressors, 241
Cigarette smoking, 138, 228
Clinical care
    alcohol consumption, 254
    death exposure, 252
    death of family member, 252
    major depressive disorder, 246, 248–250
    sleep differences, 253
Colon cancer, 112–114
Competence, 25–27
Complete blood count (CBC), 183–184
Consistent care, 31, 41
Continuous Positive Airway Pressure (CPAP) therapy, 173
C-reactive protein (CRP), 138, 152
Creatine kinase (CK), 185
Creatinine, 182–183
Criminal justice system, 254
Crohn's disease, 219, 227, 229
Cultural competence, 318
Cultural influences on pain reporting, 269
Cultural intelligence African American, 317, 318
Cultural sensitivity, 307–310

D

Daytime sleepiness, 173
Death, of family member, 252
Deep vein thrombosis (DVT), 66, 67
Depression, 147, 247
Diabetes, 81
    diet management approaches, 95–97
    fatalism, 93
    HbA1c, 90, 91, 93
    marketing competition, 97, 98
    medications, 92
    story telling, 316, 317
    type 2, 86, 88
Diet management approaches, 95, 96
Dietary differences
    adding meats to vegetables, 286
    advanced glycation end products, 289
    breakfast, 290–292
    food consumption at home, 287
    fried foods, 288, 289
    home cooking, 288
    obesity, 289, 293, 294
    pre-processed sugary beverages, 288
    processed meat, 286
    reusing cooking oils, 289
    sugar-sweetened beverages (SSBs), 292–295
Direct-acting antiviral agents (DAAs), 224
Disease-modifying antirheumatic drugs (DMARDs), 149

Disease-specific barriers, 325
DNA methylation, 6
Duffy antigen receptor for chemokines (DARC) gene, 184

E

Emergency medical care, 35
Emotional intelligence (EI)
  components, 308
  and cultural sensitivity, 308
Empagliflozin, 92
Emphysema, 166, 168
End-stage renal disease (ESRD), 134, 136, 137, 139, 150
Equitable care, 32
  African American racial differences, outcomes, 36
  cancer outcomes, 38
  emergency medical care, 35
  minority-serving hospital, 35
  stereotyping, 33
  variability, 40, 41
Erythrocyte sedimentation rate (ESR), 152, 153
Estimated average requirement (EAR), 192
Ethnicity, 7
EULAR Sjögren's Syndrome Disease Activity Index (ESSDAI), 153
Evidence-based differences, 5–7
Explicit biases, 21
Eye complications, sickle cell disease, 196

F

Fatalism, 93
Fats, 97
Florence Nightingale Pledge, 322
Folate, 190
Folate deficiency, 298
Fried food health risks, 288–289

G

Galactose, 292
Gallbladder disease, 232
Gastroenterology
  Barrett's esophagus, 230
  gallbladder disease, 232
  Helicobacter pylori infections, 231
  hepatitis B, 220–222
  hepatitis C, 222–225
  hepatocellular carcinoma, 225, 226
  inflammatory bowel diseases, 229

Gastroesophageal reflux disease (GERD), 229, 230
Gender disparities, 150
Genetic ancestry, 183
Genetic mapping, 8
Genetic predispositions, 108
Genome-wide association studies (GWAS), 45, 82, 148, 155, 186, 228
Giant cell arteritis (GCA), 154
Glomerular filtration rate (GFR), 137, 138, 182–183
Glucocorticoid receptor resistance (GCR), 244
Glucocorticoids, 152
Glucose-6-phosphate dehydrogenase (G6PD) deficiency, 91, 204
Glutton, 294
Gout, 154–156

H

HbA1c, 90, 91, 93, 327
Health-care providers, in trust, 18
Health disparities, 245
  sleep, 253
Health literacy, 324
Heart failure, 54
Heart rate variability (HRV), 251
Helicobacter pylori infections, 231
Hematocrit (HCT), 184
Hematological diseases
  benign ethnic neutropenia, 184–185
  cancer markers, 187–189
    alpha-fetoprotein, 189
    CA-125 levels, 188
    carbohydrate antigen 19-9, 189
    prostate-specific antigen, 187
  complete blood count, 183–184
  G6PD deficiency, 204
  laboratory results, 183
  lipid profile, 187
  reference range values, 183
  sickle cell disease, 193
    acute chest syndrome, 198
    aplastic crisis, 197–198
    APOL1, 193
    chronic complications, 193
    eye complications, 196
    incidence, 193
    priapism, 196–197
    pulmonary hypertension, 195
    splenic sequestration, 199
    stroke, 197
    vaso-occlusive crisis, 200–202
  thalassemia, 202–203
  thyroid stimulating hormone, 186

Hemodialysis, vascular access for, 135
Hemoglobin (HGB), 184, 198, 202
Hemoglobinopathies, 91
Hepatitis B infections, 220, 222
Hepatitis C virus (HCV) infections, 222–225
Hepatocellular carcinoma (HCC), 189, 225, 226
Hereditary transthyretin amyloidosis (hATTR), 57
High fructose-content sugar (HFCS), 293
Hippocratic morality, 322
Hippocratic oath, 322, 328
HLA-B27 genetic marker, 152
Household income, 243
Hydrochlorothiazide, 155, 326
Hydroxyurea, 200, 201
Hypertension, 50, 315, 325–327
    causes, 324
    control, 51
    management, African Americans, 315
    prevalence of, 48
    story telling, 314–316
    treatments, 324
Hypertensive nephrosclerosis, 136
Hypertensive therapy, 314
Hyperuricemia, 154, 155
Hypokalemia, 300
Hypothalamic-pituitary-adrenal (HPA) axis, 244, 245

I
Implicit biases, 21, 23
Incretin-based therapies, 92
Inflammation, stress-induced, 243, 255
Inflammatory bowel disease (IBD), 219, 227
    Crohn's disease, 229
    ulcerative colitis, 229
Interferon-based therapy, 223
Interprofessional core competencies for pain management, 270–271
Interrupted sleep, 173
Intravenous cyclophosphamide (IVC), 151
Iron deficiency, 299

J
Jackson Heart Study, 136
Johnston County Osteoarthritis Project, 147
Journal of the Academy of Nutrition and Dietetics, 290

K
Kidney
    disease, 88
    stones, 139, 140
    transplantation, 138, 139

L
Lactase-fortified milks, 292
Lactose, 292
Lactose intolerance African Americans, 292
Lecturing, 315
Life expectancy improvements African Americans, 327
Lipid profile, 187
Lipids, 57, 58
Lipoprotein lipase (LPL) gene, 187
Liraglutide, 92
Löfgren's syndrome, 171
Logistical barriers, 325
Low-dose computed tomography (LDCT), 119
Low neutrophil counts, 185
Lung cancer
    African American smoking paradox, 120, 121
    incidence, 117
    industrial exposure, 119
    low-dose computed tomography, 119
    smoking, 118
    tobacco cessation, 119
Lymphadenopathy (LAD), 150
Lysine-specific demethylase 1 (LSD-1), 49

M
Magnesium deficiency, 299
Major depressive disorder (MDD), 246, 250
Mean corpuscular hemoglobin (MCH), 184
Mean corpuscular hemoglobin concentration (MCHC), 184
Medical ethics, 323–324
Medication-specific barriers, 325
Mental health, 271
Mental illness, 245–252
Metabolic panel, 185–186
Metformin, 91
Milk, 286, 288, 291, 292
Mineral deficiencies, 299–300
Minority-serving hospitals, 35
Misunderstandings, 324
Modification of Diet in Renal Disease (MDRD), 182

Monoclonal gammopathy of undetermined significance (MGUS), 122
MTHFR 677TT genotype, 190
Multiple myeloma (MM), 121–123
Mycophenolate Mofetil (MMF), 151

N
Nephritis, 150
Nitric oxide (NO), 195
Nociceptive pain, 200
Nociplastic pain, 200
Nonmaleficence, 323
Nutritional disparities, 295

O
Oath and responsibility
  autonomy, 323
  beneficence, 323
  blood pressure, 326
  cultural misunderstanding, 324
  death rate for African Americans, 327
  diabetes medications, 326
  disease-specific barriers, 325
  Florence Nightingale Pledge, 322
  health literacy, 324
  hippocratic morality, 322
  justice, 323
  life expectancy, 327
  logistical barriers, 325
  medication-specific barriers, 325
  non-maleficence, 323
  oncologists clinicians, 323
  patient-specific barriers, 325
  quality providers, 328
  "SIMPLE" mnemonic, 326
  stress, 325
  treatment similarities, 327
Obesity, 81, 136
  asthma, 170
  dietary differences, 289, 293, 294
  obstructive sleep apnea, 173
  prevalence of, 84
  quality of life, 85
  risk factors, 84
  stress and, 244
Obstructive sleep apnea (OSA), 173–174
Oils, 97
Old-style breakfast, 290
Openness, 24
Opioid misuse, signs of, 267
Osteoarthritis (OA), 147–148

P
Pain, 201, 263, 264
  affirming care, 273
  assessment, 274
  cultural considerations, 269
  diagnosis, 274
  management
    disparities in, 277
    resourceful websites for, 279
  multimodal treatment pathway, 276
  patient advocacy, 272
  perception
    and communication of, 267–268
    deception of, 264–265
  psychosocial aspects of, 271
  screening, 275
Pain Management Best Practices Inter-Agency Task Force, 274
Patient-centered care, 8–11, 318
Patient controlled analgesia (PCA), 202
Patient-specific barriers, 325
Patient trust, in healthcare, 309
Pay-for-performance, 7
PDE8B locus, 186
Peripeteia, 313
Peripheral vascular disease (PVD), 38, 63, 65
Personalized medicine, 1
Pharmacogenomics, 1
Polymyalgia rheumatica (PMR), 154
Pramlintide, 92
Precision medicine, 1, 38
Priapism, 196–197
Primary chronic pain, 264
Primary secondary pain, 264
Processed meat, 286
Prophylactic aspirin, 62
Prostate cancer, 109, 115–117
Prostate-specific antigen (PSA), 116, 187
Proteinuria, 136, 137
Psychosocial aspects of pain, 271
Public health-human-civil rights issue, 266
Pulmonary diseases
  asthma, 169–171
  chronic obstructive pulmonary disease, 166–169
  COPD, 168
  obstructive sleep apnea, 173–174
  sarcoidosis, 171–172
Pulmonary embolism (PE), 66, 68
Pulmonary hypertension (PH), 195

Q
Q141K polymorphism, 155

R
RA, *see* Rheumatoid arthritis
Race, 2, 7
Racial bias, 264, 266
Racial concordance, 19
Racial differences, in trust, 19
Racial disparities
   in healthcare, 273
   in pain management, 265
Racism, systemic, 241
Radiographic knee OA, 147
Raynaud phenomenon, 153
Red blood cell (RBC) folate, 190
Reference intervals (RIs), 185
Renal complications, sickle cell disease, 194–195
Renal disease
   counseling, 138
   hypertensive nephrosclerosis, 136
   kidney stones, 139, 140
   kidney transplantation, 138, 139
   obesity, 136, 137
   proteinuria, 136, 137
   treatment, 137
Renal medullary carcinoma (RMC), 195
Rheumatic diseases
   ankylosing spondylitis, 152
   giant cell arteritis, 154
   gout, 154–156
   polymyalgia rheumatica, 154
   rheumatoid arthritis, 148
   scleroderma, 153
   Sjögren's syndrome, 152–153
   systemic lupus erythematosus, 149–152
Rheumatoid arthritis (RA), 148

S
Sarcoidosis, 171–172
Scleroderma, 153
Screen, Intervene, and Reconvene (SIR) cultural model, 273
Selenium and Vitamin E Cancer Prevention Trial, 298
Semaglutide, 93
Sexually transmitted diseases (STD), 220
Shift working, 253
Sickle cell disease (SCD), 193, 232
   acute chest syndrome, 198
   aplastic crisis, 197–198
   APOL1, 193
   chronic complications, 193
   eye complications, 196
   incidence, 193
   priapism, 196–197
   pulmonary hypertension, 195
   renal complications, 194–195
   splenic sequestration, 199
   stroke, 197
   vaso-occlusive crisis, 200–202
Sickle cell nephropathy, 194
Sickle cell retinopathy, 196
Sickle cell trait (SCT), 91
Sickled erythrocytes, 193
Single-nucleotide polymorphisms (SNPs), 67, 116
Sjögren's syndrome, 152–153
SLC22A12 gene, 155
SLC23A1 gene, 191
SLC2A9 gene, 155
Sleep differences, 253
Small cell carcinoma, 119
Smokers, 168
Smoking cessation, 119
Social determinants of health, 267
Social stressors, 244
Socioeconomic status (SES), 248
Sodium restriction, 50
Sodium sensitivity, 294, 295
Splenic sequestration, 199
Sports drinks African Americans, 294
Stereotyping, 33
Stigma, 246
Story telling, in medicine
   diabetes, 316, 317
   early African American culture, 311
   hypertension, 315, 316
   listener and, 310
   marketing for good health
      in clinical settings, 312
      components of good stories, 312, 313
      culture perspective, 314
      motivational clinical stories, 313
      patients goals, 311
      peripeteia, 313
      professional marketers, 312
      successful physicians, 312
      verisimilitude, 314
   patient's worldview, 317, 318
   prescription for medication, 314, 315
   qualitative research, 310
   role of storytellers, 311
   traditional, 310

Index

Stress, 241–245
    and cancer, 244
    and cardiometabolic disease, 245
    and obesity, 244
    chronic, 244, 245
Stress-induced inflammation, 243
Stressors, social, 244
Stroke, 61–63, 197
Stuttering priapism, 196
Substance abuse, 245
Sugar-sweetened beverages (SSBs), 292
    African Americans, 292–294
Suicide rates, 247
Surveillance Epidemiology and End Results (SEER)-Medicare database, 226
Sympathetic-adrenal-medullary (SAM) axis, 244
Symptomatic knee OA, 147
Syphilis, 16, 17
Systemic lupus erythematosus (SLE), 149–152
Systemic pressure, 243
Systemic racism, 241
Systemic sclerosis (SSc), 153
Systolic blood pressure (SBP), 51

T
Temporal arteritis, 154
Thalassemia, 202–203
    intermedia, 203
    major, 203
    minor, 203
Therapeutic nihilism, 322
Thiazide-type diuretics, 52, 137
Thyroid stimulating hormone (TSH), 186
Tirzepatide, 93
Tobacco smoking, 168
Total hip arthroplasty (THA), 148
Total joint arthroplasty (TJA), 148
Total knee arthroplasty (TKA), 148
Tricuspid regurgitation, 195
Triple-negative breast cancers (TNBCs), 110
Trust, 309
    differences in, 18, 19
    health outcomes, 20–24
    internists'omes, 22
Tuskegee Syphilis Study, 16, 17, 322

Type 1 diabetes, 95
Type 2 diabetes (DM2), 86, 230
Typical neutrophil count with Fy (a-b-) status, 184

U
Ulcerative colitis (UC), 219, 227–229
Unemployment rates, 242
United States Preventive Services Task Force (USPSTF), 116
Urinary tract calculi, 139
U.S. Cancer Statistics Working Group, 108, 113
Uterine fibroids, 299

V
Vaso-occlusive crisis (VOC), 200–202
Verisimilitude, 314
Vitamin A, 191
Vitamin A deficiency, 298
Vitamin B12, 190
Vitamin B12 deficiency, 298
Vitamin B9 deficiency, 298
Vitamin blood levels, 190
    folate, 190
    vitamin A, 191
    vitamin B12, 190
    vitamin C, 191
    vitamin E, 192
Vitamin C, 191
Vitamin C deficiency, 298
Vitamin D, 151
Vitamin D deficiency, 117, 170
    African Americans, 295–298
Vitamin E, 192
    supplementation, 298

W
White male smoker's disease, 168
Worldview African Americans, 317–318

Z
Zinc deficiency, 300

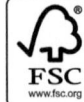

MIX
Papier aus verantwortungsvollen Quellen
Paper from responsible sources
FSC® C105338

If you have any concerns about our products,
you can contact us on
ProductSafety@springernature.com

In case Publisher is established outside the EU,
the EU authorized representative is:
**Springer Nature Customer Service Center GmbH
Europaplatz 3, 69115 Heidelberg, Germany**

Printed by Libri Plureos GmbH
in Hamburg, Germany